Infection Prevention and Control

Infection Prevention and Control

Editor: Nicholas Rodgers

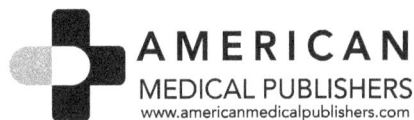

AMERICAN
MEDICAL PUBLISHERS
www.americanmedicalpublishers.com

AMERICAN
MEDICAL PUBLISHERS
www.americanmedicalpublishers.com

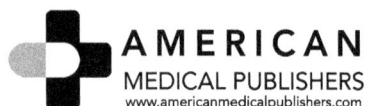

Cataloging-in-Publication Data

Infection prevention and control / edited by Nicholas Rodgers.
   p. cm.
Includes bibliographical references and index.
ISBN 978-1-63927-224-2
1. Infection. 2. Infection--Prevention. 3. Infection--Treatment. 4. Communicable diseases--Prevention.
5. Communicable diseases--Treatment. I. Rodgers, Nicholas.
RB153 .I54 2022
616.9--dc23

American Medical Publishers,
41 Flatbush Avenue,
1st Floor, New York,
NY 11217, USA

ISBN 978-1-63927-224-2 (Hardback)

Contents

Preface

This book has been a concerted effort by a group of academicians, researchers and scientists, who have contributed their research works for the realization of the book. This book has materialized in the wake of emerging advancements and innovations in this field. Therefore, the need of the hour was to compile all the required researches and disseminate the knowledge to a broad spectrum of people comprising of students, researchers and specialists of the field.

The invasion of the body tissues of an organism by disease-causing agents is known as infection. It also includes the multiplication of such agents, the toxins produced by them and their host interactions. Viruses, parasites, bacteria and arhthropods are some common infection causing agents. Infection control is associated with the prevention of nosocomial and health-care associated infection. It is related to public health practice and involves the usage of antibiotics, antibacterials, antifungals, antivirals and antiprotozoals. Infection control is based on a certain number of factors within the healthcare setting. It includes prevention, sterilization, vaccination, disinfection, monitoring of infection within a particular health-care setting and management. Sterilization uses heat, steam or liquid chemical to kill all microorganisms. Disinfection kills disease-causing microorganisms through the usage of liquid chemicals. The topics included in this book on infection prevention and control are of utmost significance and bound to provide incredible insights to readers. While understanding the long-term perspectives of the topics, the book makes an effort in highlighting their impacts as a modern tool for the growth of the discipline. The book is appropriate for students seeking detailed information in this area as well as for experts.

At the end of the preface, I would like to thank the authors for their brilliant chapters and the publisher for guiding us all-through the making of the book till its final stage. Also, I would like to thank my family for providing the support and encouragement throughout my academic career and research projects.

Editor

A prospective survey of *Pseudomonas aeruginosa* colonization and infection in the intensive care unit

Regev Cohen[1,2]*, Frida Babushkin[3], Shoshana Cohen[3], Marina Afraimov[3], Maurice Shapiro[4], Martina Uda[4], Efrat Khabra[5], Amos Adler[5,6], Ronen Ben Ami[6,7] and Svetlana Paikin[8]

Abstract

Background: *Pseudomonas aeruginosa* (PA) surveillance may improve empiric antimicrobial therapy, since colonizing strains frequently cause infections. This colonization may be 'endogenous' or 'exogenous', and the source determines infection control measures. We prospectively investigated the sources of PA, the clinical impact of PA colonization upon admission and the dynamics of colonization at different body sites throughout the intensive care unit stay.

Methods: Intensive care patients were screened on admission and weekly from the pharynx, endotracheal aspirate, rectum and urine. Molecular typing was performed using Enterobacterial Repetitive Intergenic Consensus Polymerase Chain reaction (ERIC-PCR).

Results: Between November 2014 and January 2015, 34 patients were included. Thirteen (38%) were colonized on admission, and were at a higher risk for PA-related clinical infection (Hazard Ratio = 14.6, $p = 0.0002$). Strains were often patient-specific, site-specific and site-persistent. Sixteen out of 17 (94%) clinical isolates were identical to strains found concurrently or previously on screening cultures from the same patient, and none were unique. Ventilator associated pneumonia-related strains were identical to endotracheal aspirates and pharynx screening (87–75% of cases). No clinical case was found among patients with repeated negative screening.

Conclusion: PA origin in this non-outbreak setting was mainly 'endogenous' and PA-strains were generally patient- and site-specific, especially in the gastrointestinal tract. While prediction of ventilator associated pneumonia-related PA-strain by screening was fair, the negative predictive value of screening was very high.

Keywords: *Pseudomonas aeruginosa*, Endogenous, Intensive Care unit, Surveillance, ERIC-PCR, Infection control

Background

Pseudomonas aeruginosa (PA) is a leading cause of healthcare-associated infections in intensive care units (ICUs), mainly ventilator-associated pneumonia (VAP), central line-associated bloodstream infection (CLABSI) and surgical site infection (SSI). PA colonization typically precedes infection [1]. Colonization may be endogenous, arising from the patient's own microbial repertoire [2–4], or exogenous if acquired from the hospital environment or by cross-infection from other patients [5–11]. This distinction has implications for the means needed for infection control [12]. Specifically, water fixtures and piping colonized with PA have been implicated as environmental reservoirs during outbreaks in ICUs [13, 14]. Use of point-of-care water filters was shown to effectively reduce PA infections in surgical ICUs [4].

In previous work, we studied the genetic relatedness of PA strains isolated from ventilated patients and hospital faucets. We found a clear temporal and spatial relation between patient and environmental strains [15]. In the present study we aimed to prospectively determine the clinical impact of PA colonization on admission to the

* Correspondence: regevco@gmail.com; regevc@laniado.org.il
[1]Head of Infectious diseases unit, Sanz Medical Center, Laniado hospital, Neytanya, Israel
[2]Ruth and Bruce Rappaport Faculty of Medicine, Technion, Haifa, Israel

ICU and the dynamics of colonization at different body sites throughout the ICU stay.

Methods
Study design
The study was conducted at the Sanz Medical Center, a 400-bed community hospital located in central Israel. The adult ICU is a combined medical and surgical unit with ~250 admissions (~2000 patient days) per year. The ICU is located in one room with 6 beds with no physical barrier between patients. ICU staff members were instructed to use tap water for patients bathing only, whereas sterile water was used for drinking, moistening and mouth treatment. All faucet aerators were dismantled 23 months prior to initiation of this study [15].

All patients hospitalized in the ICU from November 2014 to January 2015 were included and underwent prospective weekly PA surveillance cultures, as detailed below. Patients staying in the unit for less than 72 h were excluded from the analysis. The primary endpoint was the development of clinical infection due to PA, defined according to CDC/NHSN surveillance definitions of healthcare-associated infections [16] and American Thoracic Society criteria for VAP [17]. Secondary aims were identifying risk factors for PA colonization on admission and during ICU stay, clonal analysis of strains at each body site during the ICU stay and the concordance between the strains related to infection and those detected on weekly screening.

This study was approved by the hospital institutional review board committee (0033-14-LND). As the study was aimed for infection control and patient safety purposes, the requirement for informed consent was waived.

Clinical data
The following baseline characteristics were collected from electronic medical records: age, sex, place of residence (home or long-term care facility [LCTF]), comorbidities, hospitalization within 90 days prior to admission, surgery in the previous 30 days and duration of hospitalization before admission to the ICU. We recorded the dates of hospitalization, ICU admission and discharge, Acute Physiology and Chronic Health Evaluation (APACHE) II on ICU admission, length of stay in the ICU and in the hospital in general, ventilation duration, tracheostomy date, death in ICU and within 90 days of hospitalization and major diagnoses in ICU. We also documented the dates and sources of PA cultures (screening and clinical), and PA related diagnoses of VAP, CLABSI, SSI and catheter-associated urinary tract infection (CAUTI).

Surveillance cultures
Each patient was surveyed using standard bacterial cultures on admission (within the first 72 h) and then once a week until discharge. Cultures were collected using swabs (Transsystem, Copan®, California, USA) from 4 sites: throat, rectum, endotracheal aspirate (EA) for ventilated patients, and urine, and transferred to the laboratory within 30 min. Faucet cultures were collected weekly from the distal part of the faucet using a bacterial swab.

Swabs were inoculated on tryptic soy blood agar, chocolate agar, MacConkey agar and fluid thioglycoate medium (Hy-labs®, Rehovot, Israel). Cultures were incubated at 35° C overnight. Broth samples were subcultured to the same media plates whenever no growth was detected on the initial plates.

Bacterial identification and antimicrobial susceptibility testing were done using the VITEK 2 system (Biomerieux, Marcy l'Etoile, France) and interpreted according to CLSI criteria [18].

PA isolates were stored at -70°c for molecular analysis. Molecular typing was done by enterobacterial repetitive intergenic consensus (ERIC)-PCR. DNA was extracted using the easyMag® system (BioMerieux) and ERIC-PCR was performed as previously described [19]. PCR products were resolved using the QIAxcel capillary gel electrophoresis apparatus (QIAGEN, Hilden, Germany) [19]) and compared visually. The discriminatory power of ERIC-PCR was found to be similar to that of PFGE in PA [20].

Acquisition of PA was defined as the isolation of PA from surveillance or clinical cultures from patients not colonized within 72 h of admission. Colonization was defined as the isolation of PA from specimens taken from the rectum, catheter-urine, pharynx or EA, in the absence of clinical infection.

Statistical analysis
Patient characteristics were presented using descriptive statistics. Continuous variables were compared using the Student t test or Mann Whitney test, and two-tailed Fisher's exact test was used for categorical variables. Time to PA related infections was evaluated with the Kaplan-Meier method, with the day of ICU admission serving as day 0. Differences between curves were calculated with the two-sided logrank test. Death discharge from hospital, and PA related infection were treated as competing events. In all statistical analyses, a two-sided p-value less than 0.05 was considered significant.

Results
Faucet samples
Sixty specimens were obtained from 6 faucets over the study period. Of these, only 1 specimen (1.6%) was positive for PA, and was found to be a unique genotype.

Patient surveillance cultures

Fifty-six patients were admitted to the ICU during the study period. Eleven patients were excluded (5 hospitalized < 72h and 6 discharged prior to screening). Out of the remaining 45 patients, 34 patients were screened <72h from admission and 11 were screened ≥72h from admission. Four of the 11 patients screened late were found negative and were regarded also as negative on admission, and together comprised the study cohort of 38 patients (Fig. 1).

Of the 38 patients, 13 (34%) were colonized with PA on admission (Table 1). Advanced age (>70 years) and residency in a LTCF were significantly associated with PA colonization on admission (odds ratio (OR) 7, 95% confidence interval (CI) 1.2-38.3; $p = 0.035$; OR = 17, 95% CI 0.8–358, $p = 0.033$, respectively; Table 1). Diabetes mellitus was negatively associated with PA colonization (OR = 0.06, 95% CI 0.007–0.58; $p = 0.005$).

Of the 38 patients in the study cohort, 21 were still hospitalized on the next week, and 11 (52%) of them screened positive for PA (Table 2). The proportion of patients with positive PA screening increased with length of ICU stay, reaching 71% after 3 weeks of ICU stay (Table 2). Three (12%) of 25 patients who were negative on admission screening acquired PA during their ICU stay. In two of

them, PA was also found in clinical cultures of sputum, and in one VAP was diagnosed.

Of a total of 68 positive surveillance cultures, 33 (49%) were rectal, 17 (25%) pharynx, 16 (23%) EA, and 2 (3%) urine. Rectal screening identified 77% of colonized patients upon admission, 91% after 1 week of ICU stay, and nearly 100% thereafter.

PA genotyping

During the entire ICU stay we found 20 clonal ERIC-PCR genotypes (among 18 patients) and 11 unique genotypes from 9 patients (two patients had 2 isolates). In the clonal analysis we included cases that were excluded because of being positive on late screening.

Overall, the clonal structure was diverse. There were no dominant strains (related to many patients or to clinical cultures). Twelve patients (patients 2, 4, 5, 7, 8, 10, 12, 14, 15, 16, 17, 18 in Fig. 2) had >1 screening culture (on a following week) available for genotypic analysis (range, 1 to 10 isolates per patient). In 11 of these patients (92%) a serial identical isolate was identified on the following week (all except patient 12, in which the same genotype O was indeed found but only after 2 and 4 weeks, Fig. 2).

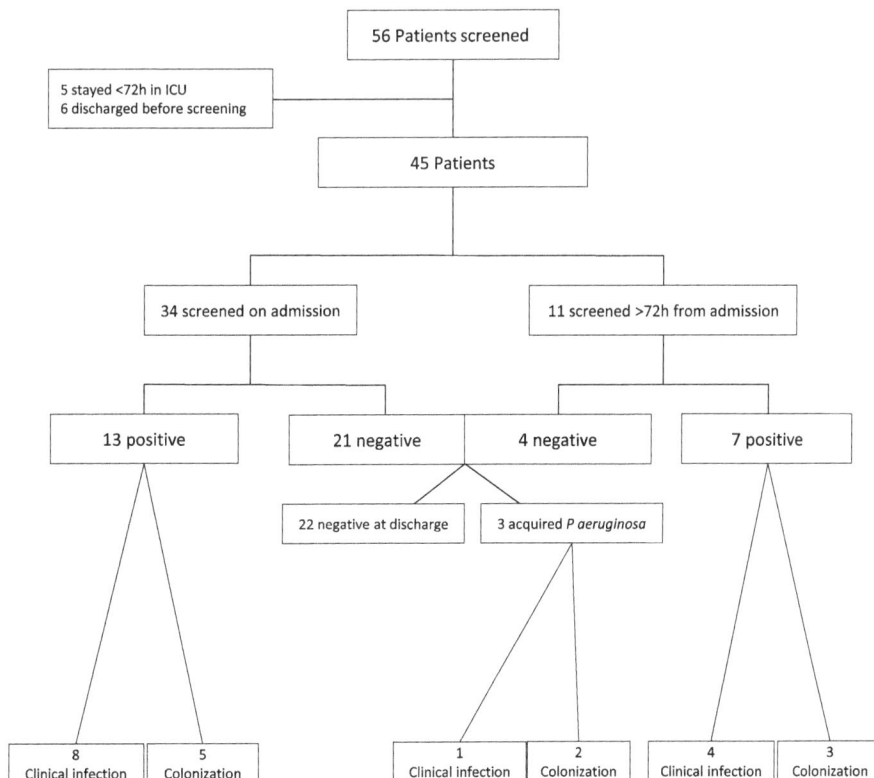

Fig. 1 Study population

Table 1 Patient characteristics according to *P. aeruginosa* carriage status on ICU admission

	All patients (n = 38)	Negative on admission (n = 25)	Positive on admission (n = 13)	P (OR, 95% CI)
Age mean (range)	70.3 (15-96)	65.6 (15-96)	79.3 (45-94)	0.0039
Age over 70 years	22 (58%)	11 (44%)	11 (84%)	0.035 (7, 1.2-38.3)
Sex				
Male	22 (58)	16 (64)	6 (46)	0.52
Female	16 (42)	9 (36)	7 (54)	0.52
LTCF residency	3 (8)	0	3 (23)	0.033 (17, 0.8-358)
APACHE II score, mean (range)	21.4 (10-42)	21.0 (10-42)	22.1 (14-34)	0.66
Days in hospital until ICU admission, mean (range)	3.7 (0-22)	3.7 (0-22)	3.7 (0-11)	0.98
Hospitalization in the last 90 days	19 (50)	11 (44)	8 (61)	0.49
Surgery in the last 30 days	14 (37)	8 (32)	6 (46)	0.48
Antimicrobials in the last 90 days	17 (45)	12 (48)	5 (38)	0.73
Prior PA in last 90 days	3 (8)	1 (4)	2 (15)	0.26
ICU LOS, mean (range)	15 (3-62)	10.6 (3-39)	23.7 (5-62)	0.0338
Hospital LOS, mean (range)	28 (6-88)	25 (6-80)	33.7 (10-88)	0.14
Ventilation days in ICU, mean (range)	17.3 (0-88)	12.8 (0-79)	26 (0-88)	0.16
COPD	11 (29)	7 (28)	4 (31)	1
IHD	15 (39)	8 (32)	7 (54)	0.29
CHF	14 (37)	7 (28)	7 (54)	0.16
Past CVA	9 (24)	6 (24)	3 (23)	1
CRF	8 (21)	5 (20)	3 (23)	1
Immunosuppression	4 (10)	4 (16)	0	0.27
Dementia	4 (10)	1 (4)	3 (23)	0.1
Active malignancy	4 (10)	3 (12)	1 (7)	1
DM type 2	15 (39)	14 (56)	1 (7)	0.005 (0.06, 0.007-0.58)
Tracheostomy in ICU	12 (31)	6 (24)	6 (46)	0.27
ICU death	5 (13)	2 (8)	3 (23)	0.31
Overall death	13 (34)	8 (32)	5 (38)	0.7

All numbers represent patients (percent), unless specified otherwise. *LTCF* long term care facility, *APACHE*, acute physiology and chronic health evaluation, *ICU* Intensive care unit, *PA P. aeruginosa*, *LOS* length of stay, *COPD* chronic obstructive pulmonary disease, *IHD* ischemic heart disease, *CHF* congestive heart failure, *CVA* cerebrovascular accident, *CRF* chronic renal failure, *DM* diabetes mellitus, *VAP* ventilator associated pneumonia, *CLABSI* central line associated blood stream infection, *CAUTI* catheter associated urinary tract infection, *OR* odds ratio, *CI* confidence interval

Table 2 *P. aeruginosa* colonization during ICU stay in 4 screening sites

	Any site (%)	Pharynx (%)	EA (%)	Urine (%)	Rectum (%)
Admission screening (n = 38)	13 (34)	3 (23)	6 (46)	1 (7)	10 (77)
Week 1 (n = 21)	11 (52)	5 (45)	3 (27)	0 (0)	10 (91)
Week 2 (n = 8)	6 (75)	4 (66)	3 (50)	0 (0)	6 (100)
Week 3 (n = 7)	5 (71)	4 (80)	4 (80)	1 (20)	4 (80)
Week 4 (n = 4)	2 (50)	0 (0)	0 (0)	0 (0)	2 (100)
Week 5 (n = 2)	1 (50)	1 (100)	1 (100)	0 (0)	1 (100)
Week 6 (n = 1)	0 (0)	0 (0)	0 (0)	0 (0)	0 (0)

ICU intensive care unit, *EA* endotracheal aspirate

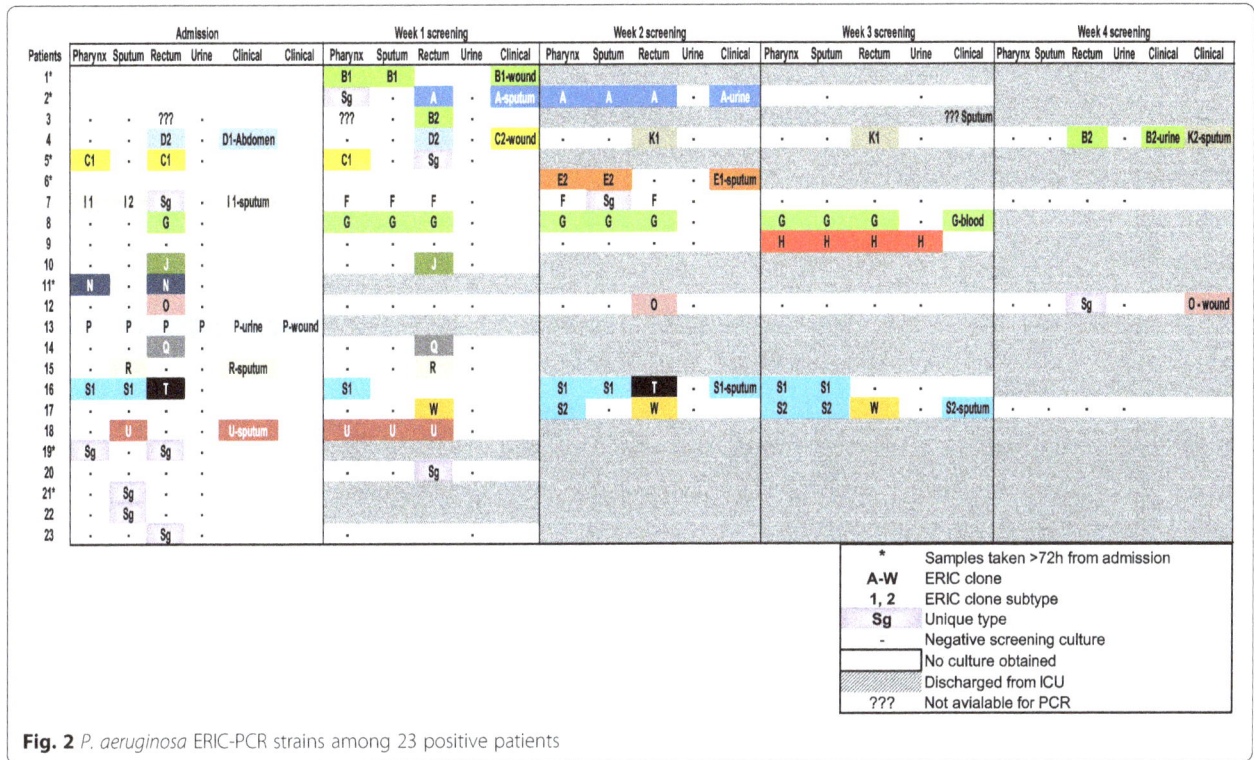

Fig. 2 *P. aeruginosa* ERIC-PCR strains among 23 positive patients

Clonal persistence vs. replacement in sequential screening

Rectum screening: 10 patients had at least 1 sequential rectal screening culture available for typing. In 9 of these (90%) the same clone persisted at least once (range 1–3 weeks). In 3 patients (30%) other strains appeared.

Pharynx screening: 5 patients had at least 1 sequential pharynx screening culture available for typing and in 4 (80%) the same clone persisted at least once (range 1–3 weeks).

AE screening: 4 patients had at least 1 sequential AE screening culture available for typing and in 3 (75%) the same clone persisted at least once (range 1–3 weeks). Cross-overs between sites and strains occurred (Fig. 2).

Calculated together, in 16 out of 19 (84%) of patients in which a sequential same-site screening cultures were available for typing, the same clone persisted. Clonal persistence was evident in all screening sites, but was most prominent in the rectum (90% vs. 80% and 75% in the pharynx and AE, respectively). Cross-overs between sites and strains occurred (Fig. 2).

In 5 patients a spread from the original site of identification to other screening sites was evident (Fig. 2). On 3 occasions the same genotype (B, C, S) was identified in different patients, indicating cross transmission.

Clinical impact of PA isolation in the ICU

Thirteen patients (29%) were diagnosed with PA infection: 10 with VAP, 4 with SSI and 1 with bloodstream infection. Ten additional patients (22%) acquired PA colonization without infection.

Patients colonized with PA on admission were at a higher risk of PA-related clinical infection, compared with patients who were PA-negative on admission [8/13 (62%) vs. 1/25 (4%), hazard ratio = 14.65, CI (3.07–47.39), $p = 0.0002$], and for PA-related VAP [hazard ratio = 7.381, CI (1.39–36.41), $p = 0.0047$], Fig. 3). PA-colonized patients also had significantly longer mean stay in the ICU (23.7 days versus 10.6 days; $p = 0.033$, Table 1). None of the 22 patients with repeated negative screening had a positive clinical culture with PA throughout their ICU stay.

Genotyping was performed on 17 clinical isolates from 12 patients (patients 1, 2, 4, 6, 7, 8, 12, 13, 15, 16, 17, 18; Fig. 2). Sixteen (94%) clinical strains were related to strains found concurrently or previously on screening cultures from the same patient and none were unique (Fig. 2, Table 3). The one exceptional clinical isolate (C2 from patient 4) was not unique since it was found in the screening cultures of patient 5. In 6 patients (50%) the clinical PA isolate could have been predicted from the screening cultures between 1 and 4 weeks earlier (genotypes A, K2, G, O, S1, S2); and in the other 6 patients the identification by screening occurred on the same week (genotypes B1, D, I,

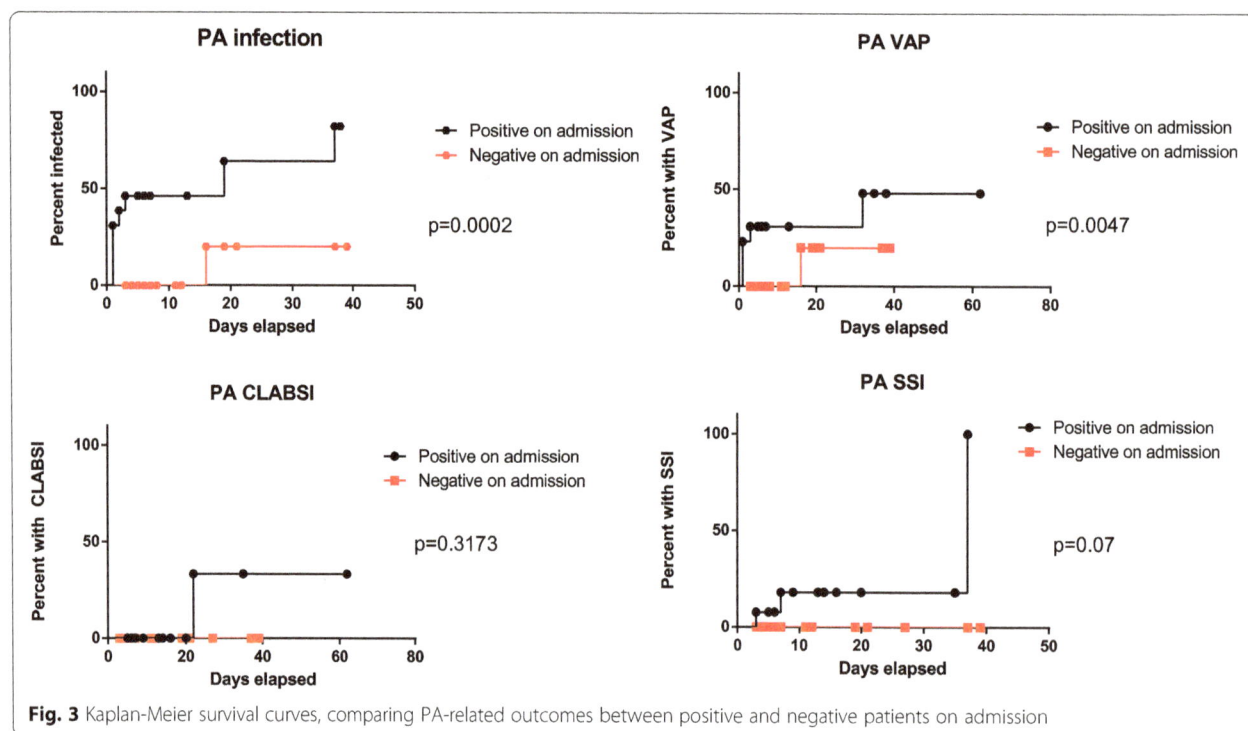

Fig. 3 Kaplan-Meier survival curves, comparing PA-related outcomes between positive and negative patients on admission

P, R, U). However, six patients (50%) had screening PA isolates that were different from a concurrent or subsequent clinical PA strain (patients 2, 4, 7, 12, 16, 17). The accuracy of (any site) surveillance cultures to predict the same genotype cultivation in a clinical sample was 76% (36/47), 75% (43/57) and 72% (45/62) when obtained on the same week or within 1 week before, 2 week before and throughout the ICU stay, respectively.

Table 4 shows the correlation of the site-specific screening culture with the infective strain according to the different diagnoses. Among 8 patients with VAP (who had clinical AE cultures available for typing), identical surveillance cultures were recovered from EA in 7 (87%), from the pharynx in 6 (75%), and from the rectum in 4 (50%). Among 4 patients with SSI, identical surveillance cultures were recovered from EA, pharynx and rectum in 2 patients (50%) each.

Discussion

We used systematic sequential screening to define the dynamics of PA colonization and infection at a general ICU. In a non-outbreak setting, we found a highly diverse population of patient-unique PA strains. Strains were often site-specific and site-persistent, particularly with regards to rectal colonization, but could also distribute between body sites, and be replaced frequently. A positive screening culture for PA was associated with an increased risk of PA related infection: there was a 50–70% likelihood of subsequent clinical infection with the same strain, depending on the timing and site of screening. Importantly, we found that when adequate infection control standards are maintained, repeated negative multi-site screening results were associated with a very low rate of subsequent clinical infection with PA.

A third of our patients were carriers of PA on admission to the ICU (26% rectal, 16% EA and 8% pharyngeal carriage). Bonten et al. reported similar figures (34%) along with striking similarities regarding the relative importance of the sites of screening: the gastrointestinal being the most sensitive (24% positivity), and pharynx and EA being positive in only 9% and 7%, respectively [3]. In a more recent study, Zorilla et al. reported similar findings (27% PA colonization on admission) [21]. Advanced age and prior hospital stay were risk factors for PA colonization on admission. Similarly, we found advanced age and residence in a LTCF as significant risk factors. Surprisingly, diabetes mellitus was associated with a low rate of PA colonization on ICU admission. In line with others [1, 22], we found that colonization often preceded infection. Specifically, patients colonized upon admission had a 14.65-fold risk of developing infection as compared with non-colonized patients.

Early and accurate antibiotic coverage in patients developing VAP in the ICU is critical to improve patient outcomes [23, 24], but the increasing rates of multidrug resistant (MDR) organisms (including PA) in ICU and non-ICU patients pose an obstacle for appropriate empiric therapy. Accurate prediction of antimicrobial resistance patterns of organisms causing VAP by using surveillance cultures in ICUs has been a matter of an ongoing debate in the literature. A recent systematic review and a meta-

Table 3 Concordance between screening and clinical ERIC-PCR strains

	Patient number	Screening culture strain	Site of screening	Clinical culture strain	Clinical culture site	Timing between screen and clinical culture
Correlated cases	1	B1	EA, P	B1	Wound	Same week
	2	A	Rc	A	EA	Same week
			Rc		Urine	1 week
			EA, P, Rc			Same week
	4	D2	Rc	D1	Abdomen	Same week
		K1	Rc	K2	EA	2 weeks
		B2	Rc	B2	Urine	Same week
	6	E2	EA, P	E1	EA	Same week
	7	I1, I2	EA, P	I1	EA	Same week
	8	G	Rc	G	Blood	3 weeks
			EA, P, Rc			2 weeks
			EA, P, Rc			1 week
			EA, P, Rc			Same week
	12	O	Rc	O	Wound	4 weeks
			Rc			2 weeks
	13	P	EA, P, Rc, U	P	Wound	Same week
					Urine	Same week
	15	R	EA	R	EA	Same week
	16	S1	EA, P	S1	EA	2 weeks
			P			1 week
			EA, P			Same week
	17	S2	P	S2	EA	1 week
			EA, P			Same week
	18	U	EA	U	EA	Same week
Uncorrelated cases	2	Sg	P	A	EA	Same week
					Urine	1 week
	4	D2	Rc	C2	Wound	1 week and same week
		B2	Rc	K2	EA	Same week
	7	Sg	Rc	I1	EA	Same week
	12	Sg	Rc	O	Wound	Same week
	16	T	Rc	S1	EA	Same week
	17	W	Rc	S2	EA	Same week

A-W – ERIC-PCR strain (a number denotes a clone subtype), Sg unique strain, *EA* endotracheal aspirate, *P* pharynx, *Rc* – rectum, *U* urine

analysis found high accuracy of surveillance cultures, with pooled sensitivities of up to 0.75 and specificities up to 0.92 in culture-positive VAP [25]. Our results support the predictive value of surveillance cultures: among patients who developed VAP, screening the EA or the pharynx accurately predicted the VAP-related strain in 75–87% of episodes. SSI-related strains were predicted by EA and pharynx screening in 50% of cases.

None of the patients who had persistently negative surveillance cultures had subsequent recovery of PA from clinical cultures. Similar findings were reported in the meta-analysis cited [25]. Hence, screening two sites weekly with negative results can provide reassurance for the physician not to initiate empirical anti-pseudomonal antibiotics in patients with suspected VAP or SSI, which are among the most frequent infections in critically ill patients. This finding may have implications for antibiotic stewardship, as it provides an evidence-based framework for limiting the use of wide-spectrum antibiotics in the ICU.

The current study is unique in providing a longitudinal assessment of PA colonization dynamics in multiple body sites throughout the ICU stay. Recently, Zorrilla et al. [1] found high rates (87%) of genotypic concordance between rectal surveillance cultures and infecting strains of PA. Our

Table 4 Prediction of clinical strain by screening sites according to diagnosis

Diagnosis	Clinical clone	Concordant screening sites				Discordant screening sites			
		EA	P	Rc	U	EA	P	Rc	U
VAP	A	+	+	+			+		
	K2			+				+	
	E1	+	+						
	I1	+	+					+	
	R	+		+					
	S1	+	+					+	
	S2	+	+					+	
	U	+	+	+					
Screen site utility for VAP (%)		7/8 (87)	6/8 (75)	4/8 (50)	NA	NA	1/8 (12)	4/8 (50)	NA
SSI	B1	+	+						
	C2							+	
	O			+				+	
	P	+	+	+	+				
Screen site utility for SSI (%)		2/4 (50)	2/4 (50)	2/4 (50)	1/4 (25)	NA	NA	2/4 (50)	NA
BSI	G	+	+	+					
IAI	D1			+					
Screen site utility for all infections (%)		10/14 (71)	9/14 (64)	8/14 (57)	1/14 (7)	NA	1/14 (7)	6/14 (43)	NA

VAP ventilator associated pneumonia, *SSI* surgical site infection, *BSI* blood stream infection, *IAI* intraabdominal infection, *EA* endotracheal aspirate, *P* pharynx, *Rc* rectum, *U* urine

results underscore the limitations of rectal screening for predicting respiratory strains, as further demonstrated in a study performed among hematopoietic stem cell recipients [26]. The high efficacy of lower airways screening to predict the strains that caused VAP is consistent with results of previous studies [3, 10].

The limitations of this study are the relatively small number of patients in a single center setting. Screening was limited to PA colonization, whereas in clinical practice empiric antimicrobial therapy often targets other MDR bacteria such as MRSA, MDR-*Acinetobacter* spp. and ESBL-producing Enterobacteriaceae. From a practical perspective, screening 3 body sites for PA only, may be expensive and labor intensive, and will miss other important causes of VAP and SSI. Another limitation is that antimicrobial susceptibility data of all screening strains was not available for comparison. Therefore, the utility of screening cultures to predict the susceptibility patterns of clinical PA strains remains to be established.

Conclusions

In this study we showed that in a non-outbreak setting of ICU, most strains were patient-unique, endogenous in origin, and cross contamination was rare. Colonization on admission was a significant risk factor for the development of infection with PA. Detection of PA on surveillance cultures may serve as a good predictor of PA clinical infection and also of the infecting clone, while negative screening is an excellent negative predictor for clinical infection. VAP-related strains are better predicted by upper airways screening than rectal screening.

Abbreviations
APACHE: Acute physiology and chronic health evaluation; CAUTI: Catheter-associated urinary tract infection; CDC: Centers for disease control and prevention; CLABSI: Central line-associated blood stream infection; EA: Endotracheal aspirate; ERIC: Enterobacterial repetitive Intergenic Consensus; ICU: Intensive care unit; LCTF: Long-term care facility; MDR: Multidrug resistant; NHSN: The national healthcare safety network; PA: *Pseudomonas aeruginosa*; PCR: Polymerase chain reaction; SSI: Surgical site infection; VAP: Ventilator associated pneumonia

Acknowledgments
None.

Funding
This study was not funded by any organization.

Authors' contributions
RC concepted the idea of the study, gathered the data, analyzed it and wrote the manuscript. BF reviewed independently the clinical cases in order to decide between infection and colonization states, and critically reviewed the manuscript. CS and AF collected the clinical and screening cultures. SM and UM treated the patients in the ICU and critically reviewed the manuscript. KE and AA performed the ERIC-PCR assays and gathered the molecular laboratory data. RBA critically reviewed the manuscript and made the statisitcal analysis. He was major contributor in writing the manuscript. PS made all the microbiology cultures and gathered all the microbiology data All authors read and approved the final manuscript.

Competing interests
The authors declare that they have no competing interests.

Consent for publication
Not applicable.

Author details
[1]Head of Infectious diseases unit, Sanz Medical Center, Laniado hospital, Neytanya, Israel. [2]Ruth and Bruce Rappaport Faculty of Medicine, Technion, Haifa, Israel. [3]Infectious diseases unit, Sanz Medical Center, Laniado hospital, Netanya, Israel. [4]Medical and Surgical intensive care unit, Sanz Medical Center, Laniado hospital, Netanya, Israel. [5]National Center of Infection Control, Ministry of Health, Tel Aviv, Israel. [6]Sackler Faculty of Medicine, Tel Aviv University, Tel Aviv, Israel. [7]Infectious diseases unit Tel Aviv Sourasky Medical Center, Tel Aviv, Israel. [8]Microbiology Laboratory, Sanz Medical Center, Laniado hospital, Netanya, Israel.

References
1. Gomez-Zorrilla S, Camoez M, Tubau F, Canizares R, Periche E, Dominguez MA, Ariza J, Pena C. Prospective observational study of prior rectal colonization status as a predictor for subsequent development of *Pseudomonas aeruginosa* clinical infections. Antimicrob Agents Chemother. 2015;59:5213–9.
2. Gruner E, Kropec A, Huebner J, Altwegg M, Daschner F. Ribotyping of *Pseudomonas aeruginosa* strains isolated from surgical intensive care patients. J Infect Dis. 1993;167:1216–20.
3. Bonten MJ, Bergmans DC, Speijer H, Stobberingh EE. Characteristics of polyclonal endemicity of *Pseudomonas aeruginosa* colonization in intensive care units. Implications for infection control. Am J Respir Crit Care Med. 1999;160:1212–9.
4. Trautmann M, Halder S, Hoegel J, Royer H, Haller M. Point-of-use water filtration reduces endemic *Pseudomonas aeruginosa* infections on a surgical intensive care unit. Am J Infect Control. 2008;36:421–9.
5. Blanc DS, Francioli P, Zanetti G. Molecular Epidemiology of *Pseudomonas aeruginosa* in the Intensive Care Units - A Review. Open Microbiol J. 2007;1:8–11.
6. Reuter S, Sigge A, Wiedeck H, Trautmann M. Analysis of transmission pathways of *Pseudomonas aeruginosa* between patients and tap water outlets. Crit Care Med. 2002;30:2222–8.
7. Thuong M, Arvaniti K, Ruimy R, de la Salmoniere P, Scanvic-Hameg A, Lucet JC, Regnier B. Epidemiology of *Pseudomonas aeruginosa* and risk factors for carriage acquisition in an intensive care unit. J Hosp Infect. 2003;53:274–82.
8. Trautmann M, Bauer C, Schumann C, Hahn P, Hoher M, Haller M, Lepper PM. Common RAPD pattern of *Pseudomonas aeruginosa* from patients and tap water in a medical intensive care unit. Int J Hyg Environ Health. 2006; 209:325–31.
9. Trautmann M, Michalsky T, Wiedeck H, Radosavljevic V, Ruhnke M. Tap water colonization with *Pseudomonas aeruginosa* in a surgical intensive care unit (ICU) and relation to Pseudomonas infections of ICU patients. Infect Control Hosp Epidemiol. 2001;22:49–52.
10. Valles J, Mariscal D, Cortes P, Coll P, Villagra A, Diaz E, Artigas A, Rello J. Patterns of colonization by *Pseudomonas aeruginosa* in intubated patients: a 3-year prospective study of 1,607 isolates using pulsed-field gel electrophoresis with implications for prevention of ventilator-associated pneumonia. Intensive Care Med. 2004;30:1768–75.
11. Venier AG, Leroyer C, Slekovec C, Talon D, Bertrand X, Parer S, Alfandari S, Guerin JM, Megarbane B, Lawrence C, et al. Risk factors for *Pseudomonas aeruginosa* acquisition in intensive care units: a prospective multicentre study. J Hosp Infect. 2014;88:103–8.
12. Petignat C, Francioli P, Nahimana I, Wenger A, Bille J, Schaller MD, Revelly JP, Zanetti G, Blanc DS. Exogenous sources of *Pseudomonas aeruginosa* in intensive care unit patients: implementation of infection control measures and follow-up with molecular typing. Infect Control Hosp Epidemiol. 2006; 27:953–7.
13. Bukholm G, Tannaes T, Kjelsberg AB, Smith-Erichsen N. An outbreak of multidrug-resistant *Pseudomonas aeruginosa* associated with increased risk of patient death in an intensive care unit. Infect Control Hosp Epidemiol. 2002;23:441–6.
14. Rogues AM, Boulestreau H, Lasheras A, Boyer A, Gruson D, Merle C, Castaing Y, Bebear CM, Gachie JP. Contribution of tap water to patient colonisation with *Pseudomonas aeruginosa* in a medical intensive care unit. J Hosp Infect. 2007;67:72–8.
15. Cohen R, Babushkin F, Shimoni Z, Cohen S, Litig E, Shapiro M, Adler A, Paikin S. Water faucets as a source of *Pseudomonas aeruginosa* infection and colonization in neonatal and adult intensive care unit patients. Am J Infect Control. 2016.
16. Horan TC, Andrus M, Dudeck MA. CDC/NHSN surveillance definition of health care-associated infection and criteria for specific types of infections in the acute care setting. Am J Infect Control. 2008;36:309–32.
17. American Thoracic S, Infectious Diseases Society of A. Guidelines for the management of adults with hospital-acquired, ventilator-associated, and healthcare-associated pneumonia. Am J Respir Crit Care Med. 2005;171:388–416.
18. CLSI. M100-S25 performance standards for antimicrobial susceptibility testing; Twenty-fifth informational supplement. 2015.
19. Wolska K, Szweda P. A comparative evaluation of PCR ribotyping and ERIC PCR for determining the diversity of clinical *Pseudomonas aeruginosa* isolates. Pol J Microbiol. 2008;57:157–63.
20. Kidd TJ, Grimwood K, Ramsay KA, Rainey PB, Bell SC. Comparison of three molecular techniques for typing *Pseudomonas aeruginosa* isolates in sputum samples from patients with cystic fibrosis. J Clin Microbiol. 2011;49:263–8.
21. Gomez-Zorrilla S, Camoez M, Tubau F, Periche E, Canizares R, Dominguez MA, Ariza J, Pena C. Antibiotic pressure is a major risk factor for rectal colonization by multidrug-resistant *Pseudomonas aeruginosa* in critically ill patients. Antimicrob Agents Chemother. 2014;58:5863–70.
22. Bertrand X, Thouverez M, Talon D, Boillot A, Capellier G, Floriot C, Helias JP. Endemicity, molecular diversity and colonisation routes of *Pseudomonas aeruginosa* in intensive care units. Intensive Care Med. 2001;27:1263–8.
23. Iregui M, Ward S, Sherman G, Fraser VJ, Kollef MH. Clinical importance of delays in the initiation of appropriate antibiotic treatment for ventilator-associated pneumonia. Chest. 2002;122:262–8.
24. Kollef M. Appropriate empirical antibacterial therapy for nosocomial infections: getting it right the first time. Drugs. 2003;63:2157–68.
25. Brusselaers N, Labeau S, Vogelaers D, Blot S. Value of lower respiratory tract surveillance cultures to predict bacterial pathogens in ventilator-associated pneumonia: systematic review and diagnostic test accuracy meta-analysis. Intensive Care Med. 2013;39:365–75.
26. Nesher L, Rolston KV, Shah DP, Tarrand JT, Mulanovich V, Ariza-Heredia EJ, Chemaly RF. Fecal colonization and infection with *Pseudomonas aeruginosa* in recipients of allogeneic hematopoietic stem cell transplantation. Transpl Infect Dis. 2015;17:33–8.

2

Antibiotic use in a tertiary healthcare facility in Ghana

Appiah-Korang Labi[1], Noah Obeng-Nkrumah[2*], Edmund Tetteh Nartey[3], Stephanie Bjerrum[4], Nii Armah Adu-Aryee[5], Yaw Adjei Ofori-Adjei[6], Alfred E. Yawson[7] and Mercy J. Newman[8]

Abstract

Background: The global rise and spread of antibiotic resistance is limiting the usefulness of antibiotics in the prevention and treatment of infectious diseases. The use of antibiotic stewardship programs guided by local data on prescribing practices is a useful strategy to control and reduce antibiotic resistance. Our objective in this study was to determine the prevalence and indications for use of antibiotics at the Korle-Bu Teaching Hospital Accra, Ghana.

Methods: An antibiotic point prevalence survey was conducted among inpatients of the Korle-Bu Teaching Hospital between February and March 2016. Folders and treatment charts of patients on admission at participating departments were reviewed for antibiotics administered or scheduled to be administered on the day of the survey. Data on indication for use were also collected. Prevalence of antibiotic use was determined by dividing the number of inpatients on antibiotics at the time of survey by the total number of patients on admission.

Results: Of the 677 inpatients surveyed, 348 (51.4%, 95% CI, 47.6–55.2) were on treatment with antibiotics. Prevalence was highest among Paediatric surgery where 20/22 patients (90.9%, 95% CI, 70.8–98.9) were administered antibiotics and lowest among Obstetrics patients with 77/214 (36%, 95% CI, 29.5–42.8). The indications for antibiotic use were 245/611 (40.1%) for community-acquired infections, 205/611 (33.6%) for surgical prophylaxis, 129/611 (21.1%) for healthcare associated infections and 33/611 (5.4%) for medical prophylaxis. The top five antibiotics prescribed in the hospital were metronidazole 107 (17.5%), amoxicillin-clavulinic acid 82 (13.4%), ceftriaxone 17(12.1%), cefuroxime 61 (10.0%), and cloxacillin 52 (8.5%) respectively. Prevalence of meropenem and vancomycin use was 12(2%) and 1 (.2%) respectively. The majority of patients 181 (52%) were being treated with two antibiotics.

Conclusion: This study indicated a high prevalence of antibiotic use among inpatients at the Korle-Bu Teaching Hospital. Metronidazole was the most commonly used antibiotic; mainly for surgical prophylaxis. There is the need to further explore factors contributing to the high prevalence of antibiotic use and develop strategies for appropriate antibiotic use in the hospital.

Keywords: Antibiotic, Ghana, Africa, Point prevalence, Antibiotic stewardship

Background

The discovery of antibiotics in the twentieth century immensely changed medical practice. It allowed for treatment of life threatening conditions and the conduct of complex medical procedures with a reduced risk of infections. Over time, global overuse of antibiotics has emerged as a major problem [1, 2], with up to 50% of patients reported to receive unnecessary antibiotics [3].

Excessive use of antibiotics leads to the development of complications such as antibiotic related diarrhoea and healthcare associated infections [4, 5]. It is also a significant contributor to the development and spread of multidrug resistant bacteria, currently regarded as global public health crisis [6–9]. Antibiotic overuse is driven by prescribing habits of practitioners, which are dynamic and likely to change over time. These habits are affected by multiple factors including pathogen related factors

* Correspondence: successfulnoahforchrist@yahoo.com
[2]Department of Medical Laboratory Sciences, School of Biomedical and Allied Health Sciences, P.O. Box KB 143, Accra, Ghana

such as changing resistance profiles [6–9], prescriber related factors [10, 11] and external factors such as pressure from the pharmaceutical industry [10–12]. It has been suggested that antibiotic consumption will increase with rising incomes in developing countries and better access to medical insurance [6, 13]. Thus efforts to promote rational antibiotic use and infection control in these regions are paramount [7]. Accurate information on the use of antibiotics are crucial to address the problem of antibiotic overuse and resistance [12]. In Africa, there are few published studies on antibiotic use among inpatients [14–16]. At the Korle-Bu Teaching Hospital (KBTH), Accra Ghana, a survey conducted in 2000 showed a 53% prevalence of antibiotic use among inpatients with metronidazole being the most commonly used antibiotic [17]. Unpublished data from a point prevalence study carried out in the Medical department of the same institution in 2012 showed that 67.9% of inpatients had been prescribed antibiotics.

Continuous evaluation of antibiotic use is important to preserve the effectiveness of antibiotics and minimize patient harm [13]. The WHO recommends surveillance of antibiotic use as a strategy for improving antibiotic use among patients and also for controlling antibiotic resistance [6]. Repeated point prevalence surveys of antibiotic use have been shown as a useful and cost effective way of evaluating antibiotic use in hospital [18, 19]. This study reports the results from a point prevalence survey of systemic antibiotic use conducted in 2016 among inpatients at the KBTH. The aim was to determine the prevalence of antibiotic use and indications for their use.

Methods

Study setting and design

The Korle-Bu Teaching Hospital is a 2000-bed tertiary referral hospital situated in Accra, Ghana with about 200 admissions per day [15]. The hospital covers all medical specialties and provides referral healthcare services to an estimated population of 24 million Ghanaians. The hospital has an estimated average bed occupancy rate of 66.1% (i.e., $n = 1321$ patients per 2000 beds) [20]. Acute care services provided by the hospital KBTH include internal medicine, general surgery, neurosurgery, orthopaedics, plastic surgery, opthalmology, ear, nose and throat, obstetrics and gynaecology, neonatal and adult intensive care, paediatrics, chest unit and cardiothoracic surgery. The point prevalence study involved the survey of inpatients records from hospital folders and was conducted in selected units of KBTH between February and March 2016. The survey instrument used in the study was adapted with modifications from the European survey of antimicrobial resistance [21]. Only folders of inpatients on admission before 8 am on the day of the survey were included in the study. The departments included in this

study were General Surgery, Orthopaedics, Paediatric Surgery, Genitourinary, Neurosurgery, Child Health (except the neonatal intensive care unit where rehabilitation works were ongoing), Medicine, Obstetrics and Gynaecology. These departments have the highest number of patient admissions per day. Wards with patients not matching the inclusion criteria and those with only day cases were excluded. As per study protocol, we excluded the Plastic Surgery & Burns Unit where patients are routinely administered long-term antibiotics on admissions.

Data collection

A multidisciplinary team of doctors and an infectious disease specialists conducted the survey at selected units. Training and piloting of the study instrument was conducted for the survey team prior to the start of the study. Briefly, the training session chaired by the lead investigator introduced survey personnel to the objectives of the study; the purpose of each item on the data collection tool including definition of terms and indicator codes; methods for assessment of individual patient data; and the roles and responsibilities of each survey personnel. The session was concluded with a 1-day pilot point-prevalence survey in a Medical ward. This session was conducted a week prior to study inception to allow for corrective action. The point prevalence survey was conducted from 8 am to 8 pm daily within a 2-week period. Data collection from each unit was completed within the 12-h period. The survey team performed retrospective data collection using standardized case report forms which primarily comprise a patient-level structured template for documenting antimicrobial use on the day of survey (Additional file 1). They reviewed patients' folders and treatment charts and collected information on antibiotic use only for the survey date. Folders of patients undergoing same day treatment or surgery were excluded. Relevant data elements such as age, sex, ward, and total number of patients on admission on survey day were retrieved. Other information collected included antibiotics administered and route of administration, their dosages, dosing intervals and number of missed doses. In addition, patients' clinical diagnosis and indications for antibiotic use (hospital- or community-acquired) were recorded. In every case, the survey team decided on clinical grounds whether the patient was infected or not according to guideline definitions [21]. Briefly, an active infection on the survey day was defined by the presence of signs and symptoms. Patients were considered infected even when signs and symptoms were no longer present but the patient was still receiving treatment for that infection on the date of the survey. The signs and symptoms were also reviewed to ascertain the indication for treatment (hospital-acquired, community-acquired, surgical prophylaxis and medical prophylaxis). The team referred to medical and nursing records and other relevant charts to determine whether the infection is a healthcare related. Clinical diagnosis of infections 48 h after admission was described as hospital-acquired infections. Infections occurring within 48 h of admission were categorized as community-acquired. The WHO anatomical therapeutic classification (ATC) of medicines was used for classifying drugs [22].

Data handling and statistical analysis

Data was entered into MS Access® and exported into statistical package for social sciences (SPSS version 21) for cleaning and analysis. The prevalence of antibiotic use was defined as a percentage of the total number of patients on any systemic antibiotic at the time of survey against the number of patients on admission. Descriptive statistics (e.g., cross-tabulations, frequencies, and proportions) were used to examine data on antibiotic use. Proportions were compared using Chi-square tests.

Results

A total 677 in-patient folders were reviewed from participating units/departments. The majority of included patients were admitted at the Obstetrics unit ($n = 214$), Child Health ($n = 111$), Medicine (106), Orthopaedics ($n = 84$), General Surgery ($n = 55$), Gynaecology ($n = 38$), Neurosurgery ($n = 23$), Urology ($n = 24$) and Paediatric Surgery ($n = 22$). The median age of included patients was 39 years and 54.2% were females. Adults (age > 15 years) comprised 71%, followed by children (29 days to 15 years old; 19.9%) and neonates (0–28 days; 9.1%).

Prevalence and type of antibiotic use

Table 1 shows the prevalence of antibiotic use in the participating hospital. In all, 348 (51.4%, 95% CI, 47.6–55.2%) of admitted patients received one or more antibiotics at the time of survey. Parenteral

formulations constituted the significant majority of all antibiotic prescriptions (59.9%, $n = 366/611$). They were administered in 32.8% ($n = 222/677$) of admitted patients. Significantly fewer patients (18.8%, $n = 127/677$) received oral antibiotics. Across hospital units, the proportion of patients on antibiotics ranged from 36% (95% CI, 29.5–42.8) in Obstetrics to 90.9% (95% CI, 70.8–98.9) in Paediatric surgery. Of 348 patients on antibiotics, 127 (36.0%, 95% CI, 31.5–41.8) were on one antibiotic, 181 (52.0%, 95% CI, 46.6–57.4) were on two antibiotics, 38 (10.9%, 95% CI, 7.9–14.8) were on three antibiotics whilst 2 (0.6%, 95% CI, 0.1–2.3) were on 4 antibiotics (Fig. 1). The median number of antibiotics per patient was 2. A total of 611 antibiotic prescriptions were recorded. The top five percentage use by drug classes (ATC level 5) were as follows: penicillin based drugs (24.9%, $n = 152$), nitroimidazoles (17.5%, $n = 107$), 3rd generation cephalosporins (13.8%, $n = 84$), 2nd generation cephalosporins (10.0%, $n = 61$), and aminoglycosides (8.8%, $n = 54$). The five most commonly used generic antibiotics (Table 2) were metronidazole (17.5%, n = 107), amoxicillin-clavulanic acid (13.4%, $n = 83$), ceftriaxone (12.1%, $n = 74$), cefuroxime (10.0%, n = 61), and cloxacillin (8.5%, $n = 50$). The obstetrics unit accounted for the highest use of metronidazole (50.5%, n = 54) and amoxicillin-clavulanic acid (58.5%, $n = 48$) respectively. Figure 2 compares the top five antibiotic prescriptions at KBTH in 2000 [17] and 2017. In 2000, the most common antimicrobial in use at KBTH was metronidazole 212(44%), followed by ampicillin/amoxicillin 199(41.6%), gentamicin 168(34%) and cloxacillin 135(28%). In 2017, only metronidazole and cloxacillin remain in the top five antibiotics prescribed, albeit with significantly reduced percentage use. Cloxacillin recorded the least reduction (19.5%) in percentage

Table 1 Prevalence rates of antibiotic use across departments/units

Department	Patients on antibiotics		Antibiotic prescriptions			
	Number	% prevalence [95% CI]	Parenteral	Oral	Total	% prevalence [95% CI]
Obstetrics (n = 214)	77	36.0 [29.5-42.8]	46 (33.8)	90 (66.2)	136	16.5[13.8-19.5]
Child Health (n = 111)	77	69.4 [59.9-77.8]	120 (85.1)	21(14.9)	141	22.5[19.5-25.9]
Medicine (n = 106)	53	50.0 [40.1-59.9]	65 (64.4)	36 (35.6)	101	16.5[13.8-19.5]
Orthopaedics (n = 84)	48	57.1 [45.9-67.9]	26 (35.6)	47 (64..4)	73	13.3[10.4-16.2
General Surgery (n = 55)	33	56.9 [43.2-69.8]	28 (58.9)	24 (46.2)	52	8.6[8.7-11.4]
Paediatric Surgery (n = 22)	20	90.9 [70.8-98.9]	32 (84.2)	6 (15.8)	38	5.8[4.2-8.6]
Gynaecology (n = 38)	17	44.7 [28.6-61.7]	17 (53.7)	13(43.3)	30	4.5[3.1-6.4]
Neuro-surgery (n = 23)	12	52.2 [30.6-73.2]	21 (87.5)	3 (12.5)	24	3.6[2.4-53.8]
Urology (n = 24)	11	45.8 [29.8-74.3]	11 (68.8)	5 (31.2)	16	2.3[1.4-3.8]
All departments (n-677)	348	51.4 [47.6-55.2]	366 (59.9)[b]	245(40.1)[a]	611	

Prevalence was determined by dividing the number of inpatients on antibiotics at the time of survey by the total of patients on admission; *CI*, confidence interval; b > a at *p* < 0.05

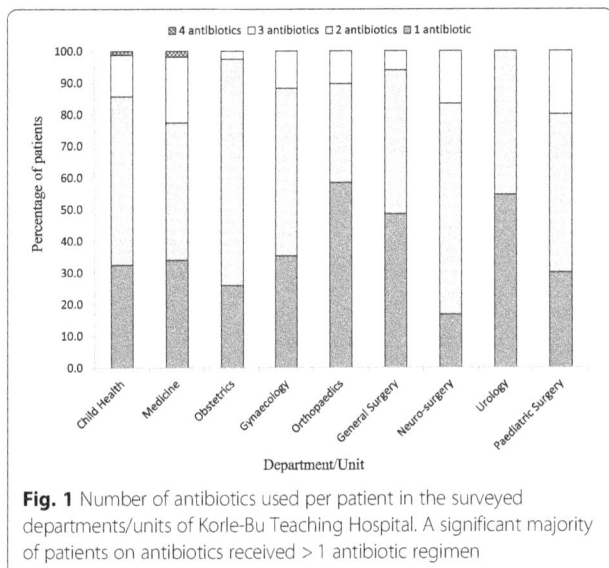

Fig. 1 Number of antibiotics used per patient in the surveyed departments/units of Korle-Bu Teaching Hospital. A significant majority of patients on antibiotics received > 1 antibiotic regimen

antibiotic use, followed by metronidazole (26.5%), gentamicin (26.6%), amoxicillin (40.0%) and ampicillin (41.1%).

Indications for antibiotic use

Overall, 245 (40.1%) of 611 prescriptions were administered for community-acquired infections, 128 (21.0%) for hospital-acquired infections, 205 (33.6%) for surgical prophylaxis and 33 (5.4%) for medical prophylaxis (Table 3). The most prescribed antibiotic for surgical prophylaxis (n = 205) was metronidazole (32.2%, n = 66), followed by amoxicillin-clavulanic acid (25.9%, n = 53) and cefuroxime (13.7%, n = 28). For community-acquired infections, the three commonly prescribed antibiotics were ceftriaxone (18.0%, n = 44), cloxacillin and gentamicin (10.6%, n = 26). Of the 128 antibiotics used for hospital-acquired infections, the top three drugs were ceftriaxone (12.5%, 16.0), metronidazole (12.5%, 16.0), and cloxacillin (11.7%, n = 15). The proportion of antibiotic use by anatomic site is presented in Table 4. About a sixth (16.0%, n = 101) of all antibiotic prescriptions were for undefined reasons. The majority of antibiotics were prescribed for genitourinary and obstetric systems (25.2%, n = 154), and skin, soft tissue, bones and joints (19.4%, n = 119). The three most prescribed antibiotics for the former were metronidazole (40.3%, n = 62/154), amoxicillin- clavulanic acid (37.0%, n = 57/154), and cefuroxime (5.2%, n = 8/154). Clindamycin (30.3%, n = 36/119), cefuroxime (22.6%, n = 27/119) and ciprofloxacin (10.9%, n = 13/119) were the most indicated antibiotics for skin, soft tissue, bones and joints.

Discussion

We conducted a point prevalence survey of antibiotic use among inpatients of the KBTH in Ghana. The study identified a high prevalence of antibiotic use with nearly 51% of

inpatients receiving antibiotics. The antibiotics were mainly used for treatment of community-acquired infections (40.1%) and surgical prophylaxis (33.6%). The prevalence level reported in this study is comparable to a prevalence rate of 53% recorded in a previous study among inpatients at KBTH in 2000 [17]. These rates may represent a relatively stable antibiotic use prevalence over the period.

The prevalence rate is however lower than 59.9% prevalence of antibiotic use recorded among out patients in primary healthcare facilities in Ghana [23]. It is also lower than 64.6 and 67.4%, which are the prevalence rates recorded in hospitals in Benin and Vietnam, countries with similar developmental profiles as Ghana [14, 24]. The prevalence of antibiotic use in this study is however comparable to the prevalence of 49.9% [13] recorded in acute care hospitals in the United States of America; and higher than antibiotic prescribing rates in Europe, which range between 30.1–35% [21, 25]. Our indicated prevalence is also lower than that reported in the ARPEC study (36.7%) which surveyed children from 226 hospitals in 41 countries across six continents [16].

High rates of antibiotic use are usually associated with inappropriate use of antibiotics and the development of antibiotic resistance and healthcare associated infections [4, 8, 26]. In Vietnam and Turkey, antibiotics were deemed to be prescribed inappropriately in 30.8 and 46.7% of cases [12, 24]. High rates of antibiotic use observed at the KBTH may be due to lack of antibiotic formulary or uniform standard protocols for managing infections for the hospital, despite presence of a national standard treatment guidelines [27]. Although this study was not designed to evaluate the appropriateness of antibiotic use, it is expected that with high prevalence of antibiotic use, a significant proportion of the use in KBTH may be inappropriate or unnecessary. This finding thus presents an opportunity to reduce antibiotic consumption in the hospital.

The prevalence of antibiotic use was highest among paediatric surgical patients (90.6%) and lowest among obstetric patients (36.0%). This fact could be explained by the high use of prophylactic antibiotics among paediatric surgical patients. The majority of patients (52%) were on two antibiotics. This is comparable to findings from the survey conducted in 2000, where 42.6% of patients in the hospital were on two antibiotics [17]. A significant proportion of prescribed antibiotics (59.9%) were administered via the parenteral route. Highest use of parenteral antibiotics was found in the neurosurgical unit, child health and paediatric surgery unit. Similar rates especially among children has been reported in other studies [16]. Such high usage of parenteral antibiotics may be associated with unsafe needle use [28]. Although the prevalence of antibiotic use in the hospital seems to be stable, the agents used are changing. In the

Table 2 Proportion of prescribed antibiotics (ATC level 5) by Departments/units

Drug name (generic)	Total	Department/Unit								
		Child Health	Medicine	Obstetrics	Gynaecology	Orthopaedics	General Surgery	Neuro-surgery	Urology	Paediatric Surgery
		n, %	n, %[1]	n, %	n, %	n, %	n, %	n, %[1]	n, %[1]	n, %[1]
Metronidazole	107 (17.5)	4 (2.8)	13 (12.9)	54 (39.7)	9 (30.0)	3 (4.1)	9 (17.3)	4 (16.7)	2 (12.5)	9 (23.7)
Amoxicillin-clavulanic acid	82 (13.4)	1 (0.7)	7 (6.9)	48 (35.3)	8 (26.7)	1 (1.4)	12 (23.1)	2 (8.3)	1 (6.3)	2 (5.3)
Ceftriaxone	74 (12.1)	20 (14.2)	27 (26.7)	4 (2.9)	4 (13.3)	1 (1.4)	2 (3.9)	7 (29.2)	1 (6.3)	8 (21.1)
Cefuroxime	61 (10.0)	6 (4.3)	2 (2.0)	13 (9.6)	5 (16.7)	28 (38.4)	5 (9.6)	1 (4.2)	–	1 (2.6)
Cloxacillin	52 (8.5)	28 (19.9)	10 (9.9)	1 (0.7)	–	5 (6.9)	–	6 (25.0)	–	2 (5.3)
Clindamycin	49 (8.0)	10 (7.1)	3 (2.9)	4 (2.9)	1 (3.3)	25 (30.1)	7 (13.5)	1 (4.2)	1 (6.3)	–
Gentamicin	46 (7.5)	30 (21.3)	3 (2.9)	2 (1.5)	1 (3.3)	1 (1.4)	2 (3.9)	1 (4.2)	–	6 (15.8)
Ciprofloxacillin	39 (6.4)	6 (4.3)	7 (6.9)	–	1 (3.3)	9 (12.3)	8 (15.4)	1 (4.2)	5 (31.3)	2 (5.3)
Azithromycin	21 (3.4)	–	13 (12.9)	5 (3.9)	1 (3.3)	1 (1.4)	–	–	1 (6.3)	–
Co-trimoxazole	14 (2.3)	7 (5.0)	7 (6.9)	–	–	–	–	–	–	
Meropenem	12 (2.0)	2 (1.4)	1 (1.0)	–	–	–	2 (3.9)	–	4 (25.0)	3 (7.9)
Amikacin	8 (1.3)	7 (5.0)	–	–	–	–	–	Q	-a	–
Ampicillin	10 (1.6)	7 (5.0)	–	–	–	–	–	–	–	3 (7.9)
Crystal penicillin	7 (1.2)	6 (4.3)	1 (1.0)	–	–	–	–	–	–	–
Cefotaxime	6 (1.0)	6 (4.3)	–	–	–	–	–	–	–	–
Levofloxacin	5 (0.8)	–	3 (3.0)	–	–	1 (1.4)	1 (1.9)	–	–	–
Erythromycin	5 (0.8)	–	1 (1.0)	4 (2.9)	–	–	–	–	–	–
Clarithromycin	3 (0.5)	–	–	–	–	–	3 (5.7)	–	–	–
Nitrofuratoin	2 (0.3)	–	–	–	–	1 (1.4)	–	–	1 (6.3)	–
Ceftazidine	2 (0.3)	–	1 (1.0)	–	–	–	–	–	–	1 (2.6)
Amoxicillin	1 (0.2)	–	–	–	–	–	1 (1.9)	–	–	–
Cefixime	1 (0.2)	–	–	1 (0.7)	–	–	–	–	–	–
Doxycycline	1 (0.2)	–	1 (1.0)	–	–	–	–	–	–	–
Cefpodoxime	1 (0.2)	–	–	–	–	–	–	–	–	1 (2.6)
Nalidixic acid	1 (0.2)	1 (0.7)	–	–	–	–	–	–	–	–
Vancomycin	1 (0.2)	–	1 (1.0)	–	–	–	–	–	–	–
Total	611	141	101	136	30	73	52	24	16	38

ATC, Anatomic therapeutic classification; n=number; %, prevalence

year 2000 the top five agents were metronidazole, followed by ampicillin/amoxicillin, gentamicin and cloxacillin [17]. In this study, 26 different antibiotics were used among inpatients with metronidazole, amoxicillin-clavulanic acid, ceftriaxone, cefuroxime and cloxacillin contributing to more than 50% of all antibiotics prescribed. These agents were mainly used for surgical prophylaxis and treatment of community-acquired infections. The apparent change in agents over the years may point to increasing reports of antibiotic resistance from Ghana over the past decades [29–31]. Use of carbapenems (2.0%) and glycopeptides (0.2%) in the hospital were

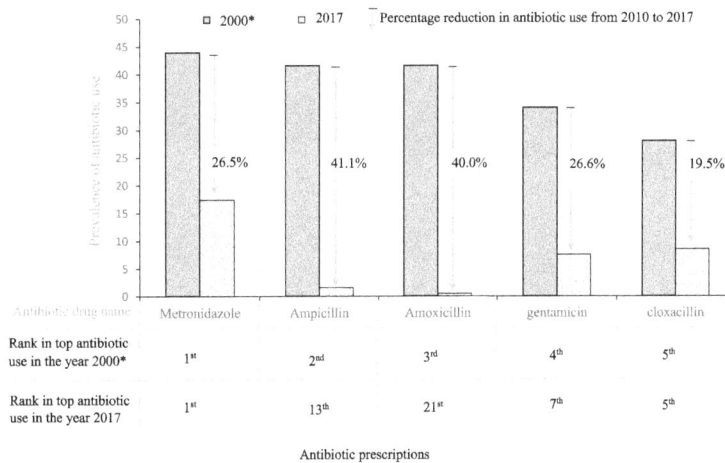

Fig. 2 Top five antibiotic use in 2000 and 2017 at KBTH. Figures on antibiotic use in 2000 based on data by Newman, 2009 [17]

Table 3 Proportion of prescribed antibiotics (ATC level 5) by indication

Drug name (generic)	Total, %	Community acquired n, %	Hospital acquired n, %	Surgical prophylaxis n, %	Medical prophylaxis n, %
Metronidazole	107 (17.5)	22 (9.0)	16 (12.5)	66 (32.2)	3 (9.1)
Amoxicillin- clavulanic acid	82 (13.4)	18 (7.4)	9 (7.0)	53 (25.9)	2 (13.4)
Ceftriaxone	74 (12.1)	44 (18.0)	16 (12.5)	13 (6.3)	1 (3.0)
Cefuroxime	61 (10.0)	24 (9.8)	7 (5.5)	28 (13.7)	2 (6.1)
Cloxacillin	52 (8.5)	26 (10.6)	15 (11.7)	8 (3.9)	3 (9.1)
Clindamycin	49 (8.0)	21 (8.6)	13 (10.2)	15 (7.3	–
Gentamicin	46 (7.5)	26 (10.6)	13 (10.2)	5 (2.4)	2 (6.1)
Ciprofloxaciin	39 (6.4)	17 (6.9)	14 (10.9)	8 (3.9)	–
Azithromycin	21 (3.4)	16 (6.5)	3 (2.3)	2 (1.0)	–
Co-trimoxazole	14 (2.3)	3 (1.2)	1 (0.8)	–	10 (30.3)
Meropenem	12 (2.0)	2 (0.8)	9 (7.0)	1 (0.5)	–
Amikacin	8 (1.3)	3 (1.2)	3 (2.3)	–	2 (6.1)
Ampicillin	10 (1.6)	7 (2.9)	–	2 (1.0)	1 (3.0)
Crystal penicillin	7 (1.2)	2 (0.8)	2 (1.6)	–	3 (9.1)
Cefotaxime	6 (1.0)	5 (2.0)	1 (0.8)	–	–
Levofloxacin	5 (0.8)	1 (0.4)	3 (2.3)	1 (0.5)	–
Erythromycin	5 (0.8)	2 (0.8)	–	–	3 (9.1)
Clarithromycin	3 (0.5)	2 (0.8)	–	1 (0.5)	–
Nitrofuratoin	2 (0.3)	–	1 (0.8)	1 (0.5)	–
Ceftazidine	2 (0.3)	–	2 (1.6)	–	–
Amoxicillin	1 (0.2)	1 (0.4)	–	–	–
Cefixime	1 (0.2)	–	–	1 (0.5)	–
Doxycycline	1 (0.2)	1 (0.4)	–	–	–
Cefpodoxime	1 (0.2)	–	1 (0.8)	–	–
Nalidixic acid	1 (0.2)	1 (0.4)	–	–	–
Vancomycin	1 (0.2)	1 (0.4)	–	–	–
Total	611(100)	245	128	205	33

ATC, Anatomic therapeutic classification, *n* number; %, prevalence

Table 4 Proportion of prescribed antibiotics (ATC level 5) by anatomic site

Drug name (generic)	Anatomic sites								
	Total	CNS	OTH	UT	GIT	SSTBJ	GUOB	RESP	Undefined
		n, %	n, %	n, %	n, %	n, %	n, %	n, %	n, %
Metronidazole	107	10 (9.3)	–	–	15 (14.0)	6 (5.6)	62 (57.9)	10 (9.3)	4 (3.7)
Amoxicillin- clavulanic acid	82	1 (1.2)	1 (1.2)	–	2 (2.4)	8 (9.8)	57 (69.5)	10 (12.2)	3 (3.7)
Ceftriaxone	74	16 (21.6)	2 (2.7)	1 (1.4)	9 (12.2)	4 (5.4)	8 (10.8)	24 (32.4)	10 (13.5)
Cefuroxime	61	1 (1.6)	–	4 (6.6)	5 (8.2)	27 (44.8)	9 (14.8)	11 (18.0)	4 (6.6)
Cloxacillin	52	13 (25.0)	1 (1.9)	–	2 (3.9)	13 (25.0)	–	–	23 (44.2)
Clindamycin	49	1 (2.0)	–	–	1 (2.0)	36 (73.5)	2 (4.1)	5 (10.2)	4 (8.2)
Gentamicin	46	3 (6.5)	2 (4.3)	1 (2.2)	3 (6.5)	6 (13.0)	1 (2.2)	5 (10.9)	25 (54.4)
Ciprofloxacin	39	1 (2.6)	–	5 (12.8)	9 (23.1)	13 (33.3)	6 (15.4)	2 (5.1)	3 (7.7)
Azithromycin	21	1 (4.8)	–	–	–	–	1 (4.8)	18 (85.7)	1 (4.8)
Co-trimoxazole	14	2 (14.3)	–	–	–	–	–	11 (78.6)	1 (7.1)
Meropenem	12	–	–	4 (33.3)	1 (8.3)	1 (8.3)	1 (8.3)	1 (8.3)	4 (33.3)
Amikacin	8	1 (12.5)	–	–	–	–	–	–	7 (87.5)
Ampicillin	10	–	–	–	2 (20.0)	–	–	3 (30.0)	5 (50.0)
Crystal penicillin	7	–	1 (14.3)	–	1 (14.3)	–	1 (14.3)	3 (42.9)	1 (14.3)
Cefotaxime	6	2 (33.3)	–	–	–	–	–	–	4 (66.7)
Levofloxacin	5	–	–	1 (25.0)	–	2 (40.0)	–	–	2 (40.0)
Erythromycin	5	–	–	–	–	1 (20.0)	4 (80.0)	–	–
Clarithromycin	3	–	–	–	3 (100)	–	–	–	–
Nitrofuratoin	2	–	–	1 (50.0)	–	1 (50.0)	–	–	–
Ceftazidine	2	–	–	1 (50.0)	–	–	–	1 (50.0)	–
Amoxicillin	1	–	–	–	1 (100)	–	–	–	–
Cefixime	1	–	–	–	–	–	1 (100)	–	–
Doxycycline	1	–	–	–	–	–	1 (100)	–	–
Cefpodoxime	1	–	–	–	–	1 (100)	–	–	–
Nalidixic acid	1	–	–	1 (100)	–	–	–	–	–
Vancomycin	1	1 (100)	–	–	–	–	–	–	–
Total	611	52	7	19	54	119	154	104	101

CNS central nervous system; OTH, others; UT urinary tract, GIT gastrointestinal tract, SSTBJ skin, soft tissue, bone and joints, GUOB genitourinary and obstetrics, RESP respiratory; n, number; %, prevalence

recorded to be low. These low rates may reflect the unavailability of these agents on the national health insurance scheme essential drug list and their association with high out-of-pocket purchase cost. It is however important to maintain low use of such agents in the hospital in the long term to avoid development of carbapenem resistant *Enterobacteriaceae* and vancomycin resistant enterococcus. Both pathogens are associated with very poor clinical outcomes [8, 32].

The majority (40%) of antibiotics were prescribed for community-acquired infections. Community- acquired infections were commonly treated with ceftriaxone (18%), with infections of the respiratory tract being in the majority (32.4%). This reflects a common clinical practice of using ceftriaxone as a first line agent for community-acquired

pneumonia. However, only moderate penicillin resistance has been reported among *Streptococcus pneumoniae* isolates in Ghana [33, 34]. Frequent use of ceftriaxone may be a contributory factor to the high prevalence of extended spectrum beta-lactamase (ESBL) producing organisms seen at the KBTH [35]. The most commonly used antibiotics were metronidazole and amoxicillin-clavulanic acid and the main indication was surgical prophylaxis. This was mainly accounted for by patients from the obstetrics and gynaecology department. Surgical prophylaxis in this group of patients is effective in reducing post-operative complications [36]. It is common practice in the hospital to give long term antibiotics to patients undergoing caesarean section as prophylaxis, although it has been found not to be beneficial [36]. High usage of anti-anaerobic antibiotics like metronidazole is associated with elimination of gut anaerobes leading to the growth promotion of nosocomial pathogens [37]. This may promote the development of hospital-acquired infections such as vancomycin resistant enterococcus infections [38]. This study supplements data on antibiotic use in the KBTH and Ghana. It sets a bench mark for which other studies may be compared with and highlights areas for possible improvement in antibiotic use if stewardship programmes are to be implemented.

Our study has some limitations. It is a one site study and results may not be extrapolated to other health facilities. The prevalence of antibiotic use may be under estimated since the survey was not conducted in every unit of the hospital. However, based on 62.5% [20] bed occupancy of the hospital and number of patients surveyed we believe our data is a good reflection on the current state of antibiotic use in the hospital.

Conclusion

In this point prevalence survey, we found a high prevalence of antibiotic use among inpatients of the KBTH with a relatively high prevalence among paediatric patients. There is high use of metronidazole and amoxicillin-clavulanic acid and low percentage use of vancomycin and meropenem. Majority of the antibiotics were used treatment of community-acquired infections and surgical prophylaxis. Attempts aimed at reducing antibiotic use in the hospital should be focused on the use of the top five antimicrobial agents as well as antibiotics used for surgical prophylaxis. There is also the need to further explore the factors contributing to the high prevalence of antibiotic use and the changing epidemiology of antibiotic use in the hospital.

Abbreviations

ATC: Anatomical therapeutic classification; CI: Confidence interval; CNS: Central nervous system; GIT: Gastrointestinal tract; GUOB: Genitourinary and obstetrics; KBTH: Korle-Bu Teaching Hospital; RESP: Respiratory; SSTBJ: Skin, soft tissue, bone and joints; UTI: Urinary tract; WHO: World Health Organization

Acknowledgements

We thank Drs. Elizabeth Agyare, Emily Boakye-Yiadom, Goldie Collinwood Williams and Okyere-Dankwa Kontor for their help with data collection. We thank the staff and patients of the departments and units where the data was collected.

Funding

The study received no external funding.

Authors' contributions

Study concept and design was by AKL, NOA, and SB. AKL, NON, ETN were responsible for data collection, analysis and interpretation. AKL and NON drafted the manuscript. The manuscript was revised for intellectual content by AKL, NON, ETN, SB, YOA, NAA, AEY, MJN. All authors read and approved the final manuscript.

Consent for publication

Not applicable. This study does not contain any individual persons data. Only hospital folders were reviewed in this study.

Competing interests

The authors declare no competing interests.

Author details

[1]Department of Microbiology, Korle-Bu Teaching Hospital, P.O. Box 77, Accra, Ghana. [2]Department of Medical Laboratory Sciences, School of Biomedical and Allied Health Sciences, P.O. Box KB 143, Accra, Ghana. [3]Centre for Tropical Clinical Pharmacology and Therapeutics, School of Medicine and Dentistry, P.O. Box 4236, Accra, Ghana. [4]Department of Infectious Diseases, Copenhagen University Hospital, Rigshospitalet, Blegdamsvej 9, 2100 Copenhagen, Denmark. [5]Department of Surgery, University of Ghana School of Medicine and Dentistry, P.O. Box 4326, Accra, Ghana. [6]Department of Medicine, Korle-Bu Teaching Hospital, P.O. Box 77, Accra, Ghana. [7]Department of Community Health, School of Public Health, College of Health Sciences, University of Ghana, Accra, Ghana. [8]Department of Medical Microbiology, School of Biomedical and Allied Sciences, P.O. Box KB 143, Accra, Ghana.

References

1. Meyer E, Gastmeier P, Deja M, Schwab F. Antibiotic consumption and resistance: data from Europe and Germany. Int J Med Microbiol. 2013;303:388–95.
2. Van Boeckel TP, Gandra S, Ashok A, Caudron Q, Grenfell BT, Levin SA, et al. Global antibiotic consumption 2000 to 2010 : an analysis of national pharmaceutical sales data. Lancet Infect Dis. 2014;14:742–50. Available from: https://doi.org/10.1016/S1473-3099(14)70780-7
3. Hecker MT, Aron DC, Patel NP, Lehmann MK, Donskey CJ. Unnecessary use of antimicrobials in hospitalized patients: current patterns of misuse with an emphasis on the antianaerobic spectrum of activity. Arch Intern Med. 2003; 163:972–8.
4. World Health Organization. Report on the Burden of Endemic Health Care-Associated Infection Worldwide. Geneva: World Health Organisation. 2011. p. 1–88.
5. Flanders SA, Saint S. WHy does antimicrobial overuse in hospitalized patients persist? JAMA Intern Med. 2014;174:661–2.
6. WHO. Antimicrobial Resistance Global Report on Surveillance. Geneva: World Health Organisation. 2014. p. 1–101.
7. Okeke IN, Laxminarayan R, Bhutta ZA, Duse AG, Jenkins P, O'Brien TF, et al. Antimicrobial resistance in developing countries. Part I: recent trends and current status. Lancet infect. Dis. 2005;5:481–93.
8. Iosifidis E, Antachopoulos C, Tsivitanidou M, Katragkou A, Farmaki E, Tsiakou M, et al. Differential correlation between rates of antimicrobial drug consumption and prevalence of antimicrobial resistance in a tertiary Care Hospital in Greece. Infect Control Hosp Epidemiol. 2008;29:615–22.
9. Holmes AH, Moore LS, Sundsfjord A, Steinbakk M, Regmi S, Karkey A, et al. Understanding the mechanisms and drivers of antimicrobial resistance. Lancet. 2016;387:176–87.
10. Hersh AL, Shapiro DJ, Pavia AT, Shah SS. Antibiotic prescribing in ambulatory pediatrics in the United States. Pediatrics. 2011;128:1053–61.
11. Vazquez-Lago JM, Lopez-Vazquez P, Lopez-Duran A, Taracido-Trunk M, Figueiras A. Attitudes of primary care physicians to the prescribing of antibiotics and antimicrobial resistance: a qualitative study from Spain. Fam Pract. 2012;29:352–60.
12. Camcioglu Y, Alhan E, Salman N, Somer A, Hatipog N, Celik U, et al. Inappropriate antimicrobial use in Turkish pediatric hospitals : a multicenter point prevalence survey. 2010;
13. Magill SS, Edwards JR, Beldavs ZG, et al. PRevalence of antimicrobial use in us acute care hospitals, may-september 2011. JAMA. 2014;312:1438–46.
14. Ahoyo T, Bankolé H, Adéoti F, Gbohoun A, Assavèdo S, Amoussou-Guénou M, et al. Prevalence of nosocomial infections and anti-infective therapy in Benin: results of the first nationwide survey in 2012. Antimicrob Resist Infect Control. 2014;3:17.

15. Versporten A, Sharland MF, Bielicki J, Drapier NB, Vankerckhoven V, Goossens H, et al. The antibiotic resistance and prescribing in European children project: a neonatal and pediatric antimicrobial web-based point prevalence survey in 73 hospitals worldwide. Pediatr Infect Dis J. 2013;32(6):e242–53.

16. Versporten A, Bielicki J, Drapier N, Sharland M, Goossens H, ARPEC project group. The worldwide antibiotic resistance and prescribing in European children (ARPEC) point prevalence survey: developing hospital-quality indicators of antibiotic prescribing for children. J Antimicrob Chemother. 2016;71:1106–17.

17. Newman MJ. Nosocomial and community acquired infections in Korle Bu teaching hospital, Accra. West Afr J Med. 2009;28:300–3.

18. Retamar P, Martín ML, Molina J, del Arco A. Evaluating the quality of antimicrobial prescribing: is standardisation possible? Enferm. Infecc Microbiol Clin. 2013;31(Suppl 4):25–30.

19. Willemsen I, Groenhuijzen A, Bogaers D, Stuurman A, van Keulen P, Kluytmans J. Appropriateness of antimicrobial therapy measured by repeated prevalence surveys. Antimicrob Agents Chemother. 2007;51:864–7.

20. Korle Bu Teaching Hospital. 2012 Annual Report. Accra: Korle-Bu Teaching Hospital; 2013.

21. Ansari F, Erntell M, Goossens H, Davey P, Ii E, Care H, et al. The European surveillance of antimicrobial consumption (ESAC) point-prevalence survey of antibacterial use in 20 European hospitals in 2006. Clin Infect Dis. 2009; 49:1496–504.

22. WHO Collaborating Centre for Drug Statistics Methodology. Guidelines for ATC classification and DDD assignment. Oslo: WHO Collaborating Centre for Drug Statistics Methodology; 2013.

23. Ahiabu M-A, Tersbol BP, Biritwum R, Bygbjerg IC, Magnussen P. A retrospective audit of antibiotic prescriptions in primary health-care facilities in eastern region, Ghana. Health Policy Plan. 2015;31(2):250–8.

24. Thu TA, Rahman M, Cof S, Mbbs H, Sakamoto J, Hung NV. Antibiotic use in Vietnamese hospitals: a multicenter point-prevalence study. Am J Infect Control. 2012;40:840–4.

25. ECDC. Point prevalence survey of healthcare-associated infections and antimicrobial use in European acute care hospitals. European Centre for Disease Prevention: Stockholm; 2013.

26. Goossens H. Antibiotic consumption and link to resistance. Clin Microbiol Infect 2009;15:12–5.

27. Ministry of Health. Ghana standard treatment guidelines. 6th ed; 2010.

28. Chowdhury AA, Roy T, Faroque A, Bachar SC, Asaduzzaman M, Nasrin N, et al. A comprehensive situation assessment of injection practices in primary health care hospitals in Bangladesh. BMC Public Health. 2011;11:779.

29. Enweronu-Laryea CC, Newman MJ. Changing pattern of bacterial isolates and antimicrobial susceptibility in neonatal infections in Korle-Bu teaching hospital, Ghana. East Afr Med J. 2007;84:164–7.

30. Newman MJ, Frimpong E, Donkor ES, Opintan JA, Asamoah-Adu A. Resistance to antimicrobial drugs in Ghana. Infect Drug Resist. 2011;4:215–20.

31. Groß U, Amuzu SK, de Ciman R, Kassimova I, Groß L, Rabsch W, et al. Bacteremia and antimicrobial drug resistance over time, Ghana. Emerg Infect Dis. 2011;17:1879–82.

32. Kirst HA, Thompson DG, Nicas TI. Historical yearly usage of Vancomycin. Antimicrob Agents Chemother. 1998;42:1303–4.

33. Dayie NT, Arhin RE, Newman MJ, Dalsgaard A, Bisgaard M, Frimodt-Møller N, et al. Penicillin resistance and serotype distribution of Streptococcus Pneumoniae in Ghanaian children less than six years of age. BMC Infect Dis. 2013;13:490.

34. Dayie NT, Arhin RE, Newman MJ, Dalsgaard A, Bisgaard M, Frimodt-Møller N, et al. Multidrug-resistant Streptococcus Pneumoniae isolates from healthy Ghanaian preschool children. Microb Drug Resist. 2015;21:636–42.

35. Obeng-Nkrumah N, Twum-Danso K, Krogfelt KA, Newman MJ. High levels of extended-Spectrum Beta-Lactamases in a major teaching Hospital in Ghana: the need for regular monitoring and evaluation of antibiotic resistance. Am J Trop Med Hyg. 2013;89:960–4.

36. Smaill FM, Grivell RM. Antibiotic prophylaxis versus no prophylaxis for preventing infection after cesarean section. Cochrane Database Syst. 2014; 10:CD007482.

37. Donskey CJ, Chowdhry TK, Hecker MT, Hoyen CK, Hanrahan JA, Hujer AM, et al. Effect of antibiotic therapy on the density of Vancomycin-resistant Enterococci in the stool of colonized patients. N Engl J Med. 2000;343:1925–32.

38. Edmond MB, Ober JF, Weinbaum DL, Pfaller MA, Hwang T, Sanford MD, et al. Vancomycin-resistant Enterococcus faecium bacteremia: risk factors for infection. Clin Infect Dis. 1995;20:1126–33.

3

No nosocomial transmission under standard hygiene precautions in short term contact patients in case of an unexpected ESBL or Q &A E. coli positive patient: a one-year prospective cohort study within three regional hospitals

Dennis Souverein[1]* [iD], Sjoerd M. Euser[1], Bjorn L. Herpers[1], Corry Hattink[2], Patricia Houtman[3], Amerens Popma[3], Jan Kluytmans[4,5], John W. A. Rossen[6] and Jeroen W. Den Boer[1]

Abstract

Background: Many Highly Resistant Gram Negative Rod (HR-GNR) positive patients are found unexpectedly in clinical cultures, besides patients who are screened and isolated based on risk factors. As unexpected HR-GNR positive patients are isolated after detection, transmission to contact patients possibly occurred. The added value of routine contact tracing in such situations within hospitals with standard hygiene precautions is unknown.

Methods: In 2014, this study was performed as a prospective cohort study. Index patients were defined as those tested unexpectedly HR-GNR positive in clinical cultures to diagnose a possible infection and were nursed under standard hygiene precautions before tested positive. After detection they were nursed in contact isolation. Contact patients were still hospitalized and shared the same room with the index patient for at least 12 h. HR-GNR screening was performed by culturing a rectal and throat swab. Clonal relatedness of HR-GNR isolates was determined using whole genome sequencing (WGS).

Results: Out of 152 unexpected HR-GNR positive patients, 35 patients (23.0%) met our inclusion criteria for index patient. ESBL E. coli was found most frequently (n = 20, 57.1%), followed by Q&A E. coli (n = 10, 28.6%), ESBL K. pneumoniae (n = 3, 8.5%), ESBL R. ornithinolytica (n = 1, 2.9%) and multi resistant P. aeruginosa (n = 1, 2.9%). After contact tracing, 69 patients were identified as contact patient of an index patient, with a median time between start of contact and sampling of 3 days. None were found HR-GNR positive by nosocomial transmission.

Conclusions: In a local setting within hospitals with standard hygiene precautions, routine contact tracing among unexpected HR-GNR positive patients may be replaced by appropriate surveillance as we found no nosocomial transmission in short term contacts.

Keywords: HR-GNRs, ESBL, Transmission, Contact tracing, Contact isolation

* Correspondence: d.souverein@streeklabhaarlem.nl
[1]Department of Epidemiology and Infection Prevention, Regional Public Health Laboratory Kennemerland, Boerhaavelaan 26, 2035 RC, Haarlem, The Netherlands

Background

Infections with Highly Resistant Gram Negative Rods (HR-GNRs) are associated with higher (hospital) costs, morbidity and mortality in comparison to susceptible micro-organisms [1–4]. Increasingly, studies report on the (colonization) prevalence of HR-GNRs, including ESBL (Extended Spectrum Beta Lactamase) producing bacteria isolated from hospitalized patients, general practitioner patients and nursing home residents [5–9]. Knowledge about regional prevalence rates is important since HR-GNR colonized patients constitute a potential reservoir for patients at risk for nosocomial infections, such as immune compromised patients and/or patients with open wounds [10–13]. Several studies showed that foreign travel is an important risk factor for HR-GNR colonization [14–16]. Therefore, in Dutch hospitals, patients who have a recent history of foreign hospital admission are actively screened and pre-emptively isolated until test results are known [17]. In addition, known HR-GNR positive patients are flagged in the Hospital Information System (HIS) and isolated when readmitted. Despite screening and isolation of high risk patients, numerous patients are found unexpectedly HR-GNR positive in clinical cultures to diagnose a possible infection [18]. Before detection these unexpected positive patients were not nursed in isolation so that transmission to other patients may have occurred since no specific infection control measures were taken except standard hygiene procedures.

Willemsen et al. showed that the nosocomial transmission rate of HR-GNRs in Dutch hospitals was 7.0%, using AFLP (Amplification Fragment Length Polymorphism) to determine the genetic relation between clinical isolates [18]. Tschudin-Sutter et al. showed that nosocomial transmission from unexpected ESBL positive patients to contact patients rarely occurs, with a transmission rate of 2.2% over a total study period of 11 years [19]. Based on these studies it could be questioned if contact tracing within hospitals with standard hygiene precautions is required as contact tracing is considered time consuming and expensive. For the development of future health policies the results of such studies are of major importance.

In the present study, the nosocomial transmission rate from unexpected HR-GNR positive patients to contact patients was studied within three regional hospitals in the Dutch region Kennemerland. In addition, we estimated the overall HR-GNR incidence including patients who were screened and pre-emptively isolated at admission.

Methods

Study design and setting

The present study was performed as a prospective cohort study. Three hospitals in the region Kennemerland participated in this study. Hospital one is a 260-bed regional hospital (37% private, 26% double and 37% multi-patient rooms), hospital two is a 400 bed teaching hospital (50% private, 25% double and 25% multi-patient rooms) and hospital three is a 400 bed teaching hospital (46% private, 37% double and 17% multi-patient rooms). A database was created including patient and laboratory information from index and contact patients. Data were collected in 2014 as part of each hospitals infection control program.

Definition of HR-GNR

HR-GNR definitions were based on the Dutch MDRO (Multi-Drug Resistant Organism) directive for hospitals [18, 20]. HR-GNRs considered in the present study were (1) Enterobacteriaceae that were Extended Spectrum Beta-Lactamase (ESBL) and/or carbapenemase positive (CPE) and/or resistant to Fluoroquinolones and Aminoglycosides (Q&A), (2) *Acinetobacter* species that were carbapenemase positive and/or resistant to Q&A, (3) *Stenotrophomonas maltophilia* resistant to co-trimoxazole and (4) multi-resistant *Pseudomonas aeruginosa*, defined as resistant to at least three of the following antibiotics or antibiotic groups: piperacillin, ceftazidime, fluoroquinolones, aminoglycosides and/or carbapenemase positive.

Definition of index patients, contact patients and infection control procedures

Independent of the sampled body site, patients who tested unexpectedly HR-GNR positive in clinical cultures were considered as index patient. Unexpected positive was defined as patients who were not earlier identified as HR-GNR carrier (not flagged in the HIS) and/or not screened because of an elevated risk at admission (history of foreign hospital admission or coming from a hospital with a known HR-GNR problem). Index patients were identified by the infection control department based on daily communicated laboratory results. Contact patients were defined as patients who were still hospitalized and shared the same room with the index patient for at least 12 h, while the index patient was nursed under standard hygiene precautions, which includes wearing gloves after entering the patients room (before performing any patient-care activity) and wearing an apron when handling contagious materials. Hand hygiene was performed according to the five moments of the WHO hand hygiene guideline [21]. Screening of contact patients was performed by sampling a rectal and throat swab (Copan eSwab including 1 mL of modified liquid Amies) supplemented with wound samples when present as soon as possible after detection of the index patient. Index patients with at least one contact patient (still hospitalized at the time of detection) were included in the study. After detection, all HR-GNR positive patients were nursed in contact isolation following the national MDRO directive [18]. Contact isolation consisted of nursing in a single room, using gloves by nursing personnel and daily disinfection of the patient room. For all HR-GNR positive patients, isolation measures were maintained during the total admission time and study period. HR-GNR positive patients were not unmarked during the study period and an alert was entered in the HIS as a warning when patients were readmitted.

Sampling of patients and laboratory techniques

All samples were processed and analysed using Standard Operating Procedures (SOPs) at the Regional Public Health Laboratory Kennemerland (RPHLK). Samples from unexpected HR-GNR positive patients (index patients) were analysed using standard microbiological procedures. When the index patient was positive for a HR-GNR (including ESBLs) rectal and throat swabs from contact patient(s) were analysed by direct culturing on both an ESBL screening agar (ChromID ESBL-ID, bioMerieux, enriched with a mixture of antibiotics, including cefpodoxime) and a CLED GM20 agar (cystine lactose electrolyte deficient agar with 20 mg/L gentamicin, Oxoid). All gram-negative rods growing on these agars were identified using MALDI-TOF (Bruker Daltonics, Germany). Antibiotic susceptibility testing was performed using the automated system VITEK2 (bioMérieux, France). All isolates suspected for the production of ESBL, defined as a VITEK 2 AES alert and/or elevated MIC (> 1 mg/L) for cefotaxime and/or ceftazidime were confirmed using the combination disk method (ceftazidime and cefotaxime or cefepime with and without clavulanic acid). Isolates with a VITEK 2 AES alert and/or elevated MIC for meropenem (> 0.25 mg/L) were suspected for carbapenemase production. Carbapenemase production was analysed using the modified Hodge test and an in-house carbapenemase PCR with targets for KPC, VIM, OXA-48 and NDM [22–24]. All HR-GNR positive isolates were stored at −80 °C.

Molecular typing of HR-GNR positive isolates

Isolates with similar micro-organism and HR-GNR type within index and contact patient(s) were genotyped using Whole Genome Sequencing (WGS) using the MiSeq instrument (Illumina) as described elsewhere [25]. De novo assembly was performed using CLC Genomics Workbench v7.0.3 (CLC bio A/S, Aarhus, Denmark) after quality trimming (Qs ≥ 28) with optimal word sizes based on the maximum N50 value. The sequence type (ST) was identified by uploading the assembled genomes to the multilocus sequence type (MLST) server (version 1.7) and the acquired resistance genes were determined with the CGE Resfinder 1.2 tool. Pairwise genetic distance between isolates was calculated

for whole genome (wgMLST) targets and core genome (cgMLST) targets by dividing the number of allele differences by the total number of targets shared by both sequences and reported as proportion. Based on previously described methods, *E. coli* isolates with a genetic distance of 0.95% or less were interpreted as clonally related [25].

Data analysis and definition of transmission

The transmission rate from index patients to contact patients was calculated by dividing the number of confirmed positive contact patients by the number of index patients, including those for whom no transmission had occurred. For every index and contact patient the following variables were calculated: contact time, defined as the period that the index patient and contact patient shared the same room; admission time; and time to sampling for the contact patient (after identification of the index patient). The overall cumulative HR-GNR incidence and incidence density for the study period was calculated by dividing the number of HR-GNR positive hospitalized patients by the total number of admissions and (hospital) patient-days. Confidence intervals (95%) for proportions were calculated using the Wilson score [26]. All statistical analyses were performed using IBM SPSS Statistics version 24.0.

Results
Characteristics of index and contact patients

Thirty-five out of 152 unexpected HR-GNR positive patients (23.0%) met our inclusion criteria and were marked as index patient. Consequently, 117 HR-GNR positive patients (77.0%) were excluded since no contact patients were identified or were already discharged. Around these index patients 69 patients were identified as contact patient (Fig. 1). Two contact patients (2.9%) were screened since they had contact on the Intensive Care Unit (ICU) with an index patient. The median number (range) of contact patients per index patient was 2 (1–5) and the median contact time (range) between index and contact patients was 2 days (0.5–9). Thirteen out of the 35 index patients (37.1%) and 44 out of the 69 contact patients (63.8%) were male and the mean age (SD) for index and contact patients was 72.1 (12.0) and 70.7 (15.2) years, respectively. The median admission time (range) for index and contact patients was 10 (2–36) and 11 (1–133) days and the median number of (hospital room) transfers (range) for index and contact patients were 3 (1–8) and 2 (1–9) transfers, respectively. The number of contact patients who used antibiotics and/or had open wounds at the time of sampling was 25 (36.2%) and 13 (18.8%) respectively. Stratified patient characteristics per hospital are shown in Table 1.

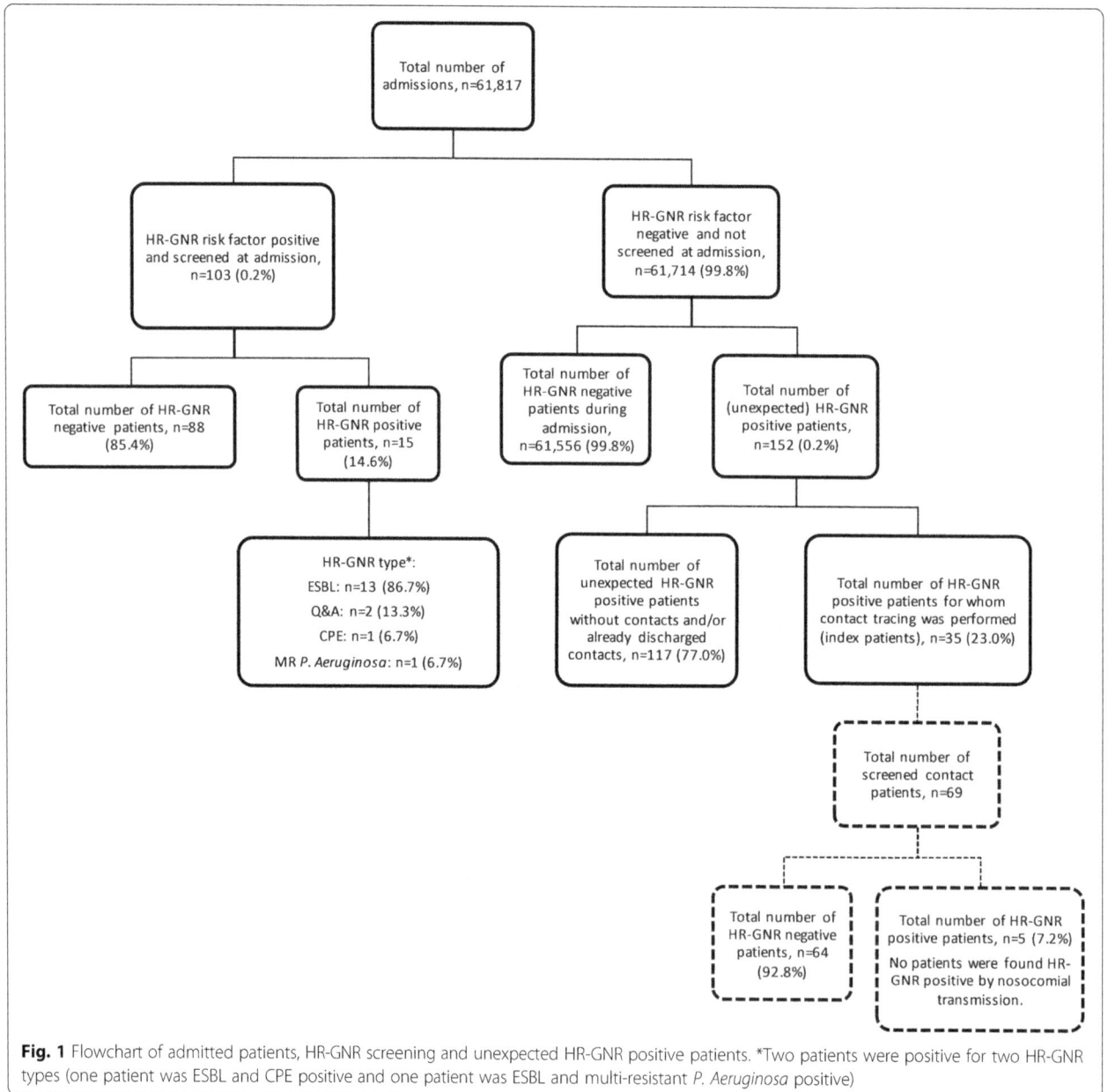

Fig. 1 Flowchart of admitted patients, HR-GNR screening and unexpected HR-GNR positive patients. *Two patients were positive for two HR-GNR types (one patient was ESBL and CPE positive and one patient was ESBL and multi-resistant *P. Aeruginosa* positive)

HR-GNR types and micro-organisms of 'index patients'

Of all 35 index patients, 20 patients were found ESBL *E. coli* positive (57.1%), followed by Q&A *E. coli* (*n* = 10, 28.6%), ESBL *K. pneumoniae* (*n* = 3, 8.5%), ESBL *R. ornithinolytica* (*n* = 1, 2.9%) and multi resistant *P. aeruginosa* (*n* = 1, 2.9%).

Transmission analysis

In total, five out of 69 contact patients (7.2%) were found HR-GNR positive. All of these contact patients were associated with a different index patient. Four of these patients were ESBL *E. coli* positive and one patient was positive for a Q&A *E. coli*. Three of the five HR-GNR positive contact patients were positive with a different HR-GNR type and/or micro-organism compared to their index patient and were therefore considered negative for nosocomial transmission. Two of the five HR-GNR positive contact patients were positive with the same HR-GNR type and micro-organism as their index patient (both ESBL *E. coli*). WGS of the ESBL *E. coli* isolates of index 1 and contact 1 showed that the isolate of index 1 was genotyped as ST 131, CTX-M-27. The isolate of contact 1 was genotyped as ST 295, SHV-12. The genetic difference between these isolates was determined using cgMLST and wgMLST and showed a genetic difference of 95.8% and 97.5% (Table 2). WGS of the ESBL *E. coli* isolates of index 2 and contact 2 showed that the isolate of index 2 was

Table 1 Characteristics of index and contact patients

	Regional		Hospital 1		Hospital 2		Hospital 3	
	Index	Contacts	Index	Contacts	Index	Contacts	Index	Contacts
Number of patients	35	69	13	35	8	13	14	21
Sex								
Male (%)	13 (37.1%)	44 (63.8%)	5 (38.5%)	21 (60.0%)	4 (50.0%)	7 (53.8%)	4 (28.6%)	16 (76.2%)
Mean age (SD)	72.1 (12.0)	70.7 (15.2)	73.3 (11.5)	74.9 (14.7)	65.9 (13.7)	70.3 (13.3)	74.5 (11.0)	64.0 (15.1)
Median number of contacts (range)	2 (1–5)	NA	3 (1–4)	NA	1 (1–5)	NA	1 (1–3)	NA
Median admission time in days (range)	10 (2–36)	11 (1–133)	10 (2–24)	10 (2–48)	11.5 (5–32)	12 (8–29)	8 (4–36)	12 (1–133)
Median number of transfers (range)	3 (1–8)	2 (1–9)	3 (2–8)	2 (1–9)	3.5 (2–8)	3 (2–6)	2 (1–4)	2 (1–5)
Median contact time in days (range)	NA	2 (0.5–9)	NA	1 (0.5–6)	NA	4 (1–6)	NA	3 (0.5–9)
Median time between end of contact and sampling (range)	NA	1 (−2–12)	NA	1 (−1–8)	NA	2 (0–12)	NA	0 (−2–7)
Wounds (%)	NA	13 (18.8%)	NA	6 (17.1%)	NA	2 (15.4%)	NA	5 (23.8%)
Antibiotic use during sampling (%)	NA	25 (36.2%)	NA	13 (37.1%)	NA	6 (46.2%)	NA	6 (28.6%)

NA not applicable

genotyped as ST 69, CTX-M-1 and the isolate of contact 2 as ST 69, CTX-M-55. The genetic difference using cgMLST was 11.6%, and 13.6% when using wgMLST (Table 2). Based on the WGS data we concluded that nosocomial transmission had not occurred in both cases. Consequently, the overall nosocomial transmission rate (95% CI) of unexpected HR-GNR and HR-GNR *E. coli* positive patients to contact patients was 0% (0–9.9) and 0% (0–11.4).

ST sequence type, *wgMLST* whole genome multilocus sequence typing, *cgMLST* core genome multilocus sequence typing

Incidence of HR-GNRs
In 2014, 15 out of 103 patients (14.6%) were HR-GNR positive as part risk factor based screening at admission (Fig. 1). In addition, 152 patients were unexpected HR-GNR positive in clinical cultures during hospitalization. Together with five positive contacts this resulted in a total of 172 HR-GNR positive patients during hospitalization. Given a total of 61,817 admissions and 223,351 (hospital) patient-days this resulted in a cumulative incidence (95% CI) and incidence density (95% CI) of 27.8 (24.0–32.3) patients per 10,000 admissions and 7.7 (6.6–8.9) patients per 10,000 (hospital) patient-days, respectively. As shown in Table 3, 68.6% (*n* = 118) of all HR-GNR positive patients tested positive for an ESBL. We expect based on the detected prevalence within contact patients (7.2%)

that 4450 admissions were with patients that were HR-GNR colonized (7.2% of 61,817 admissions).

Discussion
During a study period of 1 year, a nosocomial transmission rate of 0% from unexpected HR-GNR positive patients to contact patients was found. Out of 152 unexpected HR-GNR positive patients, 35 patients met our inclusion criteria for index patients. Around these 35 index patients, 69 contact patients were sampled, accounting for a total of 178 contact days. Although no nosocomial transmission had occurred, five contact patients were HR-GNR positive (7.2%) and four of these were ESBL *E. coli* positive (5.8%), which corresponds with earlier reported prevalence rates in Dutch hospitals [6, 27]. As expected, ESBL positive patients were found most frequently among all HR-GNR positive patients (68.6%) and index patients (68.6%). From a microorganism perspective, 85.7% of the index patients were positive for an HR-GNR *E. coli*. MRSA, VRE (Vancomycin-resistant *Enterococcus*) and PRSP (Penicillin-resistant *Streptococcus pneumoniae*) were not included in the present study.

Other studies with comparable study designs that estimated the transmission rate to contact patients are scarce, limiting the comparison with other settings. Willemsen et al. showed that the nosocomial transmission rate of HR-GNR in Dutch hospitals was 7.0% [18]. This is probably a worst-case scenario since only epidemiologically

Table 2 Index patients with possible transmission

Pair	Index	Contact	Genetic difference (wgMLST)	Genetic difference (cgMLST)	Conclusion
1	*E. coli* (ST131; CTX-M-27)	*E. coli* (ST295; SHV-12)	97.5% (3138/3219)	95.8% (2647/2764)	No nosocomial transmission
2	*E. coli* (ST69; CTX-M-1)	*E. coli* (ST69; CTX-M-55)	13.6% (439/3219)	11.6% (321/2764)	No nosocomial transmission

Table 3 Total HR-GNR incidence for 2014

	Regional	Hospital 1	Hospital 2	Hospital 3
ESBL	118	40	37	41
Q&A	54	14	20	20
CPE	3	1	0	2
S. maltophilia resistant to co-trimoxazole	1	1	0	0
MR P. aeruginosa	5	3	1	1
Total number of HR-GNR	181	59	58	64
Number unique HR-GNR positive patients[a]	172	53	57	62
Number of admissions	61,817	18,837	23,637	19,343
Number of patient days	223,351	57,749	92,070	73,533
HR-GNR incidence rate per 10.000 admissions (95% CI)	27.8 (24.0–32.3)	28.1 (21.5–36.8)	24.1 (18.6–31.2)	32.1 (25.0–41.1)
HR-GNR incidence density per 10.000 patient-days (95% CI)	7.7 (6.6–8.9)	9.2 (7.0–12.0)	6.2 (4.8–8.0)	8.4 (6.6–10.8)

[a]Represents the number of unique patients. During admission, a patient could be positive for more than one HR-GNR type. Therefore, this number is lower than the sum of all HR-GNR subgroups
HR-GNR Highly Resistant Gram Negative Rod, MR multi resistant, ESBL extended spectrum beta lactamase, Q&A enterobacteriaceae or Acinetobacter spp. resistant to fluoroquinolones and aminoglycosides, CPE carbapenemase producing enterobacteriaceae

linked clinical isolates within a time window of 4 weeks were analysed using AFLP genotyping, which is considered less discriminatory. In 2012, Tschudin-Sutter et al. studied the transmission rate from unexpected ESBL positive patients to contact patients [19]. Their results showed that during a period of 11 years two contact patients related to 93 index patients (2.2%) were ESBL positive by transmission, suggesting that nosocomial transmission rarely occurs. A study performed at the ICU in a French hospital showed an ESBL acquisition rate of 6.5% [28]. However, only one patient (out of 19) appeared to be positive by nosocomial transmission. A complicating factor for these studies (and also for our study) is the relatively high ESBL colonization prevalence in the community. We only detected 172 of these patients during our study period instead of an expected amount of 4450 admissions with HR-GNR positive patients. Consequently, expensive high resolution genotyping is needed to exclude transmission since phenotypic results, MLST, AFLP or ESBL gene are not able to discriminate enough between closely related isolates [25, 29]. Based on MLST and ESBL group alone we would have concluded that transmission had occurred between one index and a contact patient. Additional cgMLST or wgMLST analyses, as performed in the present study minimizes the chance on this kind of false conclusions. Another interesting study within a German hospital showed a nosocomial transmission rate of 2.3% for multidrug resistant E. coli based on clinical (infection) isolates using cgMLST [30]. When isolation measures of positive patients were ceased the transmission rate increased non-significantly to 5.0% and decreased on high risk wards (ICU). However, as these results were based on clinical infection cultures

only, colonized (not infected) patients were missed, underestimating the real transmission rate.

Our results and the previously mentioned studies clues that routine contact tracing in case of an unexpected HR-GNR positive patient might be replaced by appropriate surveillance in a local setting within hospitals with standard hygiene precautions. Also, since we found no nosocomial transmission, these results advocate a more flexible isolation strategy. However, (cluster) randomized controlled trials are needed to compare nosocomial transmission rates between different isolation strategies. Preferably such studies must be accompanied by adverse events that are associated with isolation (such as patient well-being) so that a balanced conclusion could be made. Because we mainly isolated HR-GNR E. coli, our results should be interpreted with caution and cannot simply be generalized for less frequently isolated HR-GNRs such as CPE or other micro-organisms than E. coli such as K. pneumoniae.

Some studies have suggested that certain sequence types of E. coli (ST 131) and K. pneumoniae (ST 258) are hyperendemic, causing outbreaks and infections [31, 32]. A recent review found evidence that E. coli ST 131 is more pathogenic than non-ST131, but the increased transmissibility or prolonged carriage could not be confirmed [33]. For K. pneumoniae ST 258, this study could not confirm or reject the increased pathogenicity, transmissibility or prolonged carriage of this sequence type [33]. As certain HR-GNR types or micro-organisms are potentially more dangerous in terms of transmissibility or pathogenicity, contact tracing can only be replaced in a local setting within hospitals where adequate standard hygiene precautions with sufficient surveillance or prevalence measurements are performed. Prevalence measurements will provide insight into local HR-GNR epidemiology and possible ongoing transmission within hospitals [27]. Appropriate surveillance could be performed by reviewing (1) clinical HR-GNR isolates, (2) patient admission data and (3) genotyping of HR-GNR isolates when transmission is suspected as performed by Mellmann et al. [30].

Comparing our overall cumulative HR-GNR incidence rate with the study of Willemsen et al. showed a lower cumulative incidence rate per 10,000 admissions (28 vs. 39) [18]. An explanation for this difference could be the large variation between hospitals, hospital types and patient populations that were included in both studies. Comparing the incidence density per 100,000 patient-days between both studies showed a higher incidence density in our study (77 vs. 55) [18]. The mean length of stay in our study was 3.6 days compared to 6.6 days, resulting in a lower denominator of patient-days. This decreasing trend of mean length of stay within Dutch hospitals was also noticed in a Dutch report published in 2013 [34].

The present study has several limitations. First, the sample size (35 index and 69 contact patients) was relatively small which is reflected by the large confidence interval of the calculated transmission rate. Future studies are necessary to confirm our results. Second, for VRE (Vancomycin-resistant *Enterococcus)* it is known that the inoculum size is related to the detection probability with culturing [35]. For HR-GNR detection it is largely unknown how much time between colonization and sampling (using culturing) is sufficient. This may have resulted in a possible underestimation of the nosocomial transmission rate in our study, as some patients could have been marked as false negative. However, the median time between start of contact and sampling in our study was 3 days (median contact time plus time between end of contact and sampling), and we therefore do not think that this has markedly influenced our results. Future studies must incorporate repeated culturing after the end of contact in order to determine the optimal culturing strategy. Third, our results cannot be solely attributed to the transmission capacity of HR-GNR type or micro-organism alone. In a setting, with other prevalence rates or infection control policies other transmission rates could be found. Fourth, we have possibly missed cases of transmission, since only admitted index and contact patients were included in our study.

Conclusion

In conclusion, our study provides evidence that the nosocomial transmission rate from unexpected HR-GNR positive patients towards short term contacts patients in a local setting within hospitals with standard hygiene precautions is low. In a local setting routine contact tracing among unexpected HR-GNR positive patients may be replaced by appropriate surveillance. As we mainly isolated ESBL *E. coli* and Q&A *E. coli*, our results cannot be extrapolated to other HR-GNR types such as CPE or other micro-organisms such as *K. pneumoniae.*

Abbreviations
AFLP: Amplification Fragment Length Polymorphism; cgMLST: Core genome multi locus sequence typing; CPE: Carbapenemase Producing Enterobacteriaceae; ESBL: Extended Spectrum Beta Lactamase; HIS: Hospital Information System; HR-GNR: Highly Resistant Gram Negative Rod; ICU: Intensive Care Unit; MDRO: Multi-Drug Resistant Organism; MRSA: Methicillin-resistant *Staphylococcus aureus*; Q&A: Resistant to Fluoroquinolones and Aminoglycosides; RPHLK: Regional Public Health Laboratory Kennemerland; S&D: Search and Destroy; SOP: Standard Operating Procedures; VRE: Vancomycin-resistant *Enterococcus*; wgMLST: Whole genome multi locus sequence typing; WGS: Whole Genome Sequencing

Acknowledgements
None.

Funding
Not applicable.

Authors' contributions
BLH, CH, PH and AP designed the study. DS, SME, BLH, CH, PH, AP, JK and JWB interpreted the results, revised the manuscript and wrote the manuscript. DS and SME performed the statistical analysis. DS, SME and BLH interpreted the results from the statistical analysis. CH, PH and AP collected patient specimens and data. JWR performed the molecular analysis of the bacterial isolates, interpreted the molecular typing results, revised the manuscript and wrote the manuscript. All authors read and approved the final manuscript.

Consent for publication
Not applicable.

Competing interests
The authors declare that they have no competing interests.

Author details
¹Department of Epidemiology and Infection Prevention, Regional Public Health Laboratory Kennemerland, Boerhaavelaan 26, 2035 RC, Haarlem, The Netherlands. ²Department of Infection Prevention, Rode Kruis Ziekenhuis, Beverwijk, The Netherlands. ³Department of Infection Prevention, Spaarne Gasthuis, Haarlem and Hoofddorp, The Netherlands. ⁴Laboratory for Microbiology and Infection Control, Amphia Hospital, Breda, The Netherlands. ⁵University Medical Center, Utrecht, The Netherlands. ⁶Department of Medical Microbiology, University of Groningen, University Medical Center Groningen, Groningen, The Netherlands.

References
1. Rottier WC, Ammerlaan HS, Bonten MJ. Effects of confounders and intermediates on the association of bacteraemia caused by extended-spectrum β-lactamase-producing Enterobacteriaceae and patient outcome: a meta-analysis. J Antimicrob Chemother. 2011;67(6):1311–20.

2. Cosgrove SE. The relationship between antimicrobial resistance and patient outcomes: mortality, length of hospital stay, and health care costs. Clin Infect Dis. 2006;42(2):S82–9.

3. Filice GA, Nyman JA, Lexau C, Lees CH, Bockstedt LA, Como-Sabetti K, et al. Excess costs and utilization associated with methicillin resistance for patients with *Staphylococcus aureus* infection. Infect Control Hosp Epidemiol. 2010;31(4):365–73.

4. Cosgrove SE, Kaye KS, Eliopoulous GM, Carmeli Y. Health and economic outcomes of the emergence of third-generation cephalosporin resistance in Enterobacter species. Arch Intern Med. 2002;162(2):185–90.

5. Reuland EA, Al Naiemi N, Kaiser AM, Heck M, Kluytmans JA, Savelkoul PH, et al. Prevalence and risk factors for carriage of ESBL-producing Enterobacteriaceae in Amsterdam. J Antimicrob Chemother. 2016;71(4):1076–82.

6. Willemsen I, Oome S, Verhulst C, Pettersson A, Verduin K, Kluytmans J. Trends in Extended Spectrum Beta-Lactamase (ESBL) Producing Enterobacteriaceae and ESBL Genes in a Dutch Teaching Hospital, Measured in 5 Yearly Point Prevalence Surveys (2010-2014). PLoS One. 2015;10(11):e0141765.

7. Kahvecioglu D, Ramiah K, McMaughan D, Garfinkel S, McSorley VE, Nguyen QN, et al. Multidrug-resistant organism infections in US nursing homes: a national study of prevalence, onset, and transmission across care settings, October 1, 2010-December 31, 2011. Infect Control Hosp Epidemiol. 2014;35(Suppl 3):S48–55.

8. Reuland EA, Overdevest IT, Al Naiemi N, Kalpoe JS, Rijnsburger MC, Raadsen SA, et al. High prevalence of ESBL-producing Enterobacteriaceae carriage in Dutch community patients with gastrointestinal complaints. Clin Microbiol Infect. 2012;19(6):542–9.

9. Balkhair A, Al-Farsi YM, Al-Muharrmi Z, Al-Rashdi R, Al-Jabri M, Neilson F, et al. Epidemiology of multi-drug resistant organisms in a teaching hospital in oman: a one-year hospital-based study. Sci World J. 2014;2014:157102.

10. Eilers R, Veldman-Ariesen MJ, Haenen A, van Benthem BH. Prevalence and determinants associated with healthcare-associated infections in long-term care facilities (HALT) in the Netherlands, May to June 2010. Euro Surveill. 2012;17(34). https://www.ncbi.nlm.nih.gov/pubmed/22939212.

11. Hopmans T, Smid EA, Wille JC, de Greeff SC. Healthcare-associated infections on readmission: 1 in 3 is linked to previous hospital admission. Ned Tijdschr Geneeskd. 2015;159:A8404.

12. van der Kooi TI, Manniën J, Wille JC, van Benthem BH. Prevalence of nosocomial infections in The Netherlands, 2007-2008: results of the first four national studies. J Hosp Infect. 2010;75(3):168–72.

13. Ider BE, Clements A, Adams J, Whitby M, Muugolog T. Prevalence of hospital-acquired infections and antibiotic use in two tertiary Mongolian hospitals. J Hosp Infect. 2010;75(3):214–9.

14. Paltansing S, Vlot JA, Kraakman ME, Mesman R, Bruijning ML, Bernards AT, et al. Extended-spectrum β-lactamase-producing enterobacteriaceae among travelers from the Netherlands. Emerg Infect Dis. 2013;19(8):1206–13.

15. von Wintersdorff CJ, Penders J, Stobberingh EE, Oude Lashof AM, Hoebe CJ, Savelkoul PH, et al. High rates of antimicrobial drug resistance gene acquisition after international travel, The Netherlands. Emerg Infect Dis. 2014;20(4):649–57.

16. Arcilla MS, van Hattem JM, Haverkate MR, Bootsma MC, van Genderen PJ, Goorhuis A, et al. Import and spread of extended-spectrum β-lactamase-producing Enterobacteriaceae by international travellers (COMBAT study): a prospective, multicentre cohort study. Lancet Infect Dis. 2017;17(1):78–85.

17. Bijzonder resistente micro-organismen (BRMO). Werkgroep Infectie Preventie (WIP). 2012. http://www.rivm.nl/dsresource?objectid=b6b99580-44e2-4b9c-8183-52871e61764f&type=org&disposition=inline. Accessed 25 Oct 2016.

18. Willemsen I, Elberts S, Verhulst C, Rijnsburger M, Filius M, Savelkoul P, et al. Highly Resistant Gram-Negative Microorganisms: Incidence Density and Occurrence of Nosocomial Transmission (TRIANGLe Study). Infect Control Hosp Epidemiol. 2011;32(4):333–41.

19. Tschudin-Sutter S, Frei R, Dangel M, Stranden A, Widmer AF. Rate of transmission of extended-spectrum beta-lactamase-producing enterobacteriaceae without contact isolation. Clin Infect Dis. 2012;55(11):1505–11.

20. Werkgroep Infectie Preventie. Meticilline-resistente *Staphylococcus aureus*. WIP. 2012. Available: http://www.rivm.nl/dsresource?objectid=3f054354-ff4a-43ef-91f9-7c6f0417be95&type=org&disposition=inline. Accessed 25 Oct 2016.

21. World Health Organization. Five moments for hand hygiene. WHO. 2009. Available: http://www.who.int/gpsc/tools/Five_moments/en/. Accessed 14 Mar 2017.

22. Yigit H, Queenan AM, Anderson GJ, Domenech-Sanchez A, Biddle JW, Steward CD, et al. Novel carbapenem-hydrolyzing beta-lactamase, KPC-1, from a carbapenem-resistant strain of *Klebsiella pneumoniae*. Antimicrob Agents Chemother. 2001;45:1151–61.

23. Lauretti L, Riccio ML, Mazzariol A, Cornaglia G, Amicosante G, Fontana R, et al. Cloning and characterization of blaVIM, a new integron-borne metallo-beta-lactamase gene from a Pseudomonas aeruginosa clinical isolate. Antimicrob Agents Chemother. 1999;43:1584–90.

24. Swayne RL, Ludlam HA, Shet VG, Woodford N, Curran MD. Real-time TaqMan PCR for rapid detection of genes encoding five types of non-metallo- (class A and D) carbapenemases in Enterobacteriaceae. Int J Antimicrob Agents. 2011;38:35-38.

25. Kluytmans-van den Bergh MF, Rossen JW, Bruijning-Verhagen PC, Bonten MJ, Friedrich AW, Vandenbroucke-Grauls CM, et al. Whole genome multilocus sequence typing of extended-spectrum beta-lactamase-producing Enterobacteriaceae. J Clin Microbiol. 2016;4(12):2919–27.

26. Wilson EB. Probable inference, the law of succession, and statistical inference. J Am Stat Assoc. 1927;22:209–12.

27. Souverein D, Euser SM, Herpers BL, Diederen B, Houtman P, van Seventer M, et al. Prevalence, risk factors and molecular epidemiology of highly resistant gram negative rods in hospitalized patients in the Dutch region Kennemerland. Antimicrob Resist Infect Control. 2016;5:8.

28. Alves M, Lemire A, Decré D, Margetis D, Bigé N, Pichereau C, et al. Extended-spectrum beta-lactamase–producing enterobacteriaceae in the intensive care unit: acquisition does not mean cross-transmission. BMC Infect Dis. 2016;16:147.

29. Voor In 't Holt AF, Wattel AA, Boers SA, Jansen R, Hays JP, Goessens WH, et al. Detection of Healthcare-Related Extended-Spectrum Beta-Lactamase-Producing *Escherichia coli* Transmission Events Using Combined Genetic and Phenotypic Epidemiology. PLoS One. 2016;11(7):e0160156.

30. Mellmann A, Bletz S, Böking T, Kipp F, Becker K, Schultes A, et al. Real-Time Genome Sequencing of Resistant Bacteria Provides Precision Infection Control in an Institutional Setting. J Clin Microbiol. 2016;54(12):2874–81.

31. Rogers BA, Sidjabat HE, Paterson DL. *Escherichia coli* O25b-ST131: a pandemic, multiresistant, community-associated strain. J Antimicrob Chemother. 2011;66(1):1–14.

32. Kitchel B, Rasheed JK, Patel JB, Srinivasan A, Navon-Venezia S, Carmeli Y, et al. Molecular epidemiology of KPC-producing *Klebsiella pneumoniae* isolates in the United States: clonal expansion of multilocus sequence type 258. Antimicrob Agents Chemother. 2009;53(8):3365–70.

33. Dautzenberg MJ, Haverkate MR, Bonten MJ, Bootsma MC. Epidemic potential of *Escherichia coli* ST131 and *Klebsiella pneumoniae* ST258: a systematic review and meta-analysis. BMJ Open. 2016;6(3):e009971.

34. Ligduurmonitor Nederlandse ziekenhuizen 2012. COPPA. 2013. http://www.coppa.nl/wp-content/uploads/2014/01/Coppa-Ligduurmonitor-2012.pdf. Accessed 25 Oct 2016.

35. D'Agata EM, Gautam S, Green WK, Tang YW. High rate of false-negative results of the rectal swab culture method in detection of gastrointestinal colonization with vancomycin-resistant enterococci. Clin Infect Dis. 2002;34(2):167–72.

4

Implementation of WHO multimodal strategy for improvement of hand hygiene: a quasi-experimental study in a Traditional Chinese Medicine hospital in Xi'an, China

Li Shen[1], Xiaoqing Wang[1]* (iD), Junming An[2], Jialu An[3], Ning Zhou[1], Lu Sun[1], Hong Chen[1], Lin Feng[4], Jing Han[3] and Xiaorong Liu[3]

Abstract

Background: Hand hygiene (HH) is an essential component for preventing and controlling of healthcare-associated infection (HAI), whereas compliance with HH among health care workers (HCWs) is frequently poor. This study aimed to assess compliance and correctness with HH before and after the implementation of a multimodal HH improvement strategy launched by the World Health Organization (WHO).

Methods: A quasi-experimental study design including questionnaire survey generalizing possible factors affecting HH behaviors of HCWs and direct observation method was used to evaluate the effectiveness of WHO multimodal HH strategy in a hospital of Traditional Chinese Medicine. Multimodal HH improvement strategy was drawn up according to the results of questionnaire survey. Compliance and correctness with HH among HCWs were compared before and after intervention. Also HH practices for different indications based on WHO "My Five Moments for Hand Hygiene" were recorded.

Results: In total, 553 HCWs participated in the questionnaire survey and multimodal HH improvement strategy was developed based on individual, environment and management levels. A total of 5044 observations in 23 wards were recorded in this investigation. The rate of compliance and correctness with HH improved from 66.27% and 47.75% at baseline to 80.53% and 88.35% after intervention. Doctors seemed to have better compliance with HH after intervention (84.04%) than nurses and other HCWs (81.07% and 69.42%, respectively). When stratified by indication, compliance with HH improved for all indications after intervention ($P < 0.05$) except for "after body fluid exposure risk" and "after touching patient surroundings".

Conclusion: Implementing the WHO multimodal HH strategy can significantly improve HH compliance and correctness among HCWs.

Keywords: Hand hygiene, Compliance, Correctness, Healthcare-associated infection

* Correspondence: w.xq1123@163.com
[1]Department of Infection Control, Xi'an Hospital of Traditional Chinese Medicine, No.69 Feng Cheng 8th Road, Weiyang District, Xi'an 710021, China

Background

Healthcare-associated infection (HAI) represents a major burden and safety issue for patients in the developing countries, with severe and greatly underestimated effect on patients and health care systems [1]. According to the survey of National HAI Surveillance System, in 2014, at least 26,972 cases of HAI arose in patients admitted to hospital in China [2]. HAI resulted in prolonged length of hospital stay, direct economic loss, morbidity and mortality among hospitalized patients [3]. A recent study in China identified that the average cost of hospitalization increased ¥13,839.16(€1792.64) due to HAI [4]. The hands of healthcare workers (HCWs) can be a major mode of transmission of microbial pathogens by touching the environment or patients' skin during healthcare delivery, which supports that hand hygiene (HH) is a critical component of a bundle approaches for preventing and controlling HAIs [5–9]. The World Health Organization (WHO) launched a multimodal strategy in 2009 to improve HH practice worldwide, which includes 5 important components: (1) system change, (2) training and education, (3) evaluation and feedback, (4) reminders in the workplace (5) institutional safety climate [10]. It has been demonstrated the implementation of WHO HH strategy is feasible and effective to enhance hand hygiene compliance, which leads to a reduction of HAI [11–14]. However, there have been few data on the implementation of the WHO multimodal HH strategy in China. We initiated this study of implementation of WHO multimodal HH strategy in order to improve awareness of HAI and enhance HH compliance and correctness among HCWs.

Methods

The study was conducted in Xi'an Hospital of Traditional Chinese Medicine (TCM), Xi'an, China, between September 2015 and August 2016. It is the largest public hospital in north Xi'an, which is the capital city of Shaanxi Province. This hospital has 1001 beds in 27 clinical departments including acupuncture and moxibustion, intensive care, emergency, surgical and TCM subspecialties with 1377 HCWs. We performed this two-part quasi-experimental study including questionnaire survey of factors affecting HH behaviors of HCWs and direct observation of compliance and correctness with HH before and after intervention.

Part I: Questionnaire survey

In this part, we did a questionnaire survey on possible factors affecting HH behaviors of HCWs. Each participant voted those factors contributing to HH noncompliance from the questionnaire. On the basis of the reasons for HH noncompliance summarized in the questionnaire, multimodal improvement strategy was developed accordingly.

Part II: Observation of compliance and correctness before and after intervention

In this part, detailed intervention measures were drawn up and then implemented according to the multimodal improvement strategy acquired from the results of questionnaire survey. We collected observational data on compliance and correctness with HH before and after intervention respectively.

Observation sessions were performed by 9 trained student nurses. The training course included HH indications and correct HH techniques recommended by WHO. A standard form was used to record the HH compliance and correctness. Observers were taught how to complete the form and record the number of HH actions and HH opportunities. We defined an opportunity as the occurrence of any indication during the observed care sequences. We recorded actions, either handwashing or hand rubbing based on WHO "My Five Moments for Hand Hygiene": before touching a patient, before clean/aseptic procedure, after body fluid exposure risk, after touching a patient, and after touching patient surroundings [15]. Since an indication for HH was related to the risk of pathogen transmission from one surface to another, we added two more WHO recommended indications in our study: if moving from a contaminated body site to a clean body site during patient care, after removing gloves [16]. An action with correct HH techniques must satisfy three criteria: (1) rub hands with 6-step HH techniques; (2) duration of the rub procedure lasts 15 s at least; (3) dry hands with disposable paper towels. Each observer monitored the HH practice of HCWs for 45–60 min.

Compliance and correctness with HH were compared before and after the implementation. HCWs including doctors, nurses, technicians, interns and cleaners were observed for HH actions and HH opportunities. Data of technicians, interns and cleaners was combined as other HCWs. We expressed HH compliance as the proportion of predefined opportunities met by HH actions. And HH correctness was regarded as the proportion of all HH actions met by HH actions with correct techniques. All the data was analyzed with SPSS version 16.0. The Chi square test was applied to test the statistical difference in HH compliance and correctness before and after the implementation. Also HH compliance stratified by professional category and indication was calculated. Results with $P < 0.05$ were considered statistically significant.

Results

Part I: Questionnaire survey

A total of 558 HCWs from 37 departments participated in this survey. Of these, 553 (99.10%) completed the baseline questionnaire. The general information of all participants was summarized in Table 1. Each participant

Table 1 The general information of 553 participants in the survey

		N (cases)	Percentage (%)	Mean (±s)
Age		553		31.78 ± 8.120
Gender	Female	433	78.30	
	Male	120	21.70	
Work experience	<1 year	104	18.81	
	1 ~ 5 years	139	25.13	
	5 ~ 10 years	155	28.03	
	≥10 years	155	28.03	
Education level	Senior high school	14	2.53	
	Junior college	181	32.73	
	College	273	49.37	
	Post graduate	85	15.37	
Profession	Doctors	191	34.54	
	Nurses	300	54.25	
	Technicians	35	6.33	
	Interns	23	4.16	
	Cleaners	4	0.72	

voted those factors contributing to HH noncompliance from the questionnaire. All the possible factors affecting HH behaviors of HCWs were arranged in descending order according to the number of votes (Fig. 1). The main reasons for HH noncompliance were classified into individual, environment and management levels. Multimodal improvement strategy was drafted accordingly (Fig. 2) and detailed intervention measures were drawn up at the same time.

For the individual reasons such as poor HH awareness, full training campaign on HH techniques among HCWs was carried out. Our management of infection control department first participated in the training of WHO "My Five Moments for Hand Hygiene" provided by Xi'an Quality Control Center of Nosocomial Infection. Then we shoot instructional videos on five key moments for HH and correct HH techniques in our hospital wards with our HCWs. After that they were called together to study HH knowledge via videos and PPT (based on WHO training slides). All the HCWs including doctors, nurses, interns, student nurses, lab technicians and cleaners should attend educational courses on HH every year. A posttest format was used to assess training efficacy after each course.

Inadequate HH supplies and inconvenient HH facilities was another cause for noncompliance with HH in our hospital. We took a series of measures to improve HH facilities: increasing supplies of pocket alcohol-based hand rub (ABHR) and disposable paper towels; making sure every wash basin equipped with disposable paper towels and poster for correct handwashing techniques; replacing water tap in nurse station with automatic electronic sensor tap; distributing skin care products to HCWs. Colorful HH posters were placed in the doctor's office in each ward with WHO "My Five Moments for Hand Hygiene". A little tip for HH was placed at the edge of the computer screen of nurse station. Visible reminders for HH were also set at the entrance of each ward. To create a better environment for HH, we offered large-scale HH improvement campaign to both HCWs

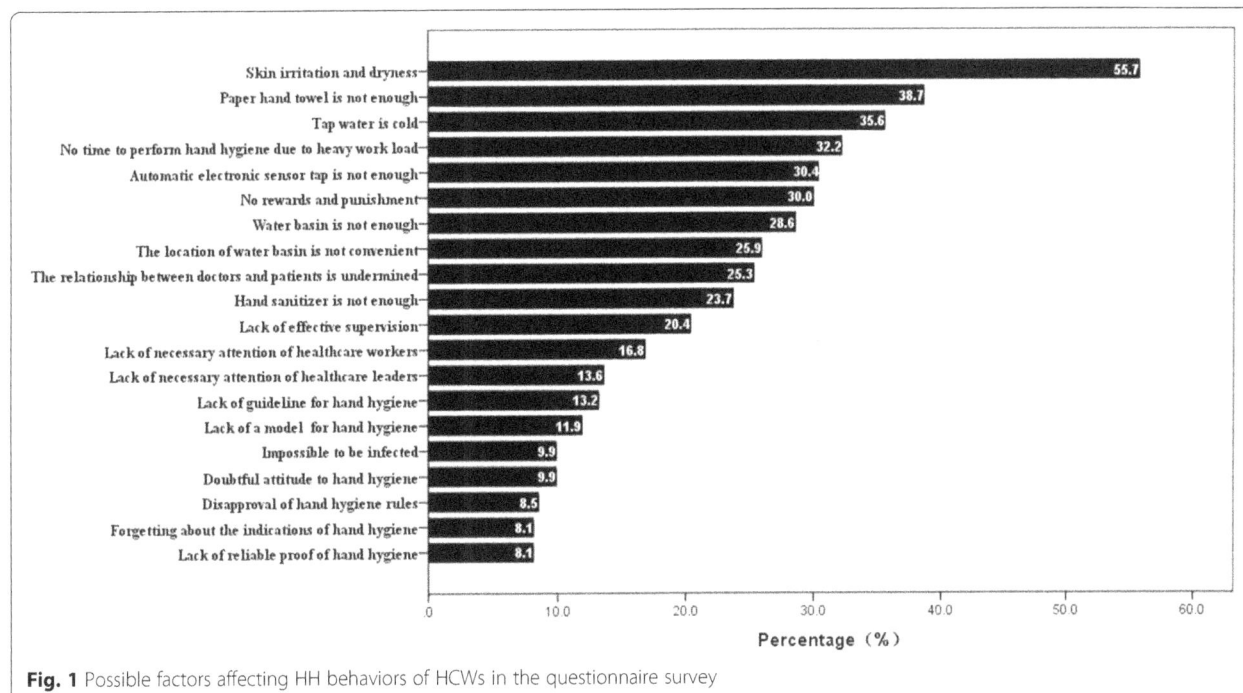

Fig. 1 Possible factors affecting HH behaviors of HCWs in the questionnaire survey

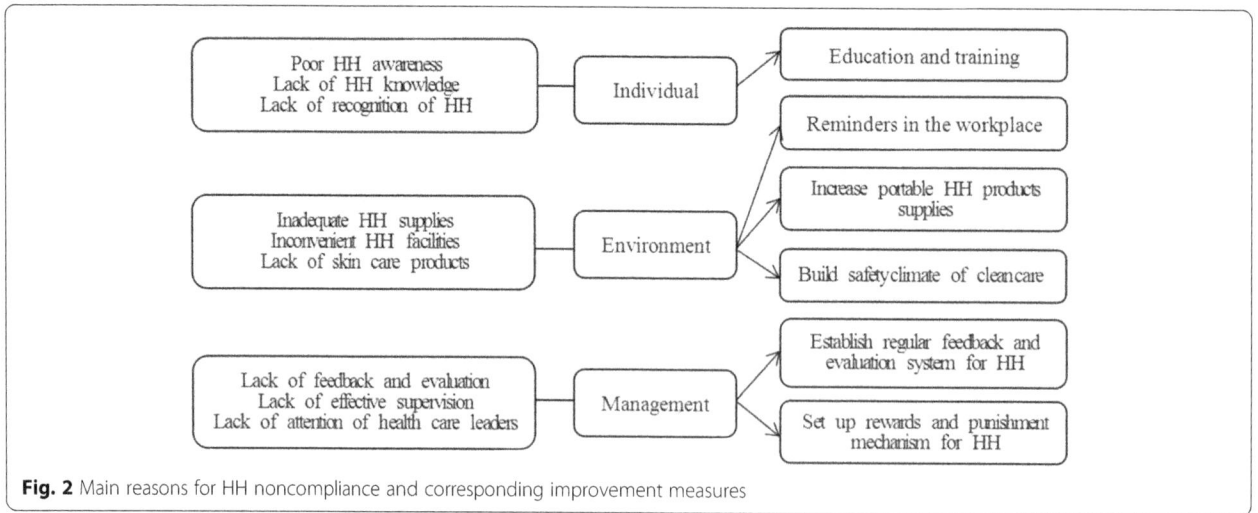

Fig. 2 Main reasons for HH noncompliance and corresponding improvement measures

and patients with knowledge contest, visible display boards, and live performance.

In order to strengthen the supervision of HH practice among HCWs, a seasonal feedback and evaluation system was established. Management of infection control department regularly reported HH compliance and HH products consumption in the meeting of Nosocomial Infection Control Management Committee, which included hospital management, department heads, head nurses and focal persons. Also HH compliance and HH products consumption was directly related to the scores of quality control of each department through HH rewards and punishment mechanism. Department with noncompliant HCWs had to pay a fine.

Part II: Observation of compliance and correctness before and after intervention

HH compliance
In our study, a total of 5044 opportunities for HH were recorded in 23 wards before and after intervention. The rate of compliance with HH improved from 66.27% at baseline to 80.53% after intervention (shown in Table 2). After implementing the improvement strategy, doctors had better HH compliance (84.04%) than nurses and other HCWs (81.07% and 69.42%, respectively). The rate

of compliance with HH was statistically increased after intervention for each professional category ($P < 0.05$).

HH correctness
A total of 2927 actions with correct HH techniques were recorded. The rate of correctness with HH improved from 47.75% to 88.35% after intervention (shown in Table 3). The increase of correctness applied for all professional categories, which was statistically significant ($P < 0.05$).

HH compliance by indication
The rate of compliance with HH was statistically elevated after intervention for all indications ($P < 0.05$) except for "after body fluid exposure risk" and "after touching patient surroundings". The highest relative improvement appeared to be indication "if moving from a contaminated body site to a clean body site during patient care", from 30.61% to 59.82% (shown in Table 4).

Discussion
Our study identified that implementation of WHO multimodal HH improvement strategy was effective to enhance HH compliance and correctness among HCWs. In the questionnaire survey, over 50% of the participants thought frequently washing hands led to hand skin

Table 2 Comparison of HH compliance of HCWs before and after intervention by professional category

	HH compliance before intervention (%)	HH compliance after intervention (%)	x^2	P
Doctors	342/459 (74.51)	279/332 (84.04)	10.362	0.001
Nurses	747/1081 (69.10)	2266/2795 (81.07)	64.538	<0.001
Other HCWs	21/135 (15.56)	168/242 (69.42)	100.58	<0.001
Overall	1110/1675 (66.27)	2713/3369 (80.53)	123.99	<0.001

Table 3 Comparison of HH correctness of HCWs before and after intervention by professional category

	HH correctness before intervention (%)	HH correctness after intervention (%)	x^2	P
Doctors	169/342 (49.42)	201/279 (72.04)	32.669	<0.001
Nurses	349/747 (46.72)	2030/2266 (89.59)	621.30	<0.001
Other HCWs	12/21 (57.14)	166/168 (98.81)	59.123	<0.001
Overall	530/1110 (47.75)	2397/2713 (88.35)	723.76	<0.001

Table 4 Comparison of HH compliance before and after intervention of HCWs by indication

	HH compliance before intervention (%)	HH compliance after intervention (%)	χ^2	P
Before touching a patient	263/489 (53.78)	766/944 (81.14)	119.121	<0.001
After touching a patient	374/489 (76.48)	737/897 (82.16)	6.420	0.011
If moving from a contaminated body site to a clean body site during patient care	15/49 (30.61)	134/224 (59.82)	13.837	<0.001
After body fluid exposure risk	65/84 (77.38)	172/209 (82.30)	0.937	0.333
Before clean/aseptic procedures	160/254 (62.99)	460/552 (83.33)	40.547	<0.001
After touching patient surroundings	150/190 (78.95)	339/415 (81.69)	0.631	0.427
After removing gloves	83/120 (69.17)	105/128 (82.03)	5.589	0.018

irritation and dryness, which was a vital cause for non-compliance with HH. In addition, irritated hands might be more vulnerable to be colonized with pathogens [17]. Since cleaning hands frequently is essential for every health care worker, it is important for health care settings to provide proper HH products. Compared with detergent and soap, ABHR has been reported to cause less skin irritation, especially those with emollient properties [18, 19]. The application of skin care products can preserve unimpaired skin, reduce the incidence of skin irritation and dryness and ensure effective hand hygiene [20]. In the last decades, there were concerns that skin care products might pose a negative influence on the efficacy of hand disinfection [21, 22]. With the wide research of well-formulated disinfectants with emollients in recent years, it seems that the efficacy of disinfectants would not be impaired when they are applied with selected, compatible skin care products [23, 24]. In our study, we provided skin care products to our HCWs to minimize the influence on HH compliance due to skin irritation and dryness. Moreover, we encourage our HCWs to use skin care products before work, cleaning and after work under recommendations [25].

Epidemiological evidence have shown that hand contamination of nurses could cause cross-infection in a direct or indirect way, especially in intensive care unit and hemodialysis unit where nurses have many patient contact opportunities [26, 27]. In our study, HH compliance of doctors seemed superior to nurses when stratified by professional category. There were far more opportunities of HH for nurses in most departments than for doctors. Then overcrowding workload of nurses made them provide clinical care to multiple patients without HH to finish their tasks faster. HH compliance in other HCWs was generally lower than doctors and nurses. Poor HH compliance was witnessed among technicians during physiotherapy [28]. Gloves were often used during cleaning work to replace HH by cleaners, which might increase the risk of transmission of bacteria via contaminated gloved hands [29, 30]. Besides, the growing mobility of cleaners and interns made it difficult

to accomplish full training on HH. All in all, HH compliance was improved in different professional categories after intervention.

Data of compliance by different HH indication was also investigated in the present study. Compliance with HH improved after intervention across all indications except for "after body fluid exposure" and "after touching patient surroundings" in the observation. We recognized that compliance rates were above 70% for these two indications before intervention, which suggested that our HCWs intended to perform HH when they thought there might be microbial contamination and infection risk. In addition, compliance rates for "before" related indications were promoted after intervention, such as "before touching a patient" and "before clean/aseptic procedures". These findings revealed that HCWs were inclined to wash their hands to protect themselves rather than protect patients from potential infection, which was noted in previous studies [31, 32]. As for indication "after touching patient surroundings", HH opportunities with this indication were most commonly associated with lower levels of compliance than following direct patient contact [33]. Traditional Chinese Medicine treatments such as acupuncture and moxibustion are often combined with diathermy machine and herb fumigation device to get better curative effect. Most of our HCWs could perform HH after therapy devices were turned off. But when there was need to adjust the setting of therapy devices, required HH practices were not performed according to our observers. Multiple studies indicated that HAI could be caused by many pathogenic organisms present in the hospital environment and objects frequently touched by patients' hands, such as bed side rail, door knob, patient record, nurse call button [34, 35]. Moreover, it was of vital importance to strengthen the effectiveness of cleaning and in order to prevent the transmission of pathogens from patient surrounding environment to HCWs and patients [36, 37].

To well acknowledge whether our HCWs mastered the standard handwashing techniques, HH correctness was investigated at the same time. In general, correctness rate was far below our standards before intervention. During the period of investigation, we found two most commonly reasons for low HH correctness rate in our hospital. Most of our HCWs knew the right HH technique procedures but the duration of rubbing hands did not meet our requirement (15 s at least). Inadequate disposable paper towel was another cause for unpleasant HH correctness rate. Therefore our infection control staff took steps to promote correct HH techniques, which included correct HH techniques training, increasing supplies of pocket ABHR and disposable paper towels. As a result, our HCWs' HH correctness rates were elevated after intervention.

In the last few years, domestic researches on improving HH practice have been reported in succession [38–44]. It is noteworthy that our study is the first observational before-and-after intervention study on improving HH compliance in Xi'an, Shaanxi province. Meanwhile it is the first study implementing WHO multimodal strategy to promote HH practice in a hospital of Traditional Chinese Medicine. HCWs have many patient contact opportunities in the process of Traditional Chinese Medicine treatments such as acupuncture and moxibustion, massage, cupping and other physical therapies. If standard HH practice were not performed, it might increase the risk of cross-infection. Our study summarized the reasons for non-compliance with HH and provided scientific evidence to promote HH practice for other hospitals of Traditional Chinese Medicine. Nevertheless, this study also had certain limitations. The entire observation of HH compliance and correctness were only carried out in general inpatient wards. We planned to observe HH practice in critical departments for infection control management such as emergency, intensive care unit and hemodialysis unit. These places are characterized by high patient volume, critically ill patients and more invasive operations. Improving HH compliance in such places would be meaningful for better infection control. Furthermore, using student nurses as observers might have an impact on observation process. These student nurses observed HH practice of HCWs in clinical wards during their clinical clerkships. Some students told us they recognized their former teaching nurses and classmates in the observation process and thus we concerned that this covert investigation might present the Hawthorn effect. In order to lessen the influence of the Hawthorn effect on HH compliance of HCWs, we plan to train every HCW in our hospital to become a competent observer for HH compliance of their co-workers. In this way every HCW could be our covert observer and we could collect reliable data of HH practice.

Conclusions
In conclusion, this intervention study has shown that implementation of WHO multimodal improvement strategy could significantly increase compliance and correctness with HH in our hospital. Further investigations with sufficient sample size and larger multicenter series are needed to validate the effectiveness of long-term persistence of HH compliance improvement strategy.

Abbreviations
ABHR: Alcohol-based hand rub; HAI: Healthcare-associated infection; HCWs: Health care workers; HH: Hand hygiene; TCM: Traditional Chinese Medicine; WHO: World Health Organization

Acknowledgements
Not applicable.

Funding
Project supported by Key Science and Technology R & D Program of Shaanxi Province, China (Grant No.2016SF-213).

Authors' contributions
LS carried out the study and drafted the manuscript. XW conceived of the study, participated in its design and coordination. JA contributed to the design of the study. JA participated in the literature review and performed statistical analysis. NZ, LS and HC provided training of hand hygiene indications and correct hand hygiene techniques for observers and collected data. LF organized workers to improve hand hygiene products and facilities. JH and XL contributed to check and enter data. All authors read and approved the final manuscript.

Consent for publication
Not applicable.

Competing interests
The authors declare that they have no competing interests.

Author details
[1]Department of Infection Control, Xi'an Hospital of Traditional Chinese Medicine, No.69 Feng Cheng 8th Road, Weiyang District, Xi'an 710021, China. [2]Department of Acupuncture and Moxibustion, Xi'an Hospital of Traditional Chinese Medicine, No.69 Feng Cheng 8th Road, Weiyang District, Xi'an 710021, China. [3]Department of Information Consultation, Library of Xi'an Jiaotong University, No.76 Yan Ta West Road, Yanta District, Xi'an 710061, China. [4]Department of Cadre Health Care, Xi'an Hospital of Traditional Chinese Medicine, No.69 Feng Cheng 8th Road, Weiyang District, Xi'an 710021, China.

References
1. Allegranzi B, Bagheri Nejad S, Combescure C, Graafmans W, Attar H, Donaldson L, et al. Burden of endemic health-care-associated infection in developing countries: systematic review and meta-analysis. Lancet. 2011;377:228–41.
2. Ren N, Wen X, Wu A. Nationwide cross-sectional survey on healthcare-associated infection in 2014. Chinese Journal of Infection Control. 2016;15:83–7.
3. Graves N, Weinhold D, Tong E, Birrell F, Doidge S, Ramritu P, et al. Effect of healthcare-acquired infection on length of hospital stay and cost. Infect Control Hosp Epidemiol. 2007;28:280–92.
4. Jia H, Hou T, Li W, Ma Q, Liu W, Yang Y, et al. Economic loss due to healthcare-associated infection in 68 general hospitals in China. Chinese Journal of Infection Control. 2016;15:637–41.

5. Allegranzi B, Pittet D. Preventing infections acquired during health-care delivery. Lancet. 2008;372:1719–20.

6. Chen P, Liu D. Epidemiological characteristics and preventive strategies of nosocomial infection outbreak incidents in China in recent 30 years. Chinese Journal of Infection Control. 2010;9:387–92,99.

7. Allegranzi B, Pittet D. Role of hand hygiene in healthcare-associated infection prevention. J Hosp Infect. 2009;73:305–15.

8. Dancer SJ. The role of environmental cleaning in the control of hospital-acquired infection. J Hosp Infect. 2009;73:378–85.

9. Weber DJ, Anderson D, Rutala WA. The role of the surface environment in healthcare-associated infections. Curr Opin Infect Dis. 2013;26:338–44.

10. WHO. Guide to implementation: a guide to the implementation of the WHO Multimodal Hand Hygiene Improvement Strategy. 2009. http://www.who.int/gpsc/5may/Guide_to_Implementation.pdf (Accessd Feb 7,2017).

11. Allegranzi B, Gayet-Ageron A, Damani N, Bengaly L, McLaws ML, Moro ML, et al. Global implementation of WHO's multimodal strategy for improvement of hand hygiene: a quasi-experimental study. Lancet Infect Dis. 2013;13:843–51.

12. Arntz PR, Hopman J, Nillesen M, Yalcin E, Bleeker-Rovers CP, Voss A, et al. Effectiveness of a multimodal hand hygiene improvement strategy in the emergency department. Am J Infect Control. 2016;44:1203–7.

13. Farhoudi F, Sanaei Dashti A, Hoshangi Davani M, Ghalebi N, Sajadi G, Taghizadeh R. Impact of WHO hand hygiene improvement program implementation: a quasi-experimental trial. Biomed Res Int. 2016;2016:7026169.

14. Pfafflin F, Tufa TB, Getachew M, Nigussie T, Schonfeld A, Haussinger D, et al. Implementation of the WHO multimodal Hand Hygiene Improvement Strategy in a University Hospital in Central Ethiopia. Antimicrob Resist Infect Control. 2017;6:3.

15. WHO. About SAVE LIVES: Clean Your Hands. 2009. http://www.who.int/gpsc/5may/background/5moments/en/ (Accessd Feb 7,2017).

16. WHO. WHO guidelines on hand hygiene in health care: a summary. 2009. http://www.who.int/gpsc/information_centre/hand-hygiene-summary/en/ (Accessd Feb 7,2017).

17. Visscher MO, Randall WR. Hand hygiene compliance and irritant dermatitis: a juxtaposition of healthcare issues. Int J Cosmet Sci. 2012;34:402–15.

18. Boyce JM, Kelliher S, Vallande N. Skin irritation and dryness associated with two hand-hygiene regimens: soap-and-water hand washing versus hand antisepsis with an alcoholic hand gel. Infect Control Hosp Epidemiol. 2000;21:442–8.

19. Larson E, Girard R, Pessoa-Silva CL, Boyce J, Donaldson L, Pittet D. Skin reactions related to hand hygiene and selection of hand hygiene products. Am J Infect Control. 2006;34:627–35.

20. Bissett L. Skin care: an essential component of hand hygiene and infection control. Br J Nurs. 2007;16:976–81.

21. Walsh B, Blakemore PH, Drabu YJ. The effect of handcream on the antibacterial activity of chlorhexidine gluconate. J Hosp Infect. 1987;9:30–3.

22. Benson L, LeBlanc D, Bush L, White J. The effects of surfactant systems and moisturizing products on the residual activity of a chlorhexidine gluconate handwash using a pigskin substrate. Infect Control Hosp Epidemiol. 1990;11:67–70.

23. Heeg P. Does hand care ruin hand disinfection? J Hosp Infect. 2001;48(Suppl A):S37–9.

24. Harnoss JC, Brune L, Ansorg J, Heidecke CD, Assadian O, Kramer A. Practice of skin protection and skin care among German surgeons and influence on the efficacy of surgical hand disinfection and surgical glove perforation. BMC Infect Dis. 2014;14:315.

25. Kampf G, Loffler H. Prevention of irritant contact dermatitis among health care workers by using evidence-based hand hygiene practices: a review. Ind Health. 2007;45:645–52.

26. Duong MC, McLaws ML. Dangerous practices in a hemodialysis unit in Vietnam identify from mixed methods. BMC Infect Dis. 2017;17:181.

27. Ghorbani A, Sadeghi L, Shahrokhi A, Mohammadpour A, Addo M, Khodadadi E. Hand hygiene compliance before and after wearing gloves among intensive care unit nurses in Iran. Am J Infect Control. 2016;44:e279–e81.

28. O'Donoghue M, Ng SH, Suen LK, Boost M. A quasi-experimental study to determine the effects of a multifaceted educational intervention on hand hygiene compliance in a radiography unit. Antimicrob Resist Infect Control. 2016;5:36.

29. McBryde ES, Bradley LC, Whitby M, McElwain DL. An investigation of contact transmission of methicillin-resistant Staphylococcus Aureus. J Hosp Infect. 2004;58:104–8.

30. Snyder GM, Thom KA, Furuno JP, Perencevich EN, Roghmann MC, Strauss SM, et al. Detection of methicillin-resistant Staphylococcus Aureus and vancomycin-resistant enterococci on the gowns and gloves of healthcare workers. Infect Control Hosp Epidemiol. 2008;29:583–9.

31. Lee A, Chalfine A, Daikos GL, Garilli S, Jovanovic B, Lemmen S, et al. Hand hygiene practices and adherence determinants in surgical wards across Europe and Israel: a multicenter observational study. Am J Infect Control. 2011;39:517–20.

32. Patel B, Engelbrecht H, McDonald H, Morris V, Smythe W. A multifaceted hospital-wide intervention increases hand hygiene compliance. S Afr Med J. 2016;106:32–5.

33. FitzGerald G, Moore G, Wilson AP. Hand hygiene after touching a patient's surroundings: the opportunities most commonly missed. J Hosp Infect. 2013;84:27–31.

34. Donskey CJ. Does improving surface cleaning and disinfection reduce health care-associated infections? Am J Infect Control. 2013;41:S12–9.

35. Weber DJ, Rutala WA, Miller MB, Huslage K, Sickbert-Bennett E. Role of hospital surfaces in the transmission of emerging health care-associated pathogens: norovirus, Clostridium Difficile, and Acinetobacter species. Am J Infect Control. 2010;38:S25–33.

36. Ramphal L, Suzuki S, McCracken IM, Addai A. Improving hospital staff compliance with environmental cleaning behavior. Proc (Bayl Univ Med Cent). 2014;27:88–91.

37. Kurashige EJ, Oie S, Furukawa H. Contamination of environmental surfaces by methicillin-resistant Staphylococcus Aureus (MRSA) in rooms of inpatients with MRSA-positive body sites. Braz J Microbiol. 2016;47:703–5.

38. Ji G, Yin H, Chen Y. Prevalence of and risk factors for non-compliance with glove utilization and hand hygiene among obstetrics and gynaecology workers in rural China. J Hosp Infect. 2005;59:235–41.

39. Li LY, Zhao YC, Jia JX, Zhao XL, Jia HX. Investigation on compliance of hand hygiene of healthcare workers. Zhongguo Yi Xue Ke Xue Yuan Xue Bao. 2008;30:546–9.

40. Chau JP, Thompson DR, Twinn S, Lee DT, Pang SW. An evaluation of hospital hand hygiene practice and glove use in Hong Kong. J Clin Nurs. 2011;20:1319–28.

41. Su D, Hu B, Rosenthal VD, Li R, Hao C, Pan W, et al. Impact of the international nosocomial infection control consortium (INICC) multidimensional hand hygiene approach in five intensive care units in three cities of China. Public Health. 2015;129:979–88.

42. Mu X, Xu Y, Yang T, Zhang J, Wang C, Liu W, et al. Improving hand hygiene compliance among healthcare workers: an intervention study in a Hospital in Guizhou Province. China Braz J Infect Dis. 2016;20:413–8.

43. Chen P, Yuan T, Sun Q, Jiang L, Jiang H, Zhu Z, et al. Role of quality control circle in sustained improvement of hand hygiene compliance: an observational study in a stomatology hospital in Shandong. China Antimicrob Resist Infect Control. 2016;5:54.

44. Cheng VC, Tai JW, Li WS, Chau PH, So SY, Wong LM, et al. Implementation of directly observed patient hand hygiene for hospitalized patients by hand hygiene ambassadors in Hong Kong. Am J Infect Control. 2016;44:621–4.

5

A twenty-four-hour observational study of hand hygiene compliance among health-care workers in Debre Berhan referral hospital, Ethiopia

Tufa Kolola* and Takele Gezahegn

Abstract

Background: Hand hygiene (HH) is recognized as the single most effective strategy for preventing health care–associated infections. In developing countries, data on hand hygiene compliance is available only for few health-care facilities. This study aimed to assess hand hygiene compliance among health-care workers in Debre Berhan referral hospital, Ethiopia.

Methods: This study employed the WHO hand hygiene observation method. Direct observation of the health care workers (HCWs) was conducted using an observation record form in five different wards. Trained and validated observers watched HCWs while they had direct contact with patients or their surroundings, and the observers then recorded all possible hand hygiene opportunities and hand hygiene actions. Observation was conducted over a 24 h period to minimize selection bias. More than 200 opportunities per ward were observed according to WHO recommendation, except in neonatal intensive care unit. HH compliance was calculated by dividing the number of times hand hygiene was performed by the total number of opportunities for hand hygiene. A 95% confidence interval (CI) was computed for compliance with the exact binomial method.

Results: A total of 917 hand hygiene opportunities were observed during the study. Overall HH compliance was 22. 0% (95% CI: 19.4–24.9). HH compliance was similar across all professional categories and did not vary by shift. Levels of compliance were lower before patient contact (2.4%; 95% CI: 0.9–5.3), before an aseptic procedure (3.6%; 95% CI: 1.6–7.6) and after contact with patient surroundings (3.3%; 95% CI: 1.2–7.9), whereas better levels of compliance were found after body fluid exposure (75.8%; 95% CI: 68.0–82.3) and after patient contact (42.8%; 95% CI: 35.2–50.7).

Conclusion: HH compliance of HCWs was found to be low in Debre Berhan referral hospital. Compliance with indications that protect patients from infection was lower than that protect the HCWs. The findings of this study indicate that HH compliance needs further improvement.

Keywords: Hand hygiene compliance, Direct observation method, Health-care worker, Debre Berhan, World health organization

* Correspondence: tufabest@gmail.com
Department of public health, Debre Berhan University, P.O.Box 445, Debre Berhan, Ethiopia

Background

Health care-associated infections (HAIs) are a major threat to patient safety worldwide [1–4]. Such infections spread between patients in the health-care settings by various means, mainly via the hands of health-care workers (HCWs) [5, 6].

Hand hygiene (HH) is the single most effective strategy for preventing HAIs [7–9]. Hand hygiene is defined as either rubbing the hands with an alcohol-based handrub or handwashing with soap and water [6]. WHO has launched a multimodal hand hygiene improvement strategy to optimize hand hygiene in health care settings [10]. This strategy is now recommended as the most reliable and evidence-based method for ensuring sustainable hand hygiene improvement around the world [11–16]. HCWs compliance with hand hygiene during routine patient care is an integral part of this strategy. HH compliance is measured in a variety of ways. These include: direct observation, handrub consumption, and survey methods [17, 18]. Direct observation of HCWs using WHO's hand hygiene observation tool is currently recognized as the gold standard for hand hygiene monitoring in the sequence of care [6, 10, 17].

World Health Organization has endorsed "My five moments for hand hygiene" approach, the moments when hand hygiene is required, to effectively interrupt the spread of HAIs [19]. This approach encourages HCWs to clean their hands, i.e., (1) before patient contact, (2) before an aseptic procedure, (3) after body fluid exposure, (4) after patient contact and (5) after contact with patient surroundings [20]. The World Health Organization (WHO) has defined these moments as hand hygiene opportunities (HHOs) to which HCWs should comply with [10, 18]. Hand hygiene opportunity exists whenever one of the indications for hand hygiene occurs. Each opportunity corresponds to hand hygiene action [18].

In developing countries with high burden of health-care-associated infections, improving HCWs compliance with hand hygiene during routine patient care is urgently needed for the patient safety [2, 21]. Despite the clear benefits of hand hygiene practices in health-care settings, compliance remains an issue in developing countries [11]. In Ethiopia, data on hand hygiene compliance is available only for few health-care facilities [14, 22]. In Debre Berhan referral hospital, HCWs compliance to the WHO's five moments for hand hygiene was not investigated so far. This study aimed to assess hand hygiene compliance among health-care workers in Debre Berhan referral hospital through direct observation of the WHO's five moments. The result of this study provides insights about hand hygiene compliance level of health care providers.

Methods

Study setting

A cross-sectional study was conducted in Debre Berhan referral hospital using the WHO hand hygiene observation method. Debre Berhan referral hospital is located in North Shoa Zone of Amhara Region which is about 130 km away from Addis Ababa to Dessie. Currently, this hospital serves as a referral centre for a population of North Shoa Zone of Amhara region and for other population from the neighbouring regions. The hospital has a total of 307 HCWs: 38 physicians, 153 nurses, 26 midwives, 7 anaesthetists, 31 laboratory technicians, 2 physiotherapists, 4 dentists, 6 radiographers, 4 optometrists and 36 pharmacists. In addition, 48 medical interns were affiliated to this hospital during data collection. This study was conducted from May 2 to 9, 2017 in the selected wards (Medical, Surgical, Paediatric, Obstetrics and gynecology, and Neonatal intensive care unit) of the hospital. All HCWs, including medical interns, having direct contact with patients or their surroundings in the selected wards were observed.

Data collection

Data were collected using standardized WHO's hand hygiene observation tool for direct observation (Additional file 1). Before conducting observation sessions, observers were trained in accordance with the WHO's hand hygiene observation method [23]. Thereafter, observers were validated by one of the authors based on Sax et al.'s [6] recommendation. In the first case, each observer engaged in an observation session during a patient care situation. Each observer completed the observation form separately while observing the same HCW and the same care sequence. Results were then compared and discordant notifications were discussed. This process was repeated until concordance is reached in terms of the number of hand hygiene opportunities and hand hygiene actions that occurred [6, 20].

In brief, three nurses directly watched 261 HCWs having direct contact with patients or their surroundings, and recorded all possible HHOs and HHAs. Observation was conducted over a 24 h period in each ward to minimize selection bias. The HCWs were unaware of being observed to minimize "Hawthorne effect". Each HCW was observed for a maximum of four HHOs during the observed care sequence. More than 200 opportunities per ward were observed according to WHO recommendation [23], except in neonatal intensive care unit (NICU). Few opportunities were observed in NICU due to the small number of HCWs working in this unit.

Data analysis

Data analysis was done using Epi Info 7 and SPSS version 21. Data set underlying the findings is available within the supplementary information files (Additional file 2). Overall compliance was calculated by dividing the number of times hand hygiene was performed by the total number of opportunities for hand hygiene. We also estimated HH compliance by professional categories, and "my five moments for hand hygiene". A 95% confidence interval (CI) was computed for compliance with the exact binomial method. Overlapping 95% confidence intervals were interpreted as not being significantly different.

Results

Hand hygiene compliance

A total of 917 opportunities for hand hygiene were observed during the study. The overall HH compliance was 22.0% (95% CI: 19.4–24.9). HH compliance was 20.6% (95% CI:16.2–25.9) for doctors, 22.9% (95% CI:19.2–27.0) for nurses, 21.2% (95% CI:13.9–30.8) for midwives, and 23.2% (95% CI: 13.4–36.7) for other HCWs. HH compliance was slightly higher in the neonatal intensive care unit (NICU) and paediatric ward compared to other wards. HH compliance varied according to the five moments for hand hygiene. Levels of compliance were lower before patient contact (2.4%%; 95% CI: 0.9–5.3), before an aseptic procedure (3.6%; 95% CI: 1.6–7.6) and after contact with patient surroundings (3.3%; 95% CI: 1.2–7.9). Better levels of compliance were found after body fluid exposure (75.8%; 95% CI: 68.0–82.3) and after patient contact (42.8%; 95% CI: 35.2–50.7) (Table 1).

Hand rubbing was performed in 95, (47.0%; 95% CI: 40.2–53.9), out of the 202 hand hygiene actions. Hand rubbing was frequently performed, (55.8%; 95% CI: 45.7–65.5), after patient contact while handwashing with soap and water was more frequent, (76.6%; 95% CI: 67.9–83.9), after body fluid exposure compared with other indications (Fig. 1).

Hand hygiene resources

In this study, sink to patient beds ratio was 1:4.9, and soap was available to 36.4% of the sinks. Alcohol-based handrub was available for 16.8% (18/107) of the patient beds.

Discussion

This study captured hand hygiene compliance of HCWs over a 24 h period. Overall hand hygiene compliance was low (22%). HH compliance was low across all professional categories and similar by shift. In line with our study, HH compliance was found low in previous studies [14, 22, 24]. In low-income and middle-income countries, HH compliance was averaged 22·4% before multimodal intervention [11]. Hand hygiene compliance was much lower in the present study compared to post- multimodal intervention studies from India (82%) [15], Kuwait (61.4%) [25], and Colombia (77%) [26].

Table 1 Hand hygiene compliance of HCWs in Debre Berhan Referral Hospital, May 2017

Characteristic	Hand hygiene opportunities (n)	Hand hygiene actions (n[a])	Compliance, % (95% CI)
Over all	917	202	22.0 (19.4–24.9)
Professional category			
Doctor	286	59	20.6 (16.2–25.9)
Nurse	476	109	22.9 (19.2–27.0)
Midwife	99	21	21.2 (13.9–30.8)
Other HCWs	56	13	23.2 (13.4–36.7)
Ward			
Medical	207	44	21.2 (16.0–27.6)
Surgical	203	38	18.7 (13.7–24.9)
Paediatric	211	56	26.5 (20.8–33.1)
OB/GYN	219	43	19.6 (14.7–25.7)
NICU	77	21	27.3 (18.0–38.8)
Shift			
Morning	369	86	23.3 (19.2–28.0)
After noon	318	74	23.3 (18.8–28.4)
Night	230	52	22.6 (17.5–28.4)
Indications			
bef. Pat	255	6	2.4 (0.9–5.3)
bef. Asept	195	7	3.6 (1.6–7.6)
aft.b.f	149	113	75.8 (68.0–82.3)
aft.pat	166	71	42.8 (35.2–50.7)
aft.p.surr	152	5	3.3 (1.2–7.9)

bef. Pat before patient contact, *bef. Asept* before an aseptic procedure, *aft.b.f* after body fluid exposure, *aft.pat* after patient contact, *aft.p.surr* after contact with patient surroundings, *HCWs* Health care workers, *n* Number of opportunities for hand hygiene, *n[a]* Number of positive hand hygiene actions, *CI* Confidence interval, *Other HCWs*, Laboratory technician, dentist and physiotherapist, *NICU* Neonatal intensive care unit, *OB/GYN*, Obstetrics and gynecology

The possible reason for low compliance in our study might be due to the WHO's multimodal HH improvement strategy which was not implemented. For instance, HH resources were deficient at the point of patient care. There were no visual reminders for hand hygiene at work place. Similarly, there was lack of HH monitoring and provision of performance feedback to HCWs. Studies have demonstrated that implementation of a multimodal strategy is globally accepted as best approach to achieve HH compliance in healthcare settings [11, 27, 28].

Hand hygiene compliance was inconsistent by the five indications for hand hygiene which might be another reason for low compliance. Lower levels of compliance were witnessed for indications before patient contact, before an aseptic procedure and after contact with patient surroundings. By contrast, compliance with hand hygiene was relatively higher after body fluid exposure

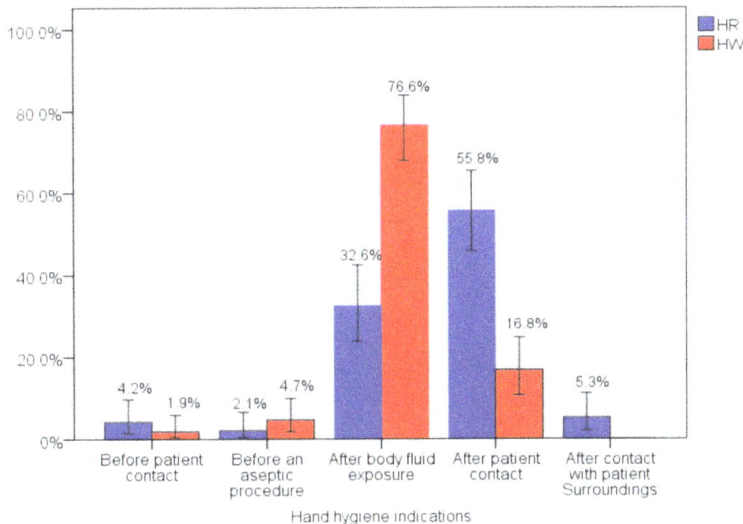

Fig. 1 Hand hygiene actions by indications among HCWs in Debre Berhan Referral Hospital, May 2017. HR: Hand rubbing with an alcohol-based handrub; HW: Handwashing with soap and water; Error bars show 95% confidence intervals around hand hygiene action; HCWs: Health care workers

followed by after patient contact. This suggests that HCWs more likely to perform HH for the indications that protect themselves from microbial contamination and infection rather than that protect patients. Self-protection tendency of HCWs has been identified in multiple studies [11, 25, 29–31].

Hand rubbing is recommended as the gold standard for hand hygiene according to the "my five moments for hand hygiene" in clinical situations [9, 21]. Particularly in resource-constrained settings, the use of alcohol based hand rubs is a practical solution to overcome constraints because they can be distributed individually to staff for pocket carriage and placed at the point of care [20, 21]. In contrary to findings from other studies [11, 12, 32], the present study revealed that hand rubbing was not the preferred means for hand hygiene. One reason could be that alcohol based hand rub was deficient at the point of care and was obstacle to performing HH according to recommendation. Ensuring availability of alcohol-based hand rubs at the point of patient care is a key factor for hand hygiene improvement in previous studies [30, 33, 34].

The strength of this study is that observation was done over a 24 h to minimize selection bias. In addition to this, the HCWs were unaware of being observed to minimize "Hawthorne effect". This study was not free of limitations. This study solely employed direct observation method. As a result, did not address why HH compliance was found to be low. The cross-sectional results of this study might not be representative of HH compliance throughout the year. This study conducted in a single hospital, and hence the generalizability of our results to other settings might be limited.

Conclusion

This study showed that HH compliance of HCWs was found to be low. Indications that are high risk to the patient have lower compliance. This suggests that the need of HH compliance improvement strategy is evident. Implementing WHO's multimodal strategy is crucial to improve HH compliance of HCWs. Access to HH resources should be emphasised as an integral part of HH improvement strategy.

Abbreviations
CI: Confidence interval; HAI: Health-care associated infection; HCW: Health care worker; HH: Hand hygiene; HHA: Hand hygiene action; HHO: Hand hygiene opportunity; HR: Hand rubbing; HW: Hand washing; NICU: Neonatal intensive care unit; OB/GYN: Obstetrics and gynecology; PSG: Patient safety goal; WHO: World Health Organization

Acknowledgements
Not applicable.

Funding
Not applicable.

Authors' contributions
TK: conception of the idea, study design, facilitation of data collection, data analysis, drafting the manuscript. TG: study design, facilitation of data collection, revising the manuscript. Both authors read and approved the final manuscript.

Consent for publication
Not applicable.

Competing interests
The authors declare that they have no competing interests.

References

1. World Health Organization (WHO). Report on the burden of endemic health care-associated infection worldwide. Geneva; 2011.
2. Allegranzi B, Nejad SB, Combescure C, Graafmans W, Attar H, Donaldson L, et al. Burden of endemic health-care-associated infection in developing countries: systematic review and meta-analysis. Lancet. 2011;377(9761):228–41.
3. Hearn P, Miliya T, Seng S, Ngoun C, Day NPJ, Lubell Y, et al. Prospective surveillance of healthcare associated infections in a Cambodian pediatric hospital. Antimicrob Resist Infect Control. 2017;6:16.
4. Ahoyo TA, Bankolé HS, Adéoti FM, Gbohoun AA, Assavèdo S, Amoussou-Guénou M, et al. Prevalence of nosocomial infections and anti-infective therapy in Benin: results of the first nationwide survey in 2012. Antimicrob Resist Infect Control. 2014;3:17.
5. Kleef Van E, Robotham JV, Jit M, Deeny SR, Edmunds WJ. Modelling the transmission of healthcare associated infections: a systematic review. BMC Infect Dis. 2013;13:294.
6. Sax H, Allegranzi B, Chraïti MN, Boyce J, Larson E, Pittet D. The World Health Organization hand hygiene observation method. Am J Infect Control. 2009;37(10):827–34.
7. Ellingson K, Haas JP, Aiello AE, Kusek L, Maragakis LL, Olmsted RN, et al. Strategies to prevent healthcare-associated infections through hand hygiene. Infect Control. 2014;35(8):937–60.
8. Septimus E, Weinstein RA, Perl TM, Goldmann DA, Yokoe DS. Approaches for preventing healthcare-associated infections: go long or go wide? Infect Control Hosp Epidemiol. 2014;35(7):797–801.
9. Allegranzi B, Pittet D. Role of hand hygiene in healthcare-associated infection prevention. J Hosp Infect. 2009;73(4):305–15.
10. Pittet D, Allegranzi B, Boyce J. The World Health Organization guidelines on hand hygiene in health care and their consensus recommendations. Geneva: Infection Control & Hospital Epidemiology; 2009.
11. Allegranzi B, Gayet-Ageron A, Damani N, Bengaly L, McLaws ML, Moro ML, et al. Global implementation of WHO's multimodal strategy for improvement of hand hygiene: a quasi-experimental study. Lancet Infect Dis. 2013;13(10):843–51.
12. Farhoudi F, Dashti AS, Davani MH, Ghalebi N, Sajadi G, Taghizadeh R. Impact of WHO hand hygiene improvement program implementation: a quasi-experimental trial. Biomed Res Int. 2016:1–7.
13. Allegranzi B, Conway L, Larson E, Pittet D. Status of the implementation of the World Health Organization multimodal hand hygiene strategy in United States of America health care facilities. Am J Infect Control. 2014;42(3):224–30.
14. Pfäfflin F, Tufa TB, Getachew M, Nigussie T, Schönfeld A, Häussinger D, et al. Implementation of the WHO multimodal hand hygiene improvement strategy in a University Hospital in Central Ethiopia. Antimicrob Resist Infect Control. 2017;6:3.
15. Chakravarthy M, Myatra SN, Rosenthal VD, Udwadia FE, Gokul BN, Divatia JV, et al. The impact of the international nosocomial infection control consortium (INICC) multicenter, multidimensional hand hygiene approach in two cities of India. J Infect Public Health. 2015;8(2):177–86.
16. Ho M, Seto W, Wong L, Wong T. Effectiveness of multifaceted hand hygiene interventions in long-term care facilities in Hong Kong: a cluster-randomized controlled trial. Infect Control Hosp Epidemiol. 2012;33(8):761–7.
17. Gould DJ, Drey NS, Creedon S. Routine hand hygiene audit by direct observation: has nemesis arrived? J Hosp Infect. 2011;77(4):290–3.
18. Steed C, Kelly JW, Blackhurst D, Boeker S, Diller T, Alper P, et al. Hospital hand hygiene opportunities: where and when (HOW2)? The HOW2 benchmark study. Am J Infect Control. 2011;39(1):19–26.
19. Sax H, Allegranzi B, Uçkay I, Larson E, Boyce J, Pittet D. "My five moments for hand hygiene": a user-centred design approach to understand, train, monitor and report hand hygiene. J Hosp Infect. 2007;67(1):9–21.
20. World Health Organization. A guide to the implementation WHO multimodal hand hygiene improvement strategy. Geneva; 2009.
21. Pittet D, Allegranzi B, Storr J, Nejad SB, Dziekan G, Leotsakos A, et al. Infection control as a major World Health Organization priority for developing countries. J Hosp Infect. 2008;68(4):285–92.
22. Schmitz K, Kempker RR, Tenna A, Stenehjem E, Abebe E, Tadesse L, et al. Effectiveness of a multimodal hand hygiene campaign and obstacles to success in Addis Ababa, Ethiopia. Antimicrob Resist Infect Control. 2014;3:8.
23. World Health Organization. Hand hygiene technical reference manual. Geneva; 2009.
24. Abdella NM, Tefera MA, Eredie AE, Landers TF, Malefia YD, Alene KA. Hand hygiene compliance and associated factors among health care providers in Gondar University. BMC Public Health. 2014;14:96.
25. Salama MF, Jamal WY, Al M a, Al-abdulghani KA, Rotimi VO. The effect of hand hygiene compliance on hospital-acquired infections in an ICU setting in a Kuwaiti teaching hospital. J Infect Public Health. 2013;6(1):27–34.
26. Barahona-guzma N, Rojas C, Rodrı M, Olarte N, Villamil-go W, Valderrama A, et al. International journal of infectious diseases impact of the international nosocomial infection control consortium (INICC) multidimensional hand hygiene approach in three cities of. Int J Infect Dis. 2014;19:67–73.
27. Storr J, Twyman A, Zingg W, Damani N, Kilpatrick C, Reilly J, et al. Core components for effective infection prevention and control programmes: new WHO evidence-based recommendations. Antimicrob Resist Infect Control. 2017;6:6.
28. Reichardt C, Königer D, Bunte-Schönberger K, van der Linden P, Mönch N, Schwab F, et al. Three years of national hand hygiene campaign in Germany: what are the key conclusions for clinical practice? J Hosp Infect. 2013;83(SUPPL. 1):11–6.
29. Wetzker W, Bunte-Schonberger K, Walter J, Pilarski G, Gastmeier P, Reichardt C. Compliance with hand hygiene: reference data from the national hand hygiene campaign in Germany. J Hosp Infect J. 2016;92:328–31.
30. Yawson A, Hesse AA. Hand hygiene practices and resources in a teaching hospital in Ghana. J Infect Dev Ctries. 2013;7(4):338–47.
31. Randle J, Arthur A, Vaughan N. Twenty-four-hour observational study of hospital hand hygiene compliance. J Hosp Infect. 2010;76(3):252–5.
32. Marra AR, Camargo TZS, Cardoso VJ, Moura DF, de Andrade EC, Wentzcovitch J, et al. Hand hygiene compliance in the critical care setting: a comparative study of 2 different alcohol handrub formulations. Am J Infect Control. 2013;41(2):136–9.
33. Allegranzi B, Sax H, Bengaly L, Richet H, Minta D, Chraiti M, et al. Successful implementation of the World Health Organization hand hygiene improvement strategy in a referral hospital in Mali, Africa. Infect Control Hosp Epidemiol. 2010;31(2):133–41.
34. Schweon SJ, Edmonds SL, Kirk J, Rowland DY, Carmen A. Effectiveness of a comprehensive hand hygiene program for reduction of infection rates in a long-term care facility. Am J Infect Control. 2013;41(1):39–44.

6

Management of a cluster of *Clostridium difficile* infections among patients with osteoarticular infections

Jacqueline Färber[1*], Sebastian Illiger[2], Fabian Berger[3], Barbara Gärtner[3], Lutz von Müller[4], Christoph H. Lohmann[2], Katja Bauer[1], Christina Grabau[5], Stefanie Zibolka[5], Dirk Schlüter[1,6] and Gernot Geginat[1]

Abstract

Background: Here we describe a cluster of hospital-acquired *Clostridium difficile* infections (CDI) among 26 patients with osteoarticular infections. The aim of the study was to define the source of *C. difficile* and to evaluate the impact of general infection control measures and antibiotic stewardship on the incidence of CDI.

Methods: Epidemiological analysis included typing of *C. difficile* strains and analysis of possible patient to patient transmission. Infection control measures comprised strict isolation of CDI patients, additional hand washings, and intensified environmental cleaning with sporicidal disinfection. In addition an antibiotic stewardship program was implemented in order to prevent the use of CDI high risk antimicrobials such as fluoroquinolones, clindamycin, and cephalosporins.

Results: The majority of CDI ($n = 15$) were caused by *C. difficile* ribotype 027 (RT027). Most RT027 isolates ($n = 9$) showed high minimal inhibitory concentrations (MIC) for levofloxacin, clindamycin, and remarkably to rifampicin, which were all used for the treatment of osteoarticular infections. Epidemiological analysis, however, revealed no closer genetic relationship among the majority of RT027 isolates. The incidence of CDI was reduced only when a significant reduction in the use of fluoroquinolones ($p = 0.006$), third generation cephalosporins ($p = 0.015$), and clindamycin ($p = 0.001$) was achieved after implementation of an intensified antibiotic stewardship program which included a systematic review of all antibiotic prescriptions.

Conclusion: The successful reduction of the CDI incidence demonstrates the importance of antibiotic stewardship programs focused on patients treated for osteoarticular infections.

Keywords: *C. difficile*, Ribotype 027, Rifampicin, Osteoarticular infections, Antibiotic stewardship

Background

Clostridium difficile is a gram-positive, anaerobic bacterium which is ubiquitously present in the gastrointestinal tract of humans and animals [1, 2]. As a spore-forming bacterium, *C. difficile* has the ability to persist and to remain infectious in the environment for extended periods of time. Spores are highly resistant to desiccation and alcohol disinfectants [1]. The main risk factors for development of *C. difficile* infection (CDI) are (i) previous antibiotic treatment, in particular with high risk antibiotics such as 3rd generation cephalosporins, clindamycin, and fluoroquinolones, (ii) long hospitalization, (iii) underlying comorbidities, and (iv) high age of patients [1, 3]. Also specific risk factors for ribotype 027 (RT027) such as selective decontamination of the digestive tract and a longer length of stay in the ICU have been reported [4]. Despite it is well established that antimicrobial therapy with clindamycin and levofloxacin results in dysbiosis and enhanced risk to develop CDI, it is suspected that simultaneous therapy with rifampicin to some degree protects patients from CDI [5–7]. The increasing incidence of severe CDI among hospitalized patients is an enormous clinical problem [8, 9]. However,

* Correspondence: jacqueline.faerber@med.ovgu.de
[1]Institute of Medical Microbiology, Infection Control and Prevention, Otto-von-Guericke University of Magdeburg, Leipziger Straße 44, 39120 Magdeburg, Germany

data on the CDI incidence among patients with prosthetic joint infections are scarce [10]. In addition, the CDI incidence among orthopedic patients after clean surgery such as primary arthroplasty of the hip or knee is very low (0.17%) [10]. A much higher CDI incidence of 7.1%, however, has been reported after open reduction and internal fixation of intertrochanteric femoral fractures, which in all cases occurred after previous antibiotic therapy [11].

Between June 2014 and December 2015 we observed an increased incidence of CDI among patients suffering from mostly implant-associated osteoarticular infections, where the majority of CDIs (57%) was caused by *C. difficile* RT027. The aims of this study were to define risk factors, possible sources of infection, and to evaluate the impact of general infection control measures and antibiotic stewardship on the incidence of CDI in this difficult to treat group of patients.

Methods

Patient population, CDI case definition, and analysis of risk-factors

The current study was initiated after recognition of a possible CDI outbreak in the first quarter 2015 on the septic ward of the department of orthopedic surgery. This department with three independent wards is part of an 1,100 bed tertiary care university hospital and acts as a regional referral center for the treatment of osteoarticular infections. Patients with osteoarticular infections stay on a specialized ward to which we refer as "septic ward".

For the study hospital-acquired CDI was defined as new onset of diarrhea 48 h after hospital admission and laboratory-confirmed detection of *C. difficile* toxin genes by PCR. Severe CDI was defined by the presence of at least one of the following symptoms: fever >38.5 °C, decreased kidney function (creatinine $>1.5 \times 10^3$ g/L) and/or high leukocyte count ($>15 \times 10^9$ cells/L). A recurrent CDI case was defined as new onset of CDI within 8 weeks after resolution of a previous CDI episode. No children were included in the study. An outbreak situation was defined as two or more CDI cases on a single ward within 28 days. Risk factors for infection with *C. difficile* RT027 were evaluated by comparing patients with CDI caused by RT027 with patients infected with non-RT027 ribotypes.

Infection control and antibiotic stewardship

Infection control measures were implemented after recognition of an enhanced CDI incedence. The infection control bundle included (i) handwashing with soap after disinfection, to reduce first vegetative forms of *C. difficile* or other bacteria and secondly spores of *C. difficile*, (ii) use of hygienic bags for bedpans, (iii) strict isolation or cohorting of infected patients, (iv) personalized use of all materials with direct contact to the patient e.g. stethoscope, and (v) disinfection of surfaces and equipment in all wards, operating rooms and physiotherapy with peracetic acid and peroxide hydrogen vaporization after discharge of patients. Intensified environmental cleaning procedures were controlled by sampling of surfaces as described below. Additionally, health care workers were educated on diagnosis, treatment and prevention of CDI and provided with an antibiotic risk checklist which groups of antibiotics in 3 risk categories (low risk: linezolid, vancomycin, metronidazole, tetracycline, trimethoprim/sulfamethoxazole, fosfomycin; daptomycin, medium risk: all beta-lactam-antibiotics with the exception of third generation cephalosporins; high risk: clindamycin, third generation cephalosporins, fluoroquinolones). Physicians were instructed to follow the in-house guidelines for antibiotic therapy and microbiological diagnostic of osteoarticular infections and to avoid the prescription of high risk antibiotics for therapy. In quarter 3/2015 an intensified antibiotic stewardship program was implemented which included a weekly review of all antibiotic prescriptions by an orthopedic surgeon and a clinical microbiologist trained in antibiotic stewardship. The organization of the team was not changed since the beginning of the intervention. If possible antibiotic therapy was adjusted in order to avoid CDI high risk antibiotics as described above.

In order to control the impact of infection control measures and antibiotic stewardship the CDI incidence was monitored as number of cases per 1,000 hospital bed days per quarter.

In addition the impact of the antibiotic stewardship intervention was controlled by quarterly monitoring of antibiotic consumption on the septic ward. Antibiotic consumption was calculated as defined daily doses (DDD) per 100 hospital bed days according to WHO standards [12].

Diagnostic specimens and CDI laboratory diagnostic testing

Diagnostic stool specimens were collected from 63 adult patients showing symptoms of diarrhea between June 2014 and December 2015. Stool diagnostic was performed as part of the routine microbiological diagnostic in a two-step algorithm.

First, clinical samples were primarily screened with a Clostridium glutamate dehydrogenase (GDH)-specific enzyme-linked immunosorbent assay (RIDASCREEN® *Clostridium difficile* GDH, R-Biopharm, Darmstadt, Germany) using the protocol provided by the manufacturer. In case of positive results ($n = 29$) DNA was extracted from the original stool sample. In brief, 100 µl stool in 900 µl sample buffer were used, followed by centrifugation at 1,000 x g for 5 min. Subsequently 400 µl supernatant was transferred into Precellys® Soil grinding SK38 tubes (Bertin Technologies, USA) and homogenized by centrifugation (5,000 x g for 75 sec) using the MagNA Lyser System (Roche Diagnostics, Mannheim, Germany). The lysate was clarified by centrifugation at 1,000 x g for 5 min and subsequent incubated for 10 min at 70 °C in a thermoshaker. DNA-extraction was performed using the QIAamp® DNA Mini Kit (Qiagen, Hilden, Germany) according to manufacturer's instructions.

Second, purified DNA samples were tested for the presence of C. difficile DNA using two commercially available real-time PCR test systems. C. difficile toxins A (tcdA) and B (tcdB) genes were detected using the RealStar® Clostridium difficile PCR Kit 1.0 (altona Diagnostics, Hamburg, Germany). The binary toxin gene and the Δ117 deletion in the tcdC gene were detected using Xpert® C. difficile/Epi PCR assay (GeneXpert, Cepheid, Sunnyvale, CA, USA). All tests were performed according to manufacturer's protocol.

Multilocus sequence typing (MLST)
MLST was performed with DNA either isolated from feces ($n = 10$) or from isolated strains ($n = 16$). The MLST was performed as described before [13], targeting 7 housekeeping genes of C. difficile: adk, atpA, dxr, glyA, recA, sod and tpi. The sequencing reactions were run on a 3130xl Genetic Analyzer (Applied Biosystems). Editing, alignment, and phylogenetic analysis of sequences were performed with the program MEGA 6.0 [14]. DNA sequences were uploaded to the MLST database and C. difficile sequence types (ST) were received from the website [15].

Clostridium difficile culture and susceptibility testing
Clostridium difficile was cultured form GDH-positive stools ($n = 16$) using a chromogenic medium (chromID™ C. difficile, bioMérieux, Marcy l'Etoile, France). The medium was inoculated with 10 µl feces and incubated anaerobically at 35 ± 1 °C for 7 days. Presumptive C. difficile colonies were confirmed by MALDI-TOF MS (VITEK® MS, bioMérieux).

The minimal inhibitory concentrations (MIC) of metronidazole, vancomycin, rifampicin, levofloxacin, and clindamycin were determined by gradient strip test (Etest, bioMérieux) on Brucella blood agar (Becton Dickinson, Heidelberg, Germany) inoculated with 100 µl solution of a 1.0 McFarland suspension of C. difficile in saline as described previously [16]. Agar plates were incubated under anaerobic conditions at 35 ± 1 °C for 48 h. For the interpretation of MIC the EUCAST epidemiological cut off values (ECOFF) were used for metronidazole (>2 mg/L), vancomycin (>2 mg/L), rifampicin

(>0.004 mg/L). No ECOFF are available for clindamycin and levofloxacin.

Enviromental sampling of inpatient environment
Sampling of the inpatient environment for the presence of C. difficile was performed as described [17]. Briefly, surface samples were taken using 25 cm² sponge swabs pre-moistened with neutralizing solution (Lab M Ltd, Heywood, United Kingdom). Frequent contact surfaces of the patient room (head/foot-end boards of patient beds, bed rail, bedside table, nurse call button, patients telephone) and the en-suite bathroom (toilet seat, toilet assist handle) were sampled. After sampling sponge swabs were placed aseptically into the sterile sample transport bag prefilled with 10 ml neutralizing solution. The laboratory bags were opened and supplemented with 40 ml sterile phosphate-buffered saline (Becton Dickinson, Heidelberg, Germany) to yield a final volume of 50 ml. Sponge bags were resealed and homogenized manually by massaging the bag for 1 min. After 10 min. incubation at room temperature the whole volume was passed through a 45 µm membrane filter (Pall GmbH Laboratory, Dreieich, Germany). Filters were aseptically put onto Brazier's CCEY agar (Oxoid, Wesel, Germany) and incubated 48 h in an anaerobic atmosphere at 35 ± 1 °C. After 48 h, suspected C. difficile colonies were further analysed by MALDI-TOF MS. Confirmed C. difficile isolates were tested for toxin production and typed by MLST.

Ribotyping and multiple-locus variable-number tandem repeat analysis (MLVA)
Ribotyping and MLVA analysis of 11 ST1 isolates was performed by the National Consultant Laboratory for C. difficile in Homburg/Saar (University of Saarland Medical Center, Homburg, Germany). PCR-ribotyping was performed for each isolate according the standard protocol (European harmonized diagnostic procedures ECDIS; http://www.ecdisnet.eu) as described earlier [18] which included capillary gel electrophoresis of fluorescent labelled fragments (Beckmann Coulter, Brea, California USA) and ribotype assignment to an institutional databank by an automated software tool (BioNumerics version 7.1, Applied Math, Sint-Martens-Latem, Belgium). MLVA was carried out as described previously [19] with BioNumerics as automated software (version 7.1, Applied Math, Sint-Martens-Latem, Belgium). The definition of clonality was based upon previous studies with a genetic difference of less than 3 repeats while a clonal cluster was defined by ≤ 2 repeat differences and genetic related isolates by ≤ 10 repeat differences [20].

Statistical analysis
Statistical analyses were performed using the Fisher's exact Test for bivariate analysis of C. difficile risk factors

(non RT027 CDI versus RT027 associated CDI) and the two-sample independent t Test for the means of antibiotic consumption data before and after intervention with a significance level of p values <0.05. The Microsoft Excel statistic tool, OpenEpi (http://www.openepi.com) was used to analyze the data. The upper and lower statistical boundaries were defined as the mean CDI incidence of the four previous quarters plus/minus standard deviation (MA ± SD).

Results

Clustering of CDI cases

Retrospective analysis showed that already in the third quarter of 2014 the CDI incidence (1.41 cases per 1,000 hospital bed days) on the septic ward, a special unit for treatment of patients with osteoarticular infections was significantly above average incidence of the whole department (0.64 cases per 1,000 hospital bed days, $p = 0.036$). Orthopedic infections in our patient cohort were associated with endoprosthesis (19/26; 65.5%), soft tissue/wound infections (4/26; 15.4%), septic spondylitis (2/26; 7.7%), and osteomyelitis (1/26; 3.8%).

In quarter 3/2014 the CDI incidence was above the mean CDI incidence of the 4 previous quarters plus SD (Fig. 1). The mean CDI incidence on the septic ward increased significantly from 0.33 infections per 1,000 hospital bed days (SD 0.25) in the period from quarter 1/2013 to 2/2014 to 2.3 infections per 1,000 hospital bed days (SD 0.98) in quarters 1/2015 to 4/2015

$(p = 7.2 \times 10^{-7})$. After implementation of an intensified antibiotic stewardship program in quarter 3/2015 the CDI incidence dropped in the first quarter 2016 to no case per quarter which was significantly below the mean CDI incidence of the 4 previous quarters minus SD of 2.13 infections per 1,000 hospital bed days (Fig. 1). Also in the second quarter 2016 no CDI case was monitored.

From June 1st 2014 to December 31th 2015 a total number of 63 patients with gastrointestinal disorders were tested for the presence of $C.\ difficile$. GDH-positive samples from 29 patients were further tested for the presence of toxin genes by PCR. CDI was confirmed by PCR in 26 patients, which also demonstrated the clinical symptoms of CDI. With exception of two samples, sequence types were determined by MLST from toxin gene-positive samples, 15 samples (57.7%) were typed as ST1 and were further identified as RT027 by CE-ribotyping. The following sequence types were identified: ST3 ($n = 2$), ST6 ($n = 2$), ST14 ($n = 2$), ST8 ($n = 1$), ST15 ($n = 1$), and ST92 ($n = 1$). In all samples both toxin encoding genes were detectable, whereas the binary toxin gene and the Δ117 in the $tcdC$ gene were only present in samples typed as ST1.

The time between admission of patients to the septic ward and diagnosis of CDI ranged from 2 to 72 days. Characteristics and co-morbidities of patients were summarized from patients records (Table 1). Renal insufficiency, treatment with gastric acid suppressors and

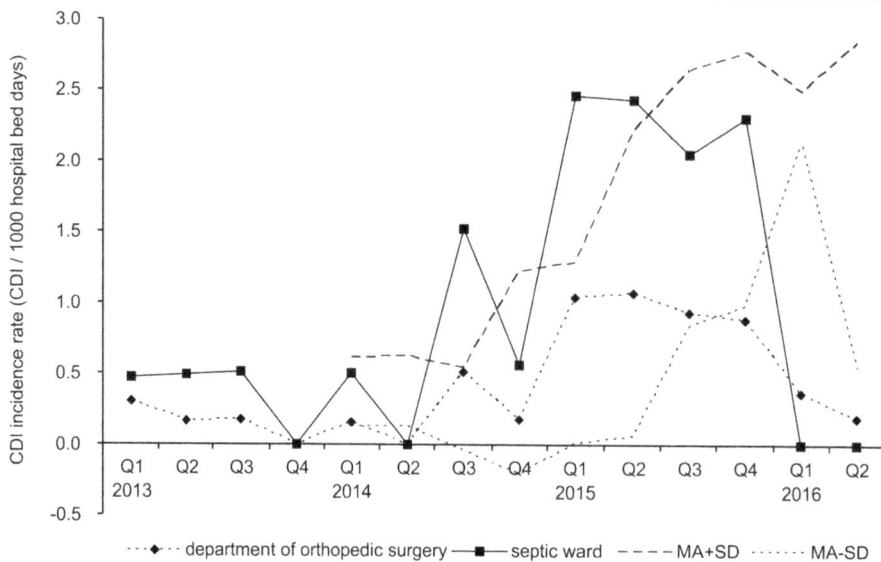

Fig. 1 Incidence of *C. difficile* infections during the study period. The CDI incidence rates (number of cases per 1000 hospital bed days per quarter) for the whole department of orthopedic surgery (diamonds) and the septic ward only (squares) are shown. For every quarter the moving average (MA) of the previous four quarters was calculated. For CDI surveillance upper (MA + SD, upper dotted line) and lower (MA-SD, lower dotted line) boundaries were defined. An increase or decrease of the CDI incidence was considered significant if the actual CDI incidence crossed the upper or lower boundaries, respectively

Table 1 Description of study cohort and assessment of potential risk factors for CDI

		CDI cases	Non-RT027	RT027	p values[a]
Median age		73.08 (range 54–87)	71.63	74.13	
Sex	female	16	6	10	0.41
	male	10	5	5	0.41
Hospitalization on septic/non-septic ward	septic ward	21	7[d]	14	0.04
	all other wards	5	4 [b,c]	1	
Primary diagnosis	periprosthetic infection	19	8	11	0.81
	soft tissue / wound infection	4	1	3	
	spondylitis	2	2	0	
	osteomyelitis	1	0	1	
Co-morbidities	renal insufficiency	12	4	8	0.41
	diabetes	11	5	6	
	pneumonia	1	0	1	
	neoplasm	2	1	1	
	hepatic disease	2	1	1	
Antimicrobial therapy	aminopenicillins	4	1	3	0.72
	ureidopenicillins	6	2	4	0.42
	fluoroquinolones	9	3	6	0.27
	cephalosporins	13	5	8	0.24
	clindamycin	7	3	4	0.81
	rifampicin	13	6	7	0.69
Gastric acid suppressors	proton pump inhibitors/H2 blockers	25	11	14	
Severity factors	creatinine ($>1.5 \times 10^3$g/L)	7	3	4	0.99
	leukocytosis ($>1.5 \times 10^9$/L)	10	4	6	0.93
Antimicrobial CDI treatment					
First episode	metronidazole po.	18	8	10	
	vancomycin po.	1	0	1	
	metronidazole iv. vancomycin po.	2	unknown	unknown	
	fidaxomicin po.	4	1	3	
	colectomy	1	0	1	
	no treatment	1	0	1	
Recurrence	vancomycin po.	5	2	3	
	metronidazole iv. + vancomycin po.	1	0	1	
	fidaxomicin po.	3	1	2	
	fecal biota transplantation	1	0	1	
Clinical outcome	cure	15	9	6	0.21
	recurrence	10	3	7	0.37
	death within 6 months	4	0	4	0.13
	death CDI attributed	1	0	1	
	death CDI contributed	3	0	3	

[a] p values were determined with Fisher's exact Test
[b] Sequence type ST 6
[c] Sequence types ST3, 14, 15
[d] Sequence types ST3, 6, 8, 14, 92, and two unknown strains

treatment with CDI high risk antibiotics were the most frequent risk factors but were not significantly different among patients infected with *C. difficile* RT027 (ST1) and non-RT027 strains. The only significant risk factor for CDI caused by RT027 was a patient's stay on the septic ward.

Outcome of CDI

Non-severe CDI was initially diagnosed in 18 from 26 patients (69.2%) and in 6 from 15 patients (40.0%) infected with RT027. Treatment of CDI was initiated in all cases according to current European Society of Clinical Microbiology and Infectious Diseases guidelines [21]. After primary CDI treatment 15 (57.7%) patients recovered, among them 6 (40%) patients with RT027. Recurrences were observed in 10 (38.5%) patients. The mortality of 15.4% (4/26) within 6 months after diagnosis of CDI was exclusively attributable to CDI due to *C. difficile* RT027.

Infection control and antibiotic stewardship

After clustering of CDI cases was first recognized in the quarter 1/2015 a primary infection control and antibiotic stewardship bundle was implemented (see methods section).

Orthopedic infections generally require a long-term (≥6 weeks) antibiotic treatment [22–24]. In most cases, antibiotic therapy of the primary orthopedic infection consisted of two or more antibiotics. The most frequently prescribed classes of antibiotics were fluoroquinolones (34.6%), cephalosporins (50.0%), clindamycin (26.9%), rifampicin (50.0%), and the penicillin/betalactamase

inhibitor combinations ampicillin/clavulanic acid (15.4%) and piperacillin/tazobactam (23.1%) (Table 1).

Initial review of antibiotic prescription data indicated an overuse of CDI high risk antibiotics (Table 2) although an in-house guideline for antibiotic therapy and infectious disease diagnostics had been in use for several years. The primary antibiotic stewardship intervention focused on information of medical doctors, who were provided with an antibiotic risk checklist which groups of antibiotics in 3 risk categories. Physicians were instructed to follow the in-house guidelines for antibiotic therapy and microbiological diagnostic of osteoarticular infections and to avoid the prescription of high risk antibiotics for therapy. An intensified antibiotic stewardship program was implemented during quarter 3/2015 which included a weekly review of all antibiotic prescriptions by a clinical microbiologist.

The quarterly analysis of antibiotic consumption between quarters 1/2013 and 2/2016 shows that fluoroquinolones, 1st and 2nd generation cephalosporins and clindamycin were the most prescribed antibiotics on the septic ward, even after the initial recommendation to avoid these antibiotics after recognition of the enhanced CDI incidence in quarter 1/2015 (Table 2).

Significant reduction of antibiotic consumption of *C. difficile* high risk antibiotics was achieved after the intensified antibiotic stewardship program for septic orthopedic patients was initiated in quarter 3/2015. This intervention led to a significant reduction (p values <0.05, Table 2, Fig. 2) of the consumption of fluoroquinolones, clindamycin, and 1st and 2nd generation cephalosporins and increased use of narrow spectrum

Table 2 Antibiotic consumption in the septic ward during quarters 1/2013 to 2/2016

| | Antibiotic consumption (DDD/100 hospital bed days) | | | | | | | | | | | | | | p^a |
| | 2013 | | | | 2014 | | | | 2015 | | | | 2016 | | |
	Q1	Q2	Q3	Q4	Q1	Q2	Q3	Q4	Q1	Q2	Q3	Q4	Q1	Q2	
Narrow spectrum penicillins[b]	8.8	20.8	16.5	26.3	6.8	11.3	8.3	15.0	26.5	19.6	13.0	34.8	35.0	52.0	0.131
Amino penicillin/BLI	7.8	3.2	0.5	1.8	6.4	4.1	15.4	4.3	7.2	10.9	16.7	16.3	10.0	7.2	0.044
Broad spectrum penicillins[c]	2.7	1.0	1.6	0.0	2.4	3.4	5.2	2.0	4.5	2.3	8.2	4.5	3.5	5.1	0.046
Cephalosprins 1st and 2nd gen.	12.2	27.2	42.3	32.3	35.5	43.3	23.0	30.5	21.5	32.8	22.2	23.0	14.0	23.5	0.016
Cephalosprins 3rd gen.	2.1	3.2	2.1	2.4	4.1	3.7	0.8	1.5	0.9	0.6	1.7	0.0	1.8	0.0	0.015
Carbapenems	4.8	3.2	5.1	2.7	7.9	3.0	4.9	5.9	3.4	5.0	5.1	10.0	2.4	6.8	0.283
Fluoroquinolones	49.7	35.0	29.7	21.6	32.6	45.1	34.3	32.0	33.6	31.2	26.0	6.6	4.3	10.6	0.006
Clindamycin	9.1	12.1	19.3	0.0	12.3	25.2	19.4	12.6	22.1	15.2	6.8	3.7	4.4	5.1	0.001
Linezolid	2.4	3.2	4.4	2.4	4.0	3.6	3.5	2.0	2.8	7.9	4.8	6.9	8.7	10.1	0.019
Glycopeptide/daptomycin	5.4	5.9	5.7	1.5	6.2	4.5	4.6	3.8	5.1	3.6	4.8	8.9	5.4	13.8	0.143
Rifampicin	18.3	14.1	19.2	0.4	9.7	9.9	0.0	0.0	3.5	10.1	4.5	17.8	12.2	13.9	0.243
Total	125.6	132.3	150.6	106.9	129.7	157.3	122.7	113.1	133.0	141.6	122.1	133.5	103.5	150.2	0.348

[a]Comparision of average antibiotic consumption before (Q1/213-Q2/2015) and after (Q3/2105-Q2/2016) implementation of an intensified antibiotic stewardship program. [b]narrow spectrum peniciliins: penicillin G, flucloxacillin, aminopenicillins, [c] broad spectrum penicillins: piperacillin, piperacillin/tazobactam aminopenicillins

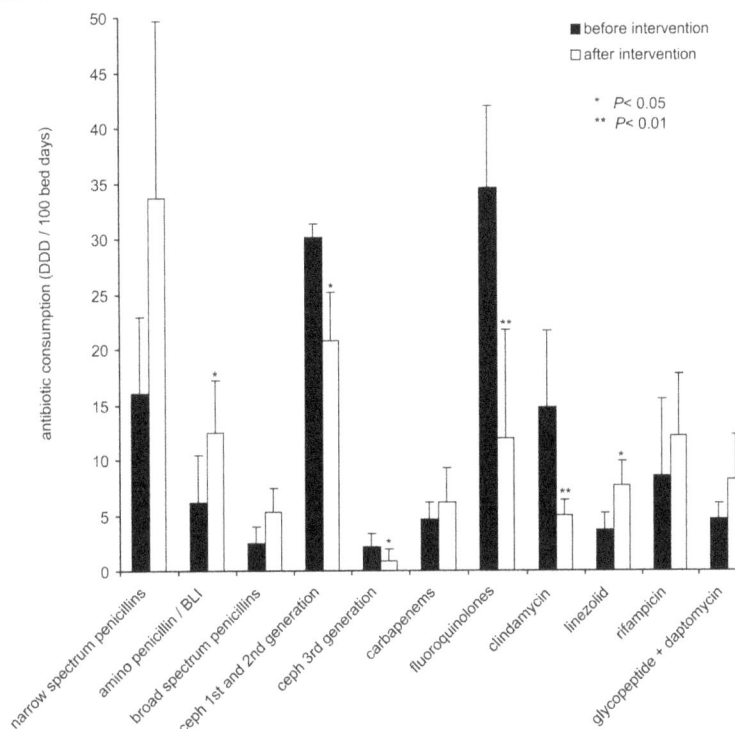

Fig. 2 Antibiotic prescription for patients of the septic ward before and after implementation of the intensified antibiotic stewardship program in quarter 3/2015. Bars indicate the mean antibiotic consumption calculated as defined daily doses (DDD) per 100 hospital bed days. For the major classes of antibiotics the mean antibiotic consumption and standard deviations were calculated for quarters 1/2013 to 2/2015 before intervention and quarters 3/2015 to 2/2016 after intervention. Narrow spectrum penicillins include benzylpenicillin, flucloxacillin, and aminopenicillins; broad spectrum penicllins include piperacillin and piperacillin/tazobactam. Asterisks indicate a significant (p values <0.05) difference of antibiotic consumption before and after intervention

penicillins (benzylpenicillin and flucloxacillin, +110%), linezolid (+111%), and rifampicin (+41%). The total average antibiotic consumption before intervention was 131.3 DDD per 100 hospital bed days and after intervention 127.3 DDD per 100 hospital bed days, respectively. Thus, although consumption of high risk antimicrobials was significantly lowered total antibiotic consumption remained on a high level after the intervention.

Antibiotic susceptibility testing of *C. difficile* isolates

In vitro antibiotic susceptibility tests were performed with 16 *C. difficile* isolates (ST1 ($n = 11$), ST6 ($n = 2$), ST8 ($n = 1$), ST14 ($n = 1$), and ST92 ($n = 1$) (Table 3). All ST1 (RT027) isolates showed an elevated MIC for multiple antibiotics including levofloxacin (MIC ≥ 32 mg/L), and rifampicin (MIC ≥ 32 mg/L). Also the MIC of clindamycin was elevated among the majority of RT027 isolates. All non-RT027 strains showed a low MIC for rifampicin (<0.002 mg/L) and the MIC of clindamycin (2.0–8.0 mg/L) was under the epidemiological cut-off value of 16.0 mg/L. The MIC of levofloxacin was 6.0 mg/L (ECOFF not available).

Epidemiological analysis

The inquiry by infection control personal yielded no noticeable epidemiological association among patients with identical non-RT027 strains (data not shown). In order to confirm a possible epidemiological association of RT027 isolates form the septic ward subtyping by MLVA was performed. The typing of 11 RT027 isolates revealed two genetically related clusters (defined as ≤ 10 repeat differences). The larger cluster comprised 9 isolates (isolates 1–4 and 7–11) and the minor cluster 2 isolates (isolates 5 and 6) (Fig. 3). Only three isolates (1, 3, and 4) showed clonal relatedness (defined as ≤ 2 repeat differences). A fourth isolate (# 3) showing three repeat differences was also closely related to this cluster. We further analyzed the possible epidemiological association of the four patients from which these genetically closely related strains (repeat differences ≤ 3) were isolated. A detailed inquiry of possible contacts, however, did not reveal any direct or indirect contacts of inpatients infected within these related RT027 isolates. As shown in Fig. 4, there were no overlaps of admission and discharge data of excluding direct contact.

Table 3 MLST types and MICs for selected antibiotics of *C. difficile* isolates

Inpatient #	MLST type	RT	MIC (mg/L)				
			Metronidazole	Vancomycin	Rifampicin	Levofloxacin	Clindamycin
1	ST1	027	1	1.5	≥32	≥32	≥256
2	ST1	027	1	1.5	≥32	≥32	≥256
3	ST1	027	1	1.5	≥32	≥32	6.0
4	ST1	027	1	1.5	≥32	≥32	2.0
5	ST1	027	1	1.5	≥32	≥32	≥256
6	ST1	027	1	1.5	≥32	≥32	≥256
7	ST1	027	1	1.5	≥32	≥32	≥256
8	ST1	027	1	1.5	≥32	≥32	≥256
9	ST1	027	1	1.5	≥32	≥32	≥256
10	ST1	027	1	1.5	≥32	≥32	≥256
11	ST1	027	1	1.5	>32	>32	≥256
12	ST1	n.d.	n.d.	n.d.	n.d.	n.d.	n.d.
13	ST1	n.d.	n.d.	n.d.	n.d.	n.d.	n.d.
14	ST1	n.d.	n.d.	n.d.	n.d.	n.d.	n.d.
15	ST1	n.d.	n.d.	n.d.	n.d.	n.d.	n.d.
16	ST3	n.d.	n.d.	n.d.	n.d.	n.d.	n.d.
17	ST3	n.d.	n.d.	n.d.	n.d.	n.d.	n.d.
18	ST6	n.d.	0.25	0.05	<0.002	6.0	3.0
19	ST6	n.d.	0.38	0.05	<0.002	6.0	8.0
20	ST8	n.d.	0.25	0.05	<0.002	6.0	2.0
21	ST14	n.d.	n.d.	n.d.	n.d.	n.d.	n.d.
22	ST14	n.d.	0.5	0.5	<0.002	6.0	2.0
23	ST15	n.d.	n.d.	n.d.	n.d.	n.d.	n.d.
24	ST92	n.d.	0.125	0.5	<0.002	6.0	8.0
25	unknown	n.d.	n.d.	n.d.	n.d.	n.d.	n.d.
26	unknown	n.d.	n.d.	n.d.	n.d.	n.d.	n.d.

n.d. not determined

In order to further exclude a remnant reservoir of viable *C. difficile* RT027 in patient rooms after discharge of the patient and cleaning of the room, environmental investigations of surfaces of patient rooms were performed. Among 60 environmental samples taken in August 2015, December 2015, and January 2016 *C. difficile* RT027 was isolated from only one sample from the telephone set of an inpatient infected with RT027, without any transmissions of this particular strain to other inpatients up to now. Thus indicating that cleaning procedures were adequate and a persistent environmental *C. difficile* reservoir in patient rooms was highly unlikely.

Discussion

Here we report an increased incidence of CDI mainly caused by *C. difficile* RT027 with an elevated MIC for rifampicin among patients suffering from osteoarticular infections and the successful control of CDI by implementation of an antibiotic stewardship program focused on this difficult to treat group of patients.

The dominance of *C. difficile* RT027 among patients with orthopedic infections observed in the current study could be due to a number of different reasons. During the primary outbreak analysis, the investigation focused on a possible common source of *C. difficile* RT027 isolates. The only risk factor for CDI caused by RT027 was a patient's stay on the septic ward neither molecular epidemiological analysis, nor analysis of inpatient contacts, nor environmental sampling suggested a possible common source of RT027 isolates. Probably, CDI was mainly restricted to the septic ward due to the higher exposure of inpatients to CDI high risk antibiotics required for the treatment of osteoarticular infections. Antibiotic consumption of high risk antibiotics on the septic ward was 2 to 3-fold higher compared to the other wards of

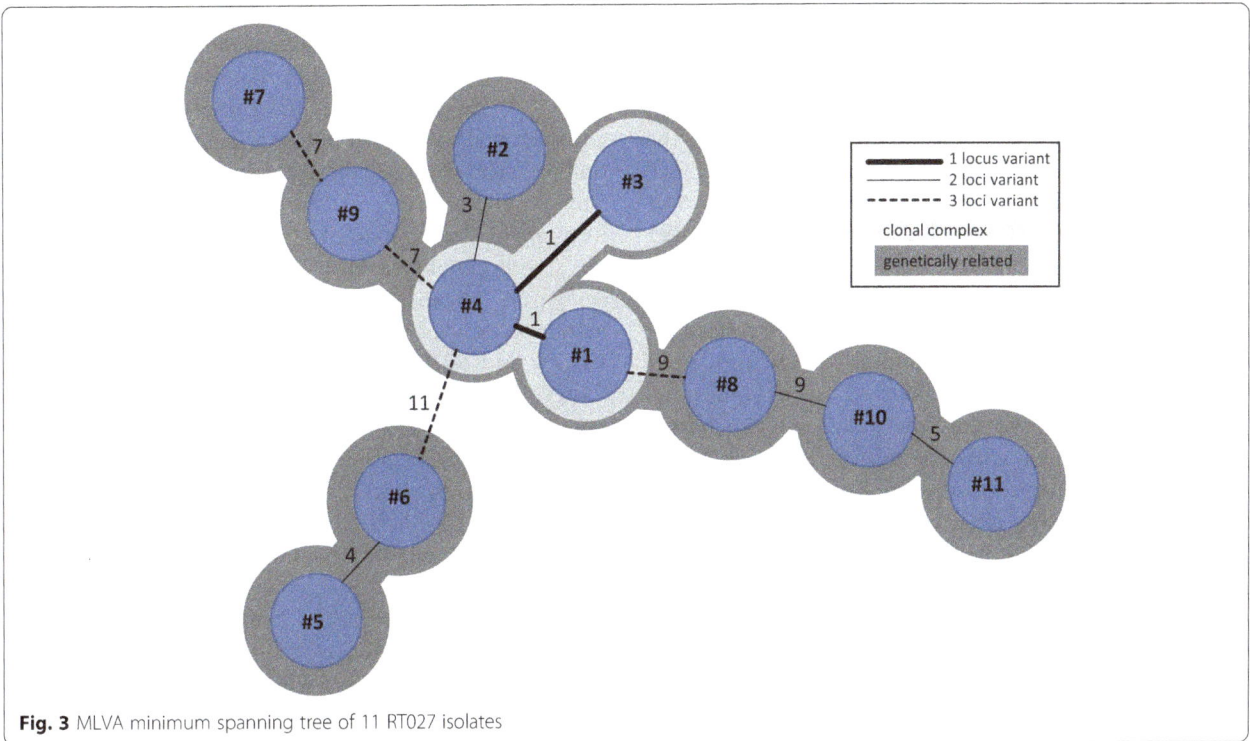

Fig. 3 MLVA minimum spanning tree of 11 RT027 isolates

the orthopedic department (data not shown). The majority of complications was associated with RT027, however due to the low number of patients the observed differences between patients infected with RT027 and non-RT027 were not significant.

The bundle of optimized antibiotic treatment, environmental cleaning procedures and education of health care workers effectively controlled nosocomial CDI thus corroborating previously published studies [10, 25–27]. Implementation of infection control measures alone, however, did not reduce the incidence of CDI, which was only achieved after drastic reduction of the consumption of *C. difficile* high risk antibiotics. The

incidence of CDI was significantly reduced only after implementation of an intensified antibiotic stewardship program which lowered the prescription of fluoroquinolones, clindamycin, and cephalosporins in favor of low risks antibiotics such as penicillins and linezolid.

Average total antibiotic consumption before intervention was 131 DDD/100 hospital bed days and after intervention 127 DDD/100 hospital bed days. The antibiotic stewardship intervention shifted antibiotic therapy towards the use of narrow spectrum penicillins (benzylpenicillin and flucloxacillin, +110%), linezolid (+111%), and rifampicin (+41%). The DDD of benzylpenicillin is 3.6 g. Treatment of serious infections, however, generally

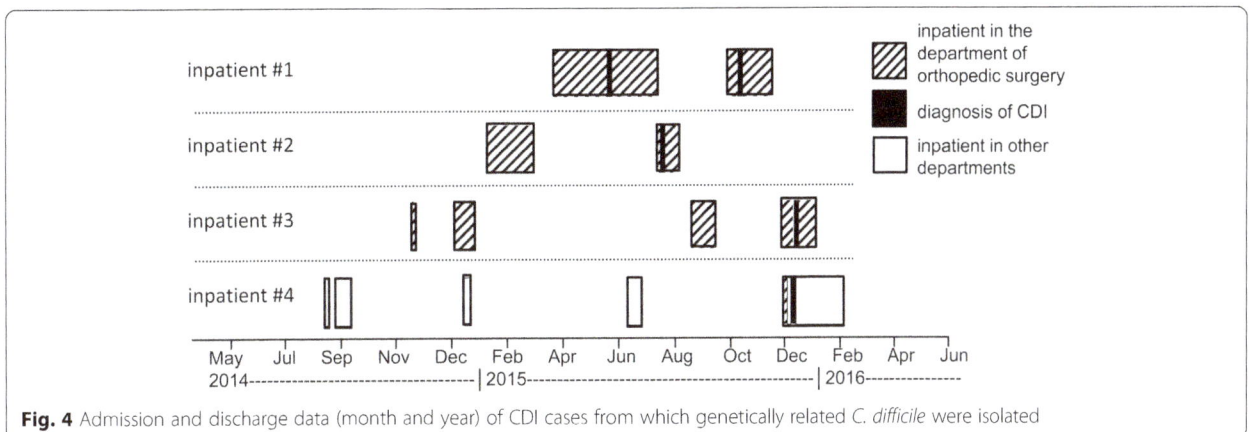

Fig. 4 Admission and discharge data (month and year) of CDI cases from which genetically related *C. difficile* were isolated

requires a dose of 12 g or even higher. Thus calculating DDD while using much higher therapeutic doses results in an overestimation of the prescribed doses [28]. If correcting this by using recommended daily doses (RDD) [28] for the calculation of antibiotic consumption the antibiotic consumption before intervention was 99.0 RDD/100 hospital bed days and after intervention 86.1 RDD/100 hospital bed days, indicating that the number of prescribed doses on the septic ward was reduced roughly 13%. Total antibiotic consumption on the septic ward, however, remained significantly above the available national benchmark data for surgical departments other than general surgery (75% quantile 56 RDD/100 hospital bed days) [28, 29]. To our knowledge no benchmark data are available for units specialized on septic orthopedic surgery like the septic ward studied here. On the septic ward inpatients often require high-dose antibiotic combination therapies which explain the significantly higher antibiotic consumption compared to general orthopedic departments.

The average consumption of fluoroquinolones was 34.5 DDD (33.3 RDD) per 100 hospital bed days before and 11.5 DDD (10.3 RDD) per 100 hospital bed days after implementation of intensified antibiotic stewardship program. Despite after the intervention roughly 70% less quinolones were used overall quinolone consumption was still significantly above the national benchmark (75% quantile 6.9 RDD/100 patient days) [28, 29]. The consumption of first and second generation cephalosporins was reduced roughly 30% by replacing them with flucloxacillin for the therapy of susceptible staphylococci and by avoiding prolonged perioperative prophylaxis.

In Germany regionally between 5.3% and 33.5% of CDI are caused by RT027 [30, 31]. In our study 66% of CDI on the septic ward were caused by RT027, suggesting selection of this particular strain. Because for the study region no data are available for the rate of asymptomatic RT027 carriers, we cannot judge the degree of selection of RT027 among our patient group.

Antimicrobial therapy of osteoarticular infections often requires prolonged antibiotic treatment for 6 to 12 weeks [22–24]. According to current guidelines an initial parenteral therapy with beta-lactam antibiotics is often followed by oral therapy with antibiotics such as fluoroquinolones and rifampicin with good bioavailability, effective tissue and bone penetration, and biofilm activity [22–24]. Nevertheless, reports indicating an enhanced CDI incidence among patients with prosthetic joint infections are scarce [10]. Our current working hypothesis is that cephalosporins, quinolones and clindamycin as high risk antibiotics trigger CDI and concurrent treatment with rifampicin protects patients from CDI caused by rifampicin-susceptible *C. difficile*. Thus

the reduced susceptibility of RT027 to rifampicin might increase the risk of CDI among patients treated with rifampicin [5, 32, 33]. However, rifampicin alone probably did not trigger CDI because less prescription of high risk antimicrobials even without reduction of the consumption of rifampicin significantly lowered the CDI incidence. The *ClosER* (*Clostridium difficile* European Resistance) study reported elevated MICs of *C. difficile* for fluoroquinolones and clindamycin among various ribotypes, whereas elevated rifampicin MICs were mainly associated with a few ribotypes such as RT027, RT018, and RT356 which are more common in South Eastern Europe [34]. It has also been shown before that long-term rifampicin treatment may result in the selection of *C. difficile* strains with an elevated rifampicin MIC [32–34]. In view of the low rifampicin MIC of the majority of *C. difficile* strains, it has been hypothesized that rifampicin might prevent CDI in osteoarticular infections [5–7].

Our study has a number of limitations. Firstly, because culture-based diagnostic of *C. difficile* was initiated by the laboratory after recognition of the epidemic situation in May 2015 the initial epidemiological analysis was performed based on PCR and MLST only. Sequence type 1 (ST1) can correspond to several ribotypes in particular RT176 [2], and the GeneXpert cannot differentiate between RT027 and RT176 [35, 36]. In Germany, however, RT176 is rather uncommon [37, 38], and ribotyping of 11 isolates confirmed that all ST1 belong to RT027. Because the discriminatory power of MLST alone is not sufficient for the analysis of the molecular epidemiology of *C. difficile* in outbreaks [39] MLVA analysis of 11 RT027 isolates was performed. The results indicated the presence of a very closely related strain in only four out of 11 patients, making a clonal outbreak caused by a common source in the hospital unlikely.

Secondly, the initially increased incidence of CDI in quarter 3/2014 correlated with the introduction of a new diagnostic test for the detection of *C. difficile*, which was switched from a toxin-specific enzyme-linked immunosorbent assay to primary screening with a GDH-specific ELISA followed by a toxin gen-specific PCR test. Thus, initially the increased number of patients with positive *C. difficile* tests was interpreted as result of the improved sensitivity of the new diagnostic test. Gould et al. reported an increase of the CDI incidence ranging from 43% to 67% after switching from toxin enzyme immunoassays to PCR-based *C. difficile* diagnostic tests [40]. Beginning with the third quarter 2014 the incidence of recurrent and severe CDI increased compared to the period before. Among all cases of CDI 28.6% of patients and among the cases of CDI caused by RT027 38,5% of patients had at least one criterion of severe CDI at the time point of laboratory diagnosis. In accordance with reported data, the CDI-associated mortality rate within 6 months was 15.4% for all CDI cases and 26.7% for RT027 cases, respectively. Severe CDI occurred mostly among elderly patients with multiple co-morbidities [10, 25, 27, 34, 41].

Third, despite the analysis of patient to patient contacts did not reveal a direct connection of our patients from which highly related RT027 were isolated we cannot strictly exclude a possible epidemiological connection. We could not exclude possible patient contacts outside the hospital and environmental screening was performed after cleaning and, therefore, the environment cannot be strictly excluded as source of infection. Also, screening of health care workers and asymptomatic patients was not performed which have been reported to act as vector for nosocomial transmission of *C. difficile* [42, 43].

Conclusion

To our knowledge, this is the first report of an enhanced incidence of CDI caused by *C. difficile* RT027 with elevated MICs for rifampicin among patients with osteoarticular infections. The successful reduction of the CDI incidence demonstrates the importance of antibiotic stewardship programs focused on patients treated for osteoarticular infections. The impact of antibiotic stewardship on the restriction of *C. difficile* high risk antimicrobials should be tightly monitored in order to ensure that antibiotic stewardship recommendations are followed.

Abbreviations
CDI: *Clostridium difficile* infection; ClosER: *Clostridium difficile* European resistance study; DDD: Defined daily doses; ECOFFs: Epidemiological cut-off value; ELISA: Enzyme-linked immunosorbent assay; GDH: Clostridium glutamate dehydrogenase; MA+/− SD: Moving average plus/minus standard deviation; MIC: Minimum inhibitory concentration; MLST: Multilocus sequence typing; MLVA: Multiple locus variable-number tandem repeat analysis; n.d.: Not determined; Q1-4: Quarter 1–4; RT027: *C. difficile* ribotype 027; ST: Sequence type; WHO: World Health Organization

Acknowledgments
We thank Lisa Fröhlich, Michael Schulz, and Silke Ehrich for expert technical assistance.

Funding
No external funding was obtained for this study.

Authors' contributions
JF and GG conceived the study, participated in its design and coordination and drafted the manuscript. JF, KB, FB, BG, LM, DS collected and compiled microbiological data. SI and CHL collected and compiled clinical data. CG, SZ, GG collected and compiled antibiotic consumption data. All authors read and approved the final manuscript.

Competing interests
The authors declare that they have no competing interests

Consent for publication
Not applicable.

Author details
[1]Institute of Medical Microbiology, Infection Control and Prevention, Otto-von-Guericke University of Magdeburg, Leipziger Straße 44, 39120 Magdeburg, Germany. [2]Department of Orthopedic Surgery, Otto-von-Guericke University of Magdeburg, Magdeburg, Germany. [3]Institute of Medical Microbiology and Hygiene, Consultant Laboratory for Clostridium difficile, University of Saarland, Saarland, Germany. [4]Institute for Laboratory Medicine, Microbiology and Hygiene, Christophorus Kliniken, Coesfeld, Germany. [5]Central pharmacy, Otto-von-Guericke University of Magdeburg, Magdeburg, Germany. [6]Organ-specific Immune Regulation, Helmholtz Centre for Infection Research, Braunschweig, Germany.

References
1. Knight DR, Elliott B, Chang BJ, Perkins TT, Riley TV. Diversity and evolution in the genome of *Clostridium difficile*. Clin Microbiol Rev. 2015;28(3):721–41.
2. Knetsch CW, Terveer EM, Lauber C, Gorbalenya AE, Harmanus C, Kuijper EJ, et al. Comparative analysis of an expanded *Clostridium difficile* reference strain collection reveals genetic diversity and evolution through six lineages. Infect Genet Evol. 2012;12(7):1577–85.
3. Buchler AC, Rampini SK, Stelling S, Ledergerber B, Peter S, Schweiger A, et al. Antibiotic susceptibility of *Clostridium difficile* is similar worldwide over two decades despite widespread use of broad-spectrum antibiotics: An analysis done at the University Hospital of Zurich. BMC Infect Dis. 2014;14:607.
4. van Beurden YH, Dekkers OM, Bomers MK, Kaiser AM, van Houdt R, Knetsch CW, et al. An outbreak of *Clostridium difficile* ribotype 027 associated with length of stay in the intensive care unit and use of selective decontamination of the digestive tract: A case control study. PLoS One. 2016;11(8):e0160778.
5. Miller MA, Blanchette R, Spigaglia P, Barbanti F, Mastrantonio P. Divergent rifamycin susceptibilities of *Clostridium difficile* strains in Canada and Italy and predictive accuracy of rifampin etest for rifamycin resistance. J Clin Microbiol. 2011;49(12):4319–21.
6. O'Connor JR, Galang MA, Sambol SP, Hecht DW, Vedantam G, Gerding DN, et al. Rifampin and rifaximin resistance in clinical isolates of *Clostridium difficile*. Antimicrob Agents Chemother. 2008;52(8):2813–7.
7. Schindler M, Bernard L, Belaieff W, Gamulin A, Racloz G, Emonet S, et al. Epidemiology of adverse events and *Clostridium difficile*-associated diarrhea during long-term antibiotic therapy for osteoarticular infections. J Infect. 2013;67(5):433–8.
8. Kato H, Ito Y, van den Berg RJ, Kuijper EJ, Arakawa Y. First isolation of *Clostridium difficile* 027 in Japan. Euro Surveill. 2007;12(1):E070111 3.
9. Kuijper EJ, Coignard B, Tull P. Emergence of *Clostridium difficile*-associated disease in North America and Europe. Clin Microbiol Infect. 2006;12 Suppl 6:2–18.
10. Maltenfort MG, Rasouli MR, Morrison TA, Parvizi J. *Clostridium difficile* colitis in patients undergoing lower-extremity arthroplasty: Rare infection with major impact. Clin Orthop Relat Res. 2013;471(10):3178–85.
11. Sharma P, Bomireddy R, Phillips S. *Clostridium difficile*-associated diarrhoea after internal fixation of intertrochanteric femoral fractures. Eur J Clin Microbiol Infect Dis. 2003;22(10):615–8.
12. Who collaborating centre for drug statistics methodology, Oslo, Norway, http://www.Whocc.No/atc_ddd_index/. Accessed 10 Jul 2016.
13. Griffiths D, Fawley W, Kachrimanidou M, Bowden R, Crook DW, Fung R, et al. Multilocus sequence typing of *Clostridium difficile*. J Clin Microbiol. 2010;48(3):770–8.
14. Tamura K, Stecher G, Peterson D, Filipski A, Kumar S. Mega6: Molecular evolutionary genetics analysis version 6.0. Mol Biol Evol. 2013;30(12):2725–9.
15. *Clostridium difficile* MLST databases. Available at: http://pubmlst.org/cdifficile/. Accessed 10 Jul 2016.
16. Erikstrup LT, Danielsen TK, Hall V, Olsen KE, Kristensen B, Kahlmeter G, et al. Antimicrobial susceptibility testing of *Clostridium difficile* using EUCAST epidemiological cut-off values and disk diffusion correlates. Clin Microbiol Infect. 2012;18(8):E266–72.
17. Ali S, Muzslay M, Wilson P. A novel quantitative sampling technique for detection and monitoring of *Clostridium difficile* contamination in the clinical environment. J Clin Microbiol. 2015;53(8):2570–4.

18. Indra A, Schmid D, Huhulescu S, Hell M, Gattringer R, Hasenberger P, et al. Characterization of clinical *Clostridium difficile* isolates by pcr ribotyping and detection of toxin genes in austria, 2006–2007. J Med Microbiol. 2008;57(Pt 6):702–8.
19. van den Berg RJ, Schaap I, Templeton KE, Klaassen CH, Kuijper EJ. Typing and subtyping of *Clostridium difficile* isolates by using multiple-locus variable-number tandem-repeat analysis. J Clin Microbiol. 2007;45(3):1024–8.
20. Marsh JW, O'Leary MM, Shutt KA, Pasculle AW, Johnson S, Gerding DN, et al. Multilocus variable-number tandem-repeat analysis for investigation of *Clostridium difficile* transmission in hospitals. J Clin Microbiol. 2006;44(7):2558–66.
21. Debast SB, Bauer MP, Kuijper EJ. European Society of Clinical Microbiology and Infectious Diseases: Update of the treatment guidance document for *Clostridium difficile* infection. Clin Microbiol Infect. 2014;20 Suppl 2:1–26.
22. Zimmerli W, Trampuz A, Ochsner PE. Prosthetic-joint infections. N Engl J Med. 2004;351(16):1645–54.
23. Osmon DR, Berbari EF, Berendt AR, Lew D, Zimmerli W, Steckelberg JM, et al. Diagnosis and management of prosthetic joint infection: Clinical practice guidelines by the Infectious Diseases Society of America. Clin Infect Dis. 2013;56(1):e1–e25.
24. Renz N, Perka C, Trampuz A. Management of periprosthetic infections of the knee. Orthopade. 2016;45(1):65–71.
25. Gulihar A, Nixon M, Jenkins D, Taylor GJ. *Clostridium difficile* in hip fracture patients: Prevention, treatment and associated mortality. Injury. 2009;40(7):746–51.
26. Lachowicz D, Szulencka G, Obuch-Woszczatynski P, van Belkum A, Pituch H. First polish outbreak of *Clostridium difficile* ribotype 027 infections among dialysis patients. Eur J Clin Microbiol Infect Dis. 2015;34(1):63–7.
27. Oleastro M, Coelho M, Giao M, Coutinho S, Mota S, Santos A, et al. Outbreak of *Clostridium difficile* PCR ribotype 027–the recent experience of a regional hospital. BMC Infect Dis. 2014;14:209.
28. Kern WV, Fellhauer M, Hug M, Hoppe-Tichy T, Forst G, Steib-Bauert M, et al. Recent antibiotic use in German acute care hospitals - from benchmarking to improved prescribing and quality care. Dtsch Med Wochenschr. 2015;140(23):e237–46.
29. Kern WV, Fellhauer M, De With K. ADKA-if-RKI Antiinfektiva-Surveillance, 5. Krankenhausvergleichsreport 2012/2013, http://www.antiinfektiva-surveillance.de.
30. von Muller L, Mock M, Halfmann A, Stahlmann J, Simon A, Herrmann M. Epidemiology of *Clostridium difficile* in Germany based on a single center long-term surveillance and German-wide genotyping of recent isolates provided to the advisory laboratory for diagnostic reasons. Int J Med Microbiol. 2015;305(7):807–13.
31. Arvand M, Bettge-Weller G. *Clostridium difficile* ribotype 027 is not evenly distributed in Hesse, Germany. Anaerobe. 2016;40:1–4.
32. Choi JM, Kim HH, Park SJ, Park MI, Moon W. Development of pseudomembranous colitis four months after initiation of rifampicin. Case Rep Gastroenterol. 2011;5(1):45–51.
33. Obuch-Woszczatynski P, Dubiel G, Harmanus C, Kuijper E, Duda U, Wultanska D, et al. Emergence of *Clostridium difficile* infection in tuberculosis patients due to a highly rifampicin-resistant pcr ribotype 046 clone in Poland. Eur J Clin Microbiol Infect Dis. 2013;32(8):1027–30.
34. Freeman J, Vernon J, Morris K, Nicholson S, Todhunter S, Longshaw C, et al. Pan-european longitudinal surveillance of antibiotic resistance among prevalent *Clostridium difficile* ribotypes. Clin Microbiol Infect. 2015;248(3):e9-48–e16.
35. Krutova M, Matejkova J, Nyc O. *C. difficile* ribotype 027 or 176? Folia Microbiol. 2014;59(6):523–6.
36. Mentula S, Laakso S, Lyytikainen O, Kirveskari J. Differentiating virulent 027 and non-027 *Clostridium difficile* strains by molecular methods. Expert Rev Mol Diagn. 2015;15(9):1225–9.
37. Krutova M, Nyc O, Kuijper EJ, Geigerova L, Matejkova J, Bergerova T, et al. A case of imported *Clostridium difficile* PCR-ribotype 027 infection within the Czech Republic which has a high prevalence of *C. difficile* ribotype 176. Anaerobe. 2014;30:153–5.
38. Pituch H, Obuch-Woszczatynski P, Lachowicz D, Wultanska D, Karpinski P, Mlynarczyk G, et al. Hospital-based *Clostridium difficile* infection surveillance reveals high proportions of PCR ribotypes 027 and 176 in different areas of Poland, 2011 to 2013. Euro Surveill. 2015;20:38.
39. Knetsch CW, Lawley TD, Hensgens MP, Corver J, Wilcox MW, Kuijper EJ. Current application and future perspectives of molecular typing methods to study *Clostridium difficile* infections. Euro Surveill. 2013;18(4):20381.
40. Gould CV, Edwards JR, Cohen J, Bamberg WM, Clark LA, Farley MM, et al. Effect of nucleic acid amplification testing on population-based incidence rates of *Clostridium difficile* infection. Clin Infect Dis. 2013;57(9):1304–7.
41. Pepin J, Valiquette L, Cossette B. Mortality attributable to nosocomial *Clostridium difficile*-associated disease during an epidemic caused by a hypervirulent strain in Quebec. CMAJ. 2005;173(9):1037–42.
42. Longtin Y, Gilca R, Loo VG. Effect of detecting and isolating asymptomatic *Clostridium difficile* carriers-reply. JAMA Intern Med. 2016;176(10):1573.
43. Longtin Y, Paquet-Bolduc B, Gilca R, Garenc C, Fortin E, Longtin J, et al. Effect of detecting and isolating clostridium difficile carriers at hospital admission on the incidence of *C. difficile* infections: A quasi-experimental controlled study. JAMA Intern Med. 2016;176(6):796–804.

7

The infection risk scan (IRIS): standardization and transparency in infection control and antimicrobial use

Ina Willemsen[1,2]* (iD) and Jan Kluytmans[1,3]

Abstract

Background: Infection control needs user-friendly standardized instruments to measure the compliance to guidelines and to implement targeted improvement actions. This abstract describes a tool to measure the quality of infection control and antimicrobial use, the Infection Risk Scan (IRIS). It has been applied in a hospital, several nursing homes and a rehabilitation clinic in the Netherlands.

Method: The IRIS consists of a set of objective reproducible measurements, combining patient- and healthcare related variables, such as: hand hygiene compliance, environmental contamination using ATP measurements, prevalence of resistant microorganisms by active screening, availability of infection control preconditions, personal hygiene of healthcare workers, appropriate use of indwelling medical devices and appropriate use of antimicrobials. Results are visualized in a spider plot using traffic light colors to facilitate the interpretation.

Results: The IRIS provided ward specific results within the hospital that were the basis for targeted improvement programs resulting in measurable improvements. Hand hygiene compliance increased from 43% to 66% (more than 1000 observations per IRIS, $p < 0.000$) and ATP levels were significantly reduced ($p < 0.000$). In the nursing homes, large differences were observed with environmental contamination as common denominator. Most remarkable were the difference in Extended Spectrum Beta-Lactamase Enterobacteriaceae (ESBL-E) prevalence (mean 11%, range 0–21%).

Conclusion: The bundle approach and visualization of the IRIS makes it a useful infection prevention tool providing standardization and transparency. Targeted interventions can be started based on the results of the improvement plot and repeated IRIS can show the effect of interventions. In that way, a quality control cycle with continuous improvement can be achieved.

Keywords: Infection prevention, Antimicrobial resistance, Guidelines, Benchmarking

Background

Healthcare-associated infections (HAI) constitute a major public health problem worldwide [1]. In the future, an increase in HAI is expected due to the growing number of vulnerable and elderly patients and the emergence in antimicrobial resistance [2, 3]. Therefore, it is of utmost importance to intensify our effort in infection control and antimicrobial stewardship [4]. There is no standard

method to measure the quality of care on these aspects. Therefore, we developed the infection Risk Scan (IRIS). This is a standardized method that assesses the quality of infection control by measuring different patient (residents in nursing home)-, department- and care related risk factors. This bundle of measurements provides a complete picture, which is visualized in an easy to understand way to give healthcare providers insight in the strengths and weakness of their performance.

We describe the IRIS-method, it's implementation and the results obtained in a hospital, several nursing homes and a rehabilitation clinic.

* Correspondence: iwillemsen@amphia.nl
[1]Laboratory for Microbiology and Infection Control, Amphia Hospital, PO Box 90158, 4800, RK, Breda, The Netherlands
[2]Center for Infectious Disease Expertise and Research (CIDER), Tilburg, The Netherlands

Method

IRIS consists of cross-sectional measurements and investigates patient/resident-, ward- and care-related variables. Patient/resident-related risks were visualized in a patient risk profile. Ward and care-related risk were visualized in an improvement spider-plot (Fig. 1). Table 1 shows an overview of the included variables, methods, outcome measures and risk stratification.

One or more point-prevalence surveys were performed by infection control practitioners according to the Dutch national surveillance protocol for hospitals (PREZIES) or nursing homes (SNIV) [5, 6]. All patient records of the included patients/residents were investigated, and if necessary, discussed with the attending physician. At least 50 patients (residents in nursing homes) were included in each IRIS.

Risk profile

The risk profile shows the vulnerability of the patient population and consist of four variables:

1. Prevalence of indwelling urethral or suprapubic catheters and intravascular devices (including a peripheral intravenous catheter not in active use) on the day of the survey. The risk classification was based on prevalence numbers from the national surveillance for hospitals as well as for nursing homes [5–8].
2. Prevalence of intravenous or oral antibacterial antimicrobial therapy on the day of the survey [9]. Inhalation medication, cement beads, topical

antibiotics, antiviral and antifungal therapy, were not included, nor did we include antibiotic prophylaxis administrated in the operating theater. The risk classification was based on prevalence obtained from the national surveillance for hospitals as well as for nursing homes [5, 6, 8, 9].

3. Prevalence of rectal carriage of Extended Spectrum Beta-Lactamase (ESBL)-producing Enterobacteriaceae (ESBL-E), detected through perianal swab culture (Table 1) [10, 11]. Rectal ESBL-carriage is common in the population. In Dutch nursing homes a range in ESBL-E prevalence between zero and 21% was found [8, 12]. The average prevalence in the Amphia hospital was 5% in the last 4 years, with a high variability in genotypes [13]. Considering the inaccuracy of the measurement, a prevalence of 7% or lower was interpreted as low.
4. Expected mortality and comorbidity, expressed in a graph showing the distribution in McCabe scores in hospitals, or dependency in activities of daily living in nursing homes according to the Katz Index [14, 15].

Improvement plot

The improvement plot shows 7 ward- and care-related risk factors, both process- as well as outcome variables. These factors can be influenced by the healthcare professional or organization.

1. Appropriate use of indwelling medical devices

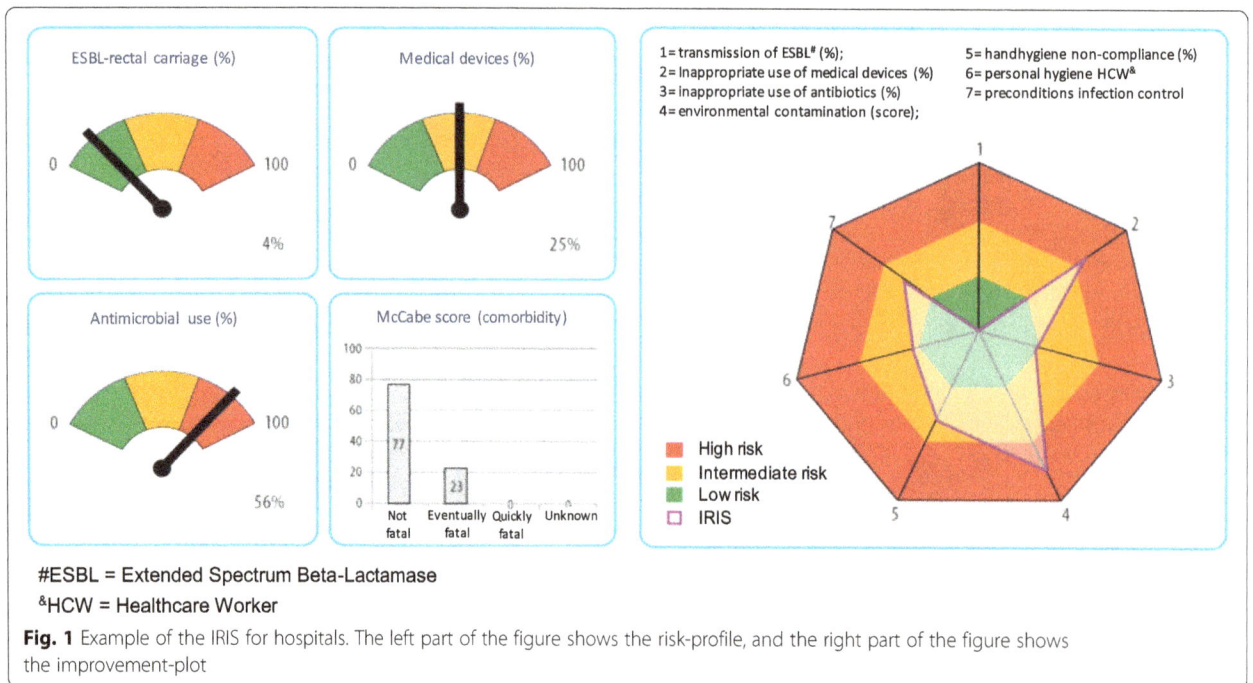

#ESBL = Extended Spectrum Beta-Lactamase

&HCW = Healthcare Worker

Fig. 1 Example of the IRIS for hospitals. The left part of the figure shows the risk-profile, and the right part of the figure shows the improvement-plot

Table 1 Overview of all collected variables, the method used, outcome variables that are visualized in the risk profile and improvement plot, and breakpoints for the risk classification

variables	Hospital	NH[^]	method	Outcome variable	Risk classification Low	Intermediate	High
Risk profile							
Severity of underlying diseases, according to the McCabe score	X		Prevalence survey (file research & interview)	The percentage per category is presented in the risk profile	N.A.[&]		
Independency scale according to Katz-score		X	Prevalence survey (file research & interview)	The percentage per category is presented in the risk profile	N.A.[&]		
indwelling medical devices, including venflon not in use	X		Prevalence survey (file research & interview)	Percentage (n=total number inclusions)	≤15 ≤5	>15 and ≤50 >5 and ≤10	>50 >10
Antibiotic use	X	X	Prevalence survey (file research & interview)	Percentage (n=total number inclusions)	≤15 ≤5	>15 and ≤50 >5 and ≤10	>50 >10
Rectal carriage of ESBL-E[‡] and CPE[##]	X	X	Prevalence survey (culture of faeces or perianal swab)	Percentage (n=total number patients of whom faeces was cultured)	≤7	>7 and ≤11	>11
Improvement plot							
Inappropriate use of medical devices	X	X	Prevalence survey (file research & interview)	Percentage (n=total number of patients with medical devices in use)	≤15	>15 and ≤25	>25
Inappropriate use of antibiotics	X	X	Prevalence survey (file research & interview)	Percentage (n=total number of patients administered one or more antibiotics)	≤15	>15 and ≤25	>25
Transmission of ESBL-E and CPE	X	X	Prevalence survey (molecular typing of ESBL-E and CPE)	Transmission = 2 or more identical ESBL-E and CPE with an epidemiological link	No transmission	No transmission	Transmission
Hand hygiene non-compliance	X		Direct observations of hand hygiene moments per unit	% non-compliance overall (n>200 moments)	≤ 40	>40 and ≤60	>60
Environmental contamination	X	X	ATP detection on pre-defined surfaces/objects per ward. Per tested surface/object, RLU is converted to a score (1, 2, 3 or 4)	Total score per ward/setting (in case of multiple wards within 1 setting, breakpoints will be adjusted as needed)	≤ 4 ≤ 3	>4 and ≤12 >3 and ≤9	>12 ZH >9 VH
Shortcomings in infection control preconditions	X	X	10 preconditions are observed per ward	Score from 1 to 10	≤ 1	>1 and ≤3	>3
Personal hygiene of healthcare workers	X	X	20 nurses and other healthcare employees, per ward, were checked for compliance with the dress code.	Score from 1 to 20 (in case of less observations, breakpoints will be adjusted as needed)	≤ 1	>1 and ≤4	>4

[^]NH = Nursing Home;
[&]N.A.=not applicable; [‡] ESBL-E = Extended Spectrum Beta-Lactamase producing Enterobacteriaceae
[##]CPE-E = Carbapenemase producing Enterobacteriaceae

Appropriateness of the indication for intravascular devices was judged based on local guidelines. The appropriateness of the indication of urethral catheters was judged according to the flowchart used in the national Dutch prevalence survey for HAI [5]. The proportion of patients with a medical device that was considered inappropriate was presented in the improvement plot. The cutoff points for classification are based on "expert opinion" as there are no reference values available.

2. Appropriate use of antimicrobial therapy

Appropriateness of treatment (indication and choice of antimicrobial) was judged against the local antibiotic formulary using a standardized method [9]. The following classifications were used: appropriate use (i.e. justified use and appropriate choice), inappropriate use (i.e. unjustified use and/or justified use, but inappropriate choice), or insufficient information. The proportion of patients with antimicrobial therapy that was considered unjustified and/or inappropriate choice was presented in the improvement plot.

3. Clonal relatedness of ESBL-E

Clonal relatedness was determined based on the microbiological cultures, ESBL gene detection using the Check-MDR CT103 microarray (Check-Points, Wageningen, Netherlands), and molecular typing using Amplified Fragment Length Polymorphism (AFLP) and epidemiological investigation [11, 16]. When two or more identical ESBL-E strains, with identical resistance genes were detected in two or more patients from one prevalence survey within the same epidemiological setting, this was judged as indicative for transmission. We assumed that one case per cluster was the index.

4. Environmental contamination

Detection of Adenosine Triphosphate (ATP) was used to identify the level of environmental contamination with organic material [17, 18]. Samples were taken, using an ATP device (3 M Inc., St. Paul, MN, US), from a fixed amount of pre-defined objects or surfaces, within each unit, at least two hours after the routine cleaning and in accordance to the manufacturer's guidelines (Table 2). In hospitals and in nursing homes, 20 and 15 items were tested, respectively. These test points were selected because they met the following criteria: frequently touched objects/instruments by the nursing staff, frequently touched objects/surfaces by the patient; the immediate surroundings of the patients or items that should always be clean. For each test point, the amount of RLU was converted to a score:

Table 2 Overview of all tested surfaces and objects for environmental contamination in the hospital and nursing home

Testpoints	Hospital	Nursing Home
Bedrail (twice, in two rooms)	X	X
Over bed table	X	X
Washstand	X	X
Shower chair	X	
Support bar in the toilet room	X	X
Toilet seat (sitting area)	X	X
Door handle nursing office	X	
Patient alarm bell	X	
I.V. pole (most frequently touched part of the pole)	X	
Keyboard P.C. in the nursing office	X	X
Telephone	X	X
Control panel bedpan washer	X	
Bedside commode	X	X
Cabinet for medical supply & bandages	X	X
Blood pressure cuff	X	
Ear thermometer (ear tip)	X	X
Glucometer	X	X
Work surface of the bench for drug preparation	X	
Keyboard computer on wheels (COW)	X	
Table living room		X
Supply room "sterile" materials		X
Door handle living room		X
Patient lift, client handle		X

< 1500 RLU = 0 points; > 1500 and ≤3000 RLU = 1 point; > 3000 and ≤10.000 RLU = 2 points; and > 10.000 RLU = 3 points. The total score of all measured objects tested within the unit was presented in the risk plot. If more than one ward was monitored, results were adjusted proportionally (Table 1). The classification is based on an analysis of previous measurements.

5. Shortcomings in infection prevention preconditions

Several preconditions are essential for an effective infection control policy. The tested items are listed in Table 3, scoring and breakpoints are shown in Table 1.

6. Personal hygiene of healthcare workers

At least 20 healthcare workers (10 nurses, 5 staff physicians or house officers and 5 other hospital employees in hospitals; in NHs at least 20 healthcare workers overall) were tested for the basic hygiene rules: no rings, no watch or wrist jewelry present, forearms uncovered (bare

Table 3 Overview of all tested infection control preconditions in the hospital and nursing home

Infection control preconditions	Hospital	Nursing Home
Trash bin(s) are closed and foot-operated (entire department)	X	X
The (clean) linen is stored in a clean place, protected against dust and moisture	X	X
The bed-pan washer meets the following requirement: Disinfection with steam or hot water of at least 80 ° C (for at least 60 s)	X	X
Sterile medical devices (catheters, IVs) are kept in a closed cabinet	X	
Sterile medical devices are kept separated in a closed cabinet		X
Medical supply and bandages are kept in closed cabinets	X	
Needle waste container (UN3291) is presence		X
Halter aprons to protect clothing are present at the ward	X	X
Surgical masks are present at the division	X	X
Non-sterile gloves (NEN-EN 420 + A1, NEN-EN374, NEN-EN) are present in every patient room	X	
Non-sterile gloves (NEN-EN 420 + A1, NEN-EN374, NEN-EN) are present in every ward		X
Hand alcohol (is present in every patient room and at point of care (EN1500)	X	
No fabric chairs or benches are present in the patient and / or treatment room	X	
No fabric chairs or benches are present in the common areas		X

below the elbow), uniform worn correctly and coat closed (Table 1).

7. Hand hygiene compliance

In the hospital, the hand hygiene compliance was determined by performing direct observation on the ward according to the World Health Organization 5 moments method. The observations were performed by trained nurses during routine handlings. The classification is based on scientific publications [19–21].

8. Presence of local infection prevention protocols

In the nursing homes, the presence of 20 essential infection prevention protocols was investigated (Table 4). These protocols contain essential basic principles of infection prevention. The rating is assigned based on "expert opinion" where one deviation is accepted.

The selection of risk factors was based on the importance, as judged by a group of experienced infection control practitioners, as well as the possibility of an objective and reproducible assessment. The current set of risk factors are considered to be important for current infection control, however the IRIS is a flexible model in which risk factors can be added or switched.

For each risk factor, breakpoints were set to distinguish low, intermediate and high categories (Table 1). Breakpoints were based on scientific publications or based on expert opinion if no such data were available, shown in Table 1.

To visualize all surveillance data in one graph, data were converted into a scale from 0 to 100 using an

Table 4 Overview of the infection prevention protocols, tested for local presence

Infection control protocols
Accidental blood contact
Collection and transport of waste and used linen
Hand hygiene
Pets (including assistance dogs)
Infectious diseases healthcare workers
Catheterization
Legionella management plan
Body care of the client
Recommendation for prevention & control of influenza
Recommendation for prevention & control of norovirus
Recommendation for prevention & control of Scabies
Recommendation for screening of Multi Drug Resistant Organisms (including screening of risk-population on admission[#])
Recommendation for prevention & control of MRSA (including screening of risk-populations on admission[#])
Storage of "sterile" materials
Personal Protection Materials (PPM)
Personal hygiene of healthcare workers
Cleaning, disinfection and sterilization
Administering medication
Urination and bowel movement (defecation)
Wound-care

risk population as defined by the Dutch Working Infection Control Party

algorithm. The algorithm included breakpoints for the 3 categories: low risk from 0 to 33%; intermediate risk from 34 to 66%; and high risk from 67 to 100%. Each axis of the plot represents an outcome variable or risk factor. If the results were in the high (red) risk-area, in-depth research and improvement activities were strongly recommended.

The risk profile and improvement plot were reported to the management of the hospital ward or healthcare setting. Management itself is responsible for the distribution of the results to all employees and for the implementation of improvement actions. The infection control department had a coaching and consulting role during the improvement programs. The figure of the improvement plot, in combination with the patient profile, gives direction to the improvement activities and helps to set priorities. The risk profile provides background information about the population. This is helpful for the interpretation of the improvement-plot and subsequent improvement activities. In a high risk population, with high prevalence of medical devices and severity of underlying diseases, environmental contamination and low compliance of hand hygiene is more critical than in a low risk population.

Results
IRIS in a hospital
IRIS was implemented in 5 wards within 5 different medical specialties during the period 2013–2015. Three cycles

of measurements, improvements and measurements were performed during this period with an interval of 6–8 months. Differences were found in the figures of the improvement plots of the different wards. However, high levels of environmental contamination were found in all 5 wards (Fig.2).

Based on the results, targeted actions were performed resulting in a considerable improvement (hand hygiene dispensers at point of care, hand hygiene campaign for and by nurses, definition of cleaning responsibilities). Especially, hand hygiene compliance improved from an average of 43% to 66% ($p < 0.001$), and the measured ATP levels reduced significantly ($p < 0.001$) meaning a cleaner environment. Of all tested patients ($n = 439$), 16 (3.6%) were proven to be carrier of a ESBL-E in the perianal culture. In two patients, an identical strain was found. No carbapenemase-producing Enterobacteriaceae were isolated. No improvement was detected in the use of antimicrobials.

IRIS in a nursing home
IRIS was performed in 19 nursing homes in the southern part of The Netherlands. Large differences were found between the nursing homes and again the common denominator was the environmental contamination. Furthermore, in most of the nursing homes, availability of hand disinfectants was

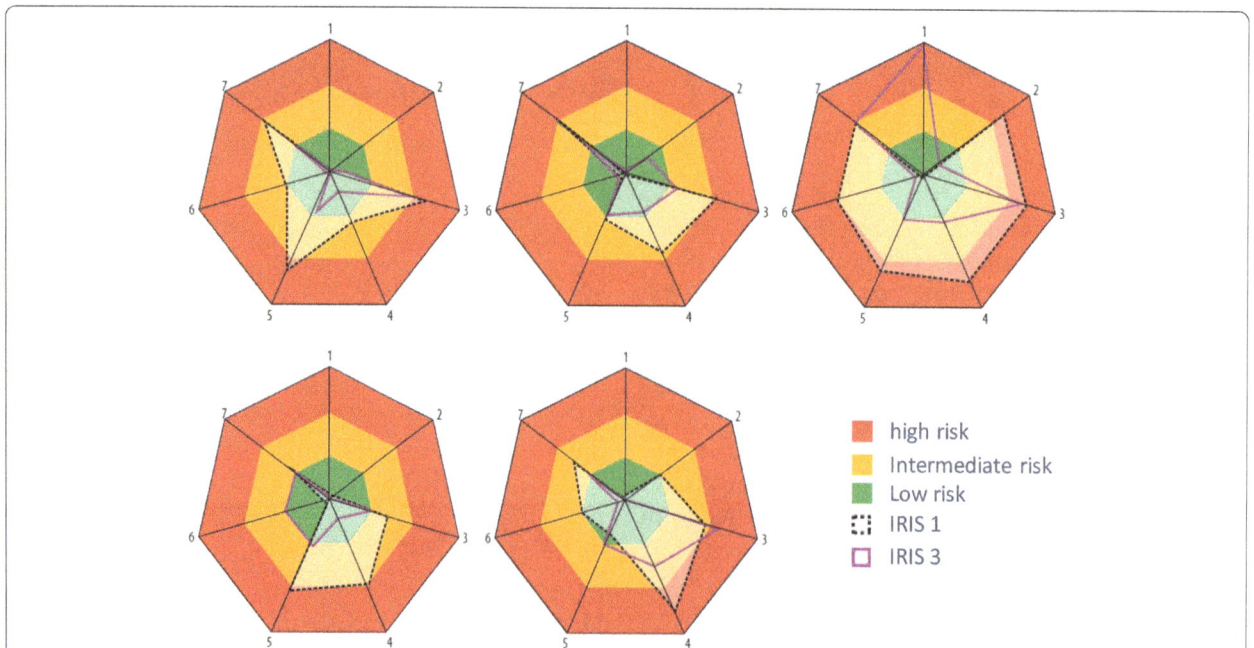

Fig. 2 The Improvement-plots from 5 hospital units, from 5 different medical specialties. Three IRIS-cycle were performed with an interval of 6 up to 8 months. The dotted black line shows the results from the first IRIS, the purple line shows the results from the third IRIS. 1= Transmission of ESBL (%); 2= Inappropriate use of medical devices (%); 3= Inappropriate use of antibiotics (%); 4= Environmental contamination (score); 5= Hand hygiene non-compliance (%); 6= Personal hygiene Healthcare workers (%); 7= Preconditions infection control (score)

insufficient and the separation between clean and dirty material was lacking. The most remarkable finding was the difference in ESBL-E prevalence, mean 11% (range 0–21%). A large outbreak was detected in one nursing home, involving more than 21 residents in different departments, with an identical *Escherichia coli* ST131 strain. [12]

IRIS in a rehabilitation center

In this center, 12 out of 71 (17%) cultured residents proved to be a carrier of ESBL-E. The molecular typing revealed that all ESBL-E were unique cases, no clonal clusters could be detected. In this center, all variables in the IRIS improvement plot were in the "green" zone. Environmental contamination was minimal, infection prevention preconditions were good and local protocols were available.

Implementation of the IRIS

The time needed to perform an IRIS depends on the size, setting and condition of (electronic) patient records. To complete an IRIS in a hospital ward with 50 beds and electronic patient records takes approximately 5 days, of which 3 days are for the measurements and 2 days for analyses and feedback. An IRIS in a nursing home with 100 residents takes about one day for preparation and execution of the prevalence survey, one day for audits, and one day for analysis and feedback. This does not include the time investment for the hand hygiene observations. Our experience reveals that during the morning routine, on average, 20 hand hygiene moments take place per hour.

Management and healthcare workers were very positive about the IRIS process. The healthcare workers on each ward implemented changes based on the IRIS results and the collaboration between the infection control department and the ward staff was considered constructive. In the hospital, infection prevention workgroups were developed to improve shortcomings together. This resulted in significant improvement in all departments.

Discussion

We describe the implementation and first results of the IRIS, an infection prevention tool that uses a bundle approach and provides transparency in the performance of infection control and use of antimicrobial therapy. Measurements are objective, reproducible, and include the most relevant indicators of infection control and antimicrobial resistance. The IRIS has been performed in 19 nursing homes, 1 rehabilitation center and 5 wards within one hospital.

The difference in improvement plots revealed that each hospital ward or healthcare setting has specific issues that need improvement. Targeted interventions were undertaken based on the IRIS results. The second and third IRIS showed an overall improvement in the hospital, with the exception being the appropriateness of antimicrobial use. This can be explained by the fact that no stewardship activities were initiated except for feedback of the results. A more intensive approach will be needed to obtain measurable improvement.

In the nursing homes, significant variation in the IRIS components was found, most remarkable were the differences found in ESBL prevalence. In one setting, a large outbreak was detected. The use of diagnostic tests, such as microbiological cultures, is limited in most nursing homes. This could result in a possible reservoir for multidrug-resistant microorganisms. Prevalence surveys, like the prevalence survey in the IRIS, are useful tools to detect the possible clusters of ESBL-E at an early stage.

The IRIS components are not new, and well known of infection prevention and antibiotic stewardship programs. However, bringing these various components together, like a bundle, results in stronger effect than those of the individual interventions. Furthermore, the multifactorial measurements are objective and reproducible, which makes comparison between healthcare settings possible.

The color codes make the results straightforward and easy to understand, for professionals who need to implement the improvements and for the managers who should promote and monitor the activities. The simplicity of the visualization creates co-ownership of the problem and provides support for interventions.

In the current IRIS, hand hygiene compliance was measured by performing direct observations of healthcare workers during the morning routine. Direct observations can lead to unrealistic high compliance, known as the Hawthorne effect. Furthermore, it gives information about a very small portion of the healthcare workers during a small time-frame of the day. We recognize these limitations, however, it is not easy to solve this issue. The use of consumption volumes of hand sanitizer could be an alternative; however, this first needs to be validated.

In the IRIS, appropriateness of use of medical devices and antimicrobial therapy were judged based on local guidelines. Local guidelines may vary and this may limit the use of this method when comparisons are made between centers. Standardization of guidelines is needed to be able to use IRIS or similar methods on a larger scale.

Furthermore, thresholds were, where possible, based on data from surveillance programs or peer-reviewed publications, but when no references were available thresholds were chosen arbitrary by a group of experts. In these cases previous results were used to define thresholds. The threshold values should be evaluated periodically and adjusted if necessary.

Conclusion

In conclusion, the bundle approach and visualization of the IRIS makes it a complete and useful infection prevention tool. It provides transparency in the quality of infection control and antimicrobial use. Targeted interventions can be started based on the results of the improvement plot and the effect of interventions can be shown by repeating the IRIS. In that way, a quality control cycle with continuous improvement can be achieved. The broader implementation of IRIS can raise the standard of infection control and make it more transparent in various healthcare settings, E.g. Nursing homes.

Abbreviations
AFLP: Amplified Fragment Length Polymorphism; ATP: Adenosine Triphosphate; ESBL: Extended Spectrum Beta-Lactamase; ESBL: Extended Spectrum Beta-Lactamase; HAI: Healthcare Associated Infections; IRIS: Infection Risk Scan

Acknowledgements
We thank the infection control practitioners, microbiologist, healthcare workers and nursing home management for their participation in this study.

Funding
The IRIS was funded by the participating healthcare facilities.

Authors' contributions
IW and JK conceived and planned the project, analyzed and interpreted the collected data and wrote the manuscript. Both authors read and approve the final manuscript.

Ethics approval and consent to participate
According to the Dutch regulation for research with human subjects, neither medical nor ethical approval was required to conduct the surveillance since it was part of the local hospital/nursing home policy, patients/residents provided oral informed consent and all data were processed anonymously. The, non-invasive, perianal swabs were collected as part of the local hospital policy which is considered routine care. The periodically performed surveys for the presence of multi drug resistant micro-organisms are part of the infection control policy in our hospital. This includes contact tracing, active search in patients with risk factors and routinely check-ups like the yearly prevalence survey. Swabs were not specifically collected for the purposes of this publication.

Consent for publication
Not applicable

Competing interests
The interest declare that they have no competing interests.

Author details
[1]Laboratory for Microbiology and Infection Control, Amphia Hospital, PO Box 90158, 4800, RK, Breda, The Netherlands. [2]Center for Infectious Disease Expertise and Research (CIDER), Tilburg, The Netherlands. [3]Julius Center for Health Sciences and Primary Care, UMC Utrecht, Utrecht, the Netherlands.

References
1. Allegranzi B, Nejad S, Combescure C, Graafmans W, Attar H, Donaldson L, Pittet D. Burden of endemic health-care-associated infection in developing countries: systematic review and meta-analysis. Lancet. 2011;377:228–41.
2. European commision, Europe in figures, eurostat yearbook 2010. http://ec. europa.eu/eurostat/documents/3217494/5721265/KS-CD-10-220-EN.PDF/ e47b231c-c411-4d4e-8cd6-e0257be4f2e6?version=1.0 Accessed 1st Nov 2017.
3. Strausbaugh LJ. Emerging health care-associated infections in the geriatric population. Emerg Infect Dis. 2001;7(2):268–71.
4. Moro ML, Gagliotti C. Antimicrobial resistance and stewardship in long-term care settings. Future Microbiol. 2013;8(8):1011–25.
5. PREZIES. Prevalentieonderzoek Ziekenhuizen: Protocol & dataspecificatie, versie maart/oktober 2016. Bilthoven: RIVM; 2016.
6. SNIV Surveillance Netwerk Infectieziekten Verpleeghuizen: Protocol & dataspecificatie versie april/november 2016. Bilthoven: Rijksinstituut voor Volksgezondheid en Milieu; 2016. [in Dutch].
7. Eilers R, Veldman-Ariesen MJ, Haenen A, Van Benthem BH. Prevalence and Determinants associated with healthcare-associated infections in long-term care facilities (HALT) in the Netherlands, may to June 2010. Euro Surveill. 2012;17(34):1-8.
8. Willemsen I, Nelson-Melching J, Hendriks Y, et al. Measuring the quality of infection control in Dutch nursing homes using a standardized method; the infection prevention risk scan (IRIS). Antimicrob Resist Infect Control. 2014;3:26.
9. Willemsen I, Groenhuijzen A, Bogaers D, Stuurman A, van Keulen P, Kluytmans J. Appropriateness of antimicrobial therapy measured by repeated prevalence surveys. Antimicrob Agents Chemother. 2007;51:864–7.
10. Kluytmans-van den Bergh MK, Verhulst C, Willemsen LE, Verkade E, Bonten MJ, Kluytmans JA. Rectal carriage of extended-spectrum-beta- lactamase-producing enterobacteriaceae in hospitalized patients: selective preenrichtment increases yield of screening. J Clin Microbiol. 2015;53:2709–12.
11. Bernards AT, Bonten MJM, Cohen Stuart J, et al. NVMM guideline: laboratory detection of highly resistant microorganisms (HRMO). Leeuwarden: Nederlandse Vereniging voor Medische Microbiologie; 2012.
12. Willemsen I, Nelson J, Hendriks Y, et al. Extensive dissemination of extended spectrum Beta-lactamase producing Enterobacteriaceae in a Dutch nursing home. Infect Control Hosp Epidemiol. 2015;36:394–400.
13. Willemsen I, Oome S, Verhulst C, Pettersson A, Verduin K, Kluytmans J. Trends in extended Spectrum Beta-lactamase (ESBL) producing Enterobacteriaceae and ESBL genes in a Dutch teaching hospital, measured in 5 yearly point prevalence surveys (2010-2014). PLoS One. 2015;10(11):e0141765.
14. Reilly JS, Coignard B, Price L, Godwin J, Cairns S, Hopkins S, et al. The reliability of the McCabe score as a marker of co-morbidity in healthcare-associated infection point prevalence studies. J Infect Prev. 2015;20(8):127-29.
15. Katz S, Ford AB, Moskowitz RW, Jacksons BE, Jaffe MW. Studies of illness in the aged: the index of ADL: a standardized measure of biological and psychosocial function. J Am Med Assoc. 1963 Sep;195(2):914–9.
16. Mohammadi T, Reesink HW, Pietersz RN, Vandenbroucke-Grauls CM, Savelkoul PH. Amplified-fragment length polymorphism analysis of Propionibacterium isolates implicated in contamination of blood products. Br J Haematol. 2005;131(3):403–9.
17. Sherlock L, O'Connell N, Creamer E, Humphreys HP. Is it really clean? An evaluation of the efficacy of four methods for determining hospital cleanliness. J Hosp Infect. 2009;72:140–6.
18. Boyce JM, Havill NL, Dumigan DG, Golebiewski M, Balogun O, Rizvani R. Monitoring the effectiveness of hospital cleaning practices by use of an adenosine triphosphate bioluminescence assay. Infect Control Hosp Epidemiol. 2009;30:678–84.
19. Pittet D, Hugonnet S, Harbarth S, Mourouga P, Sauvan V, Touveneau S, et al. Effectiveness of a hospital-wide programme to improve compliance with hand hygiene. Infection Control Programme Lancet. 2000;356(9238):1307–12.
20. Cooper BS, Medley GF, Scott GM. Preliminary analysis of the transmission dynamics of nosocomial infections: stochastic and management effects. J Hosp Infect. 1999;43(2):131–47.
21. McBryde ES, Pettitt AN, McElwain DL. A stochastic mathematical model of methicillin resistant Staphylococcus Aureus transmission in an intensive care unit: predicting the impact of interventions. J Theor Biol. 2007;245(3):470–81.

8

"First-person view" of pathogen transmission and hand hygiene – use of a new head-mounted video capture and coding tool

Lauren Clack[†], Manuela Scotoni[†], Aline Wolfensberger and Hugo Sax[*] ⓘ

Abstract

Background: Healthcare workers' hands are the foremost means of pathogen transmission in healthcare, but detailed hand trajectories have been insufficiently researched so far. We developed and applied a new method to systematically document hand-to-surface exposures (HSE) to delineate true hand transmission pathways in real-life healthcare settings.

Methods: A head-mounted camera and commercial coding software were used to capture ten active care episodes by eight nurses and two physicians and code HSE type and duration using a hierarchical coding scheme. We identified HSE sequences of particular relevance to infectious risks for patients based on the WHO 'Five Moments for Hand Hygiene'. The study took place in a trauma intensive care unit in a 900-bed university hospital in Switzerland.

Results: Overall, the ten videos totaled 296.5 min and featured eight nurses and two physicians. A total of 4222 HSE were identified (1 HSE every 4.2 s), which concerned bare (79%) and gloved (21%) hands. The HSE inside the patient zone (n = 1775; 42%) included mobile objects (33%), immobile surfaces (5%), and patient intact skin (4%), while HSE outside the patient zone (n = 1953; 46%) included HCW's own body (10%), mobile objects (28%), and immobile surfaces (8%). A further 494 (12%) events involved patient critical sites. Sequential analysis revealed 291 HSE transitions from outside to inside patient zone, i.e. "colonization events", and 217 from any surface to critical sites, i.e. "infection events". Hand hygiene occurred 97 times, 14 (5% adherence) times at colonization events and three (1% adherence) times at infection events. On average, hand rubbing lasted 13 ± 9 s.

Conclusions: The abundance of HSE underscores the central role of hands in the spread of potential pathogens while hand hygiene occurred rarely at potential colonization and infection events. Our approach produced a valid video and coding instrument for in-depth analysis of hand trajectories during active patient care that may help to design more efficient prevention schemes.

Keywords: Video, Transmission risk, Hand hygiene, Observation

* Correspondence: hugo.sax@usz.ch
[†]Equal contributors
Division of Infectious Diseases and Hospital Epidemiology, University Hospital
Zurich, University of Zurich, Raemistrasse 100, CH-8091 Zurich, Switzerland

Background

Healthcare-associated infections, including surgical site infections, ventilator-associated pneumonia, urinary tract infections, and catheter-associated bloodstream infections, prolong length of hospital stay and increase cost, morbidity and mortality [1–3]. Additionally, antibiotic resistance is emerging worldwide as a serious health threat [4].

Transmission of potential pathogens between patients occurs primarily via healthcare worker (HCW) hands when hand hygiene (HH) is omitted at critical moments [5, 6]. Such hand-to-surface exposures (HSE) occur frequently [7], resulting each time in a bi-directional exchange of microorganisms between the hand and the touched surface [6]. In consequence, hands transport microorganisms sequentially between surfaces [6]. Depending on the nature of the microorganisms and of the receiving surface, this can result in patient harm. If microorganisms feature antibiotic resistance, their transmission to a patient can result in prolonged carriage. If the microorganisms are virulent and the receiver surface is a skin lesion or an invasive device such as a central venous line, the transmission may result in healthcare-associated infection.

Several studies show that infectious microorganisms can survive on human skin long enough to be cross-transmitted and that hand hygiene using alcohol-based handrub is an effective way to decrease this transmission [8, 9]. With the WHO "My five moments for hand hygiene", a user-centered concept based on education, training, monitoring and reporting of hand hygiene has been introduced with the goal to bridge the gap between scientific evidence and daily healthcare practice [10]. Yet, HCWs still fail to consistently apply hand hygiene. The lack of awareness regarding what people touch during their routine work may play an important role in this failure to adhere to established rules [11]. Today's gold standard to monitor HH performance consists of direct observation of healthcare workers by trained observers during patient care [5, 12–14]. This method may not capture every HSE during fast-paced care and thus, underestimates the true risk of pathogen transmission [7, 15]. On the other hand, automated electronic hand hygiene monitoring systems still fall short of detecting all hand hygiene opportunities [16].

To better understand the nature of microbial hand-transmission in a real-life intensive healthcare setting, we built and pilot-tested a new observation and coding system that would consistently capture every HSE, and thus allow to study true transmission risks via HCWs' hands.

Methods

Setting up and offsite-testing of the system

We opted for a mobile, head-mounted action camera (GoPro® Hero 4 Black edition, GoPro Inc., San Mateo,

CA) worn by HCW during patient care. The camera was positioned on the forehead of the HCW by means of a head-strap and was oriented facing slightly downwards. With the help of an iPad mini (Apple, Cupertino, CA) the researcher could control the optimal orientation of the camera through a Wi-Fi connection. The camera was oriented to keep the participant's hands in its visual field. In a first round, we tested and adjusted the camera in the medical high-fidelity simulator of our institution. After resolving all technical issues, we proceeded to video-tape real-life care activity in three intensive care units (ICUs) specialized in trauma, cardiology, and visceral surgery at the University Hospital Zurich (USZ), Switzerland. The USZ is a 900-bed university-affiliated tertiary care center with a well-established infection prevention and control (IPC) group, weekly IPC rounds, and a designated IPC nurse consultant for each hospital ward.

Participants and onsite-use of the system

A convenience sample of 10 participants was recruited among ICU nurses and physicians. Each participant wore the head-mounted camera during his/her morning shift for about 70 min. Morning shifts were chosen purposefully to guarantee that patient care activity took place. Subsequently, HCW continued their care activity without further interruptions by the researcher, who left the area.

Video coding

The videos were exported from the camera and stored on a secured server. Episodes of ~30 min direct patient care were purposefully selected from each of the 10 videos for further processing. Within each of these video episodes, the occurrence, duration, and type of every HSE was systematically coded by a trained coder (MS) and supervised by a second person (LC) using the behavioral observation software INTERACT® (Mangold international, Arnstorf, Germany) together with a structured, hierarchical coding system (Fig. 1).

The observation and coding system aimed to capture the duration and nature of all HSE, defined as contact between the observed healthcare worker's hand and any other surface. The hierarchical coding system consisted of 4 levels, of which the first two indicate the nature of the hand (gloved vs. bare and right vs. left), and the latter two indicate the nature of the surface (location relative to patient zone and type of surface) involved in the hand-to-surface exposure (Fig. 1). In line with the WHO patient zone concept [10] and observation method [15] the third coding level distinguished between surfaces "inside patient zone", "outside patient zone", and "critical sites". "Inside patient zone" was defined as the patient him–/herself and all items in the immediate environment likely to be colonized with patient flora [10]. The

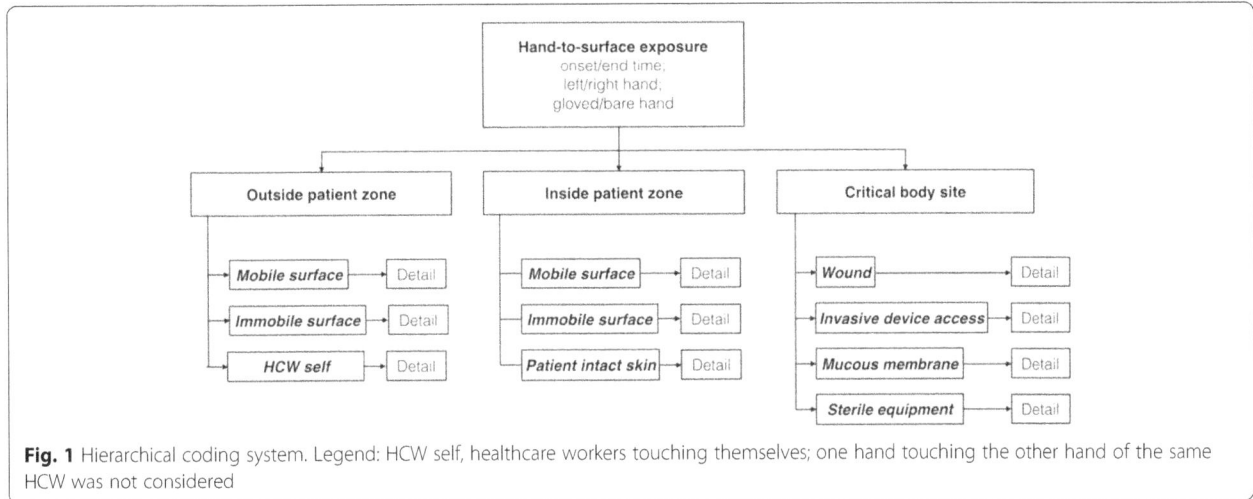

Fig. 1 Hierarchical coding system. Legend: HCW self, healthcare workers touching themselves; one hand touching the other hand of the same HCW was not considered

"outside patient zone" contained other patients with their respective zones, the HCW's own body and professional apparel ("HCW Self"), and all the other areas and surfaces outside the patient zone [10]. "Critical sites" included clean sites such as medical devices or patient's body parts that have to be protected against microbial colonization in order to avoid infections [10]. Hand hygiene actions were registered as specific events and coded as either "hand washing" or "hand disinfection" with alcohol-based handrub. Patient zones were established a-priori for each ICU setting to ensure accurate and consistent coding (Fig. 2).

Data analysis

To assess the utility of the observation and coding system, we performed a descriptive analysis of frequency and duration of HSE. Coded event data were exported

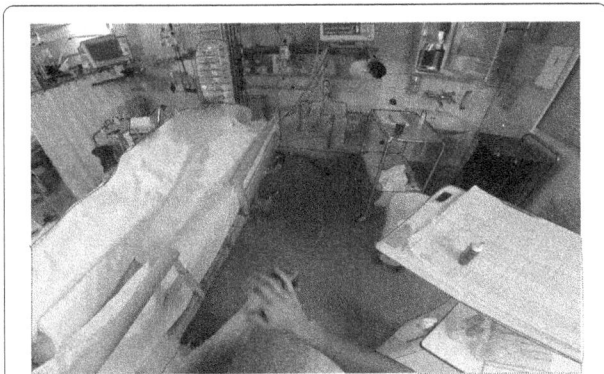

Fig. 2 Typical visual field of the head mounted GoPro® action camera and color-coded patient zone. Legend: This screenshot demonstrates the first-person view recorded from the head camera. Objects and surfaces belonging to the patient zone are colored with a green overlay and dotted outline

as comma separate values (.cvs) files, merged and edited in Excel (Microsoft, Redmond, WA) and analyzed in STATA special edition 12.0 (StataCorp, College Station, TX). Sequential analysis was additionally conducted to identify HSE sequences of particular relevance to infectious risks, as informed by the WHO 'Five Moments for Hand Hygiene' [10]. We defined sequences of touching a surface outside the patient zone followed by touching any surface inside a patient zone as a *'colonization event'* and a sequence of touching any surface, except a critical site, followed by touching a critical site as an *'infection event'* (Table 1). A *colonization event* would correspond to a modified WHO "Five Moments" concept's Moment 1 "Before touching a patient" but include touching any surface inside the patient zone and not only the patient. This modification of Moment 1 was made to capture more precisely colonization risk of the patient by hospital flora that is brought into the immediate vicinity of the patient and from there to the patient. An *infection event* would correspond to WHO "Five Moments" concept's Moment 2 "Before clean/aseptic procedure". According to Sax et al., "Critical sites for infectious risks" included breaks in the patient's intact skin such as wounds and catheter insertion sites, any patient mucous membrane, invasive devices in-situ if the lumen was accessed such as vascular or urinary catheters, and semi-critical or critical medical devices ready to be used on the patient [10].

Results

The 10 active care video sequences totaled 296.5 min and featured eight nurses of whom seven were female and two physicians of whom one was female, all right handed. Overall, 4222 HSE occurred, translating in an overall density of 14.2 HSE per minute or one HSE every 4.2 s. Exemplarily, Fig. 3 demonstrates the coding timeline of all

Table 1 Events associated with the risk of patient cross-colonization or infection

		Origin HSE surface		Destination HSE surface
Patient Colonization Event; corresponding to WHO moment 1[a]		Any HSE outside patient zone	→	Any surface inside patient zone (including fomites and intact patient skin, excluding critical sites)
	Examples	Door handle, keyboard of mobile computer	→	Patient bedside monitor, patient arm
Patient Infection Event; corresponding to WHO moment 2[a]		Any HSE (except the same critical site as arrival HSE surface)	→	Any critical site
	Examples	Patient arm, bedside monitor	→	Central venous catheter insertion site, wound, sterile needle to be used on the patient

Legend: *HSE* hand-to-surface exposure. The symbol → denotes the direct sequence of two HSE. [a]WHO moment 1 with the modification that touching a surface inside the patient zone with or without touching the patient counts as Patient Colonization Event

HSE and hand hygiene actions in the first 3 min of video #7. Details on the frequency and nature of HSE and hand hygiene actions overall and per each video sequence appear in Table 2.

The mean and median duration of the 97 observed hand hygiene actions were 12.9 (SD, 8.7) and 11 (range, 2–48) seconds, respectively. Patient *colonization events* occurred overall 291 times, 139 for the left and 152 for the right hand. Patient *infection events* were observed overall 217 times, 103 for the left and 114 for the right hand. Importantly, 117 (61%) of *colonization events* and seven (2.3%) *infection events* occurred after HCWs touching their own body. HCWs touched themselves 439 times (10% of all HSE), including their clothes 165 (38%), personal protective equipment 21 (5%), their face 24 (6%), and remaining bare skin or hair 229 (52%) times; 13 (3%) times with gloved hands.

Hand hygiene occurred prior to 14 of the 191 *colonization events* and three of the 217 *infection events*, resulting in a hand hygiene 'adherence' of 5% and 1%, respectively.

Discussion

This unique video observation and coding approach, that considers each single HSE by both HCW hands,

revealed a surprising reality of transmission opportunities during real-world intensive care. The overall density of 14.2 HSE per minute with which HCWs' hands touched surfaces during active patient care is high, suggesting that hands acquire and deposit – and thus likely transmit – potentially harmful microorganisms every 4 s onto patients and surfaces in the care environment. We identified sequences of particular interest for infection prevention, such as patient zone entries and transitions to critical sites, which each occurred roughly every 2 min of active patient care in an ICU. Hand hygiene was performed on average 19.6 times per hour, which equals one hand hygiene action every 3 min. It is not surprising that participants only sustained hand rubbing for a median of 11 s against the recommended 20–30 s [17]. In fact, if meeting the recommended duration for hand rubbing, almost one fifth of active patient care time would have been spent on this activity. Recent data indicating that 15 s might suffice are comforting in this respect [18].

The approach used in this study is in line with a human factors task analysis, whose underlying principle is to break down a task to study its individual elements [19]. In doing so, we aim to understand the factors that influence the way work is being done and, ultimately,

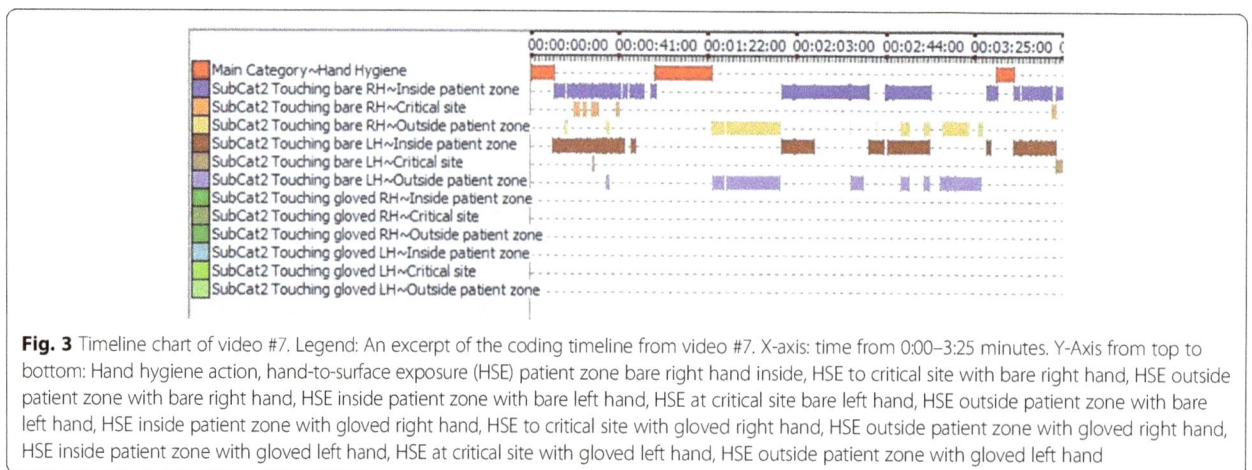

Fig. 3 Timeline chart of video #7. Legend: An excerpt of the coding timeline from video #7. X-axis: time from 0:00–3:25 minutes. Y-Axis from top to bottom: Hand hygiene action, hand-to-surface exposure (HSE) patient zone bare right hand inside, HSE to critical site with bare right hand, HSE outside patient zone with bare right hand, HSE inside patient zone with bare left hand, HSE at critical site bare left hand, HSE outside patient zone with bare left hand, HSE inside patient zone with gloved right hand, HSE to critical site with gloved right hand, HSE outside patient zone with gloved right hand, HSE inside patient zone with gloved left hand, HSE at critical site with gloved left hand, HSE outside patient zone with gloved left hand

Table 2 Hand-to-surface exposures and hand hygiene actions

Video	#1	#2	#3	#4	#5	#6	#7	#8	#9	#10	Overall
ICU specialty	Trauma	Trauma	Trauma	Trauma	Cardio-surgery	Cardio-surgery	Cardio-surgery	General surgery	Cardio-surgery	General surgery	
Length of coded care sequence; min:sec	34:50	34:50	34:50	36:20	31:17	32:38	33:31	16:39	32:19	16:32	296:30
Gender	M	F	F	F	F	F	M	M	F	F	
Profession	N	N	N	N	N	N	N	P	N	P	
HSE; n	494	472	314	495	474	671	553	176	526	47	4222
HSE density; n/min	14.2	13.6	9.0	13.6	15.2	20.6	16.5	10.6	16.3	2.8	14.2
Mean HSE duration (SD); sec	8.9 (16.0)	6.8 (10.0)	11.7 (17.0)	8.1 (18.5)	7.0 (14.9)	5.3 (10.5)	5.6 (11.8)	11.7 (15.1)	6.8 (10.7)	11.8 (26.5)	7.44 (14.1)
Hand											
Right hand (%)	273 (55.3)	254 (53.8)	173 (55.1)	277 (56.0)	250 (52.7)	358 (53.4)	304 (55.0)	93 (52.8)	292 (55.5)	25 (53.2)	2299 (54.5)
Left hand (%)	221 (44.7)	218 (46.2)	141 (44.9)	218 (44.0)	224 (47.3)	313 (46.7)	249 (45.0)	83 (47.2)	234 (44.5)	22 (46.8)	1923 (45.6)
Gloves worn during HSE											
No (%)	355 (71.9)	420 (89.0)	221 (70.4)	214 (43.2)	406 (85.7)	671 (100)	334 (60.4)	176 (100)	474 (90.1)	47 (100)	3318 (78.6)
Yes (%)	139 (28.1)	52 (11.0)	93 (29.6)	281 (56.78)	68 (14.4)	0	291 (39.6)	0	52 (9.9)	0	904 (21.4)
Any surface inside patient zone (% of all HSE)	289 (58.5)	222 (47.0)	196 (62.4)	133 (26.9)	131 (27.6)	134 (20.0)	225 (40.7)	122 (69.3)	278 (52.85)	45 (95.7)	1775 (42.0)
Patient intact skin (% of HSE inside patient zone)	12 (4.2)	30 (13.5)	12 (6.1)	13 (9.8)	0	15 (11.2)	45 (20.0)	8 (6.6)	29 (10.4)	14 (31.1)	178 (10.0)
Mobile object inside patient zone (% of HSE inside patient zone)	241 (83.4)	163 (73.4)	130 (66.3)	112 (84.2)	117 (89.3)	80 (59.7)	168 (74.7)	109 (89.3)	234 (84.2)	29 (64.4)	1383 (77.9)
Immobile surface inside patient zone (% of HSE inside patient zone)	36 (12.5)	29 (13.1)	54 (27.6)	8 (60.2)	14 (10.7)	39,829.1	12 (5.3)	5 (4.1)	15 (5.4)	2 (4.4)	214 (12.1)
Any surface outside patient zone (% of all HSE)	148 (30.0)	220 (46.6)	89 (28.3)	350 (70.7)	322 (67.9)	506 (75.4)	115 (20.8)	53 (30.1)	148 (28.1)	2 (4.3)	1953 (46.3)
HCW own body (outside patient zone) (% of HSE outside patient zone)	7 (4.7)	36 (16.4)	25 (28.1)	47 (13.4)	60 (18.6)	107 (21.2)	79 (68.7)	50 (94.3)	28 (18.9)	0	439 (22.5)
Mobile object outside patient zone (% of HSE outside patient zone)	114 (77.0)	160 (72.7)	49 (55.1)	235 (67.1)	175 (54.4)	346 (68.4)	18 (15.7)	3 (5.7)	92 (62.2)	2 (100)	1194 (61.1)
Immobile surface outside patient zone (% of HSE outside patient zone)	27 (18.2)	24 (10.9)	15 (16.9)	68 (19.4)	87 (27.0)	53 (10.5)	18 (15.7)	0	28 (18.9)	0	320 (16.4)
Any critical site (inside patient zone) (% of all HSE)	57 (11.5)	30 (6.4)	29 (9.2)	12 (2.4)	21 (4.4)	31 (4.6)	213 (38.5)	1 (0.6)	100 (19.0)	0	494 (11.7)
Sterile equipment (% of HSE at critical site)	1 (1.8)	0	0	0	0	0	123 (57.8)	1 (100)	82 (82.0)	0	207 (41.9)
Invasive device access (% of HSE at critical site)	55 (96.5)	30 (100)	29 (100)	9 (75.0)	21 (100)	21 (67.7)	65 (30.5)	0	8 (8.0)	0	238 (48.2)
Mucous membrane (% of HSE at critical site)	1 (1.8)	0	0	3 (25.0)	0	0	0	0	0	0	4 (0.8)
Wound (% of HSE at critical site)	0	0	0	0	0	10 (32.3)	25 (11.7)	0	10 (10.0)	0	45 (9.1)
Infectious risk events	41	42	43	26	44	80	117	31	72	2	508
Patient colonization events	13	26	23	16	25	54	65	30	37	2	291
Patient infection events	38	16	20	10	19	26	52	1	35	0	217
Hand hygiene actions; n	8	13	14	7	11	9	15	4	11	5	97

Table 2 Hand-to-surface exposures and hand hygiene actions *(Continued)*

Video	#1	#2	#3	#4	#5	#6	#7	#8	#9	#10	Overall
Hand hygiene action at colonization event; n (% of patient colonization events, i.e. 'adherence')	0	3 (11.5)	2 (8.7)	1 (6.2)	3 (12.0)	2 (3.7)	0	2 (6.7)	1 (2.7)	0	14 (4.8)
Hand hygiene action at infection event; n (% of patient infection events, i.e. 'adherence')	0	0	0	0	0	0	2 (3.9)	0	1 (2.9)	NA	3 (1.4)
Average density of hand hygiene actions; n/hour	13.8	22.4	24.1	11.6	21.1	16.5	26.9	14.4	20.4	18.1	19.6
Mean duration of hand hygiene actions (SD); sec	8.6 (4.7)	14.9 (6.6)	22.2 (11.0)	18.8 (7.4)	11.7 (4.5)	9.2 (4.8)	10.5 (9.6)	16.3 (12.0)	7.9 (3.7)	11.6 (6.2)	13.2 (8.6)

Legend: *HSE* hand-to-surface exposure; *ICU* intensive care unit; *F* female; *M* male; *N* nurse; *P* physician; *NA* not applicable; *SD* standard deviation. Definition for *patient colonization event* and *patient infection event* s. main text what can be done to improve it [20, 21]. In doing so, the moments we report here are more frequent than those usually reported in direct hand hygiene observation studies. For example, tasks such as a dressing change are typically seen as constituting one single hand hygiene opportunity with an indication 'Before clean/aseptic procedure' before the task and 'After body fluid exposure risk' at the end of the task [10]. In the current approach, each care task is split into multiple HSEs, taking into account both mobile objects [22] and the HCWs own body, each scrutinized for potential hand contamination and transmission. Furthermore, traditional hand hygiene models are based on the assumption that surfaces within the patient zone are colonized primarily with the patient's own flora. Our results [11], however, demonstrate that frequent transitions of hands into the patient zone without hand hygiene may lead to contamination of the patient zone with foreign microorganisms. Such lapses lead to an unsafe system state, which creates ambiguity [23] and may result in unintentional patient harm.

Our approach revealed further noteworthy realities. We considered the HCW's own body as an 'Outside patient zone' surface. More than half of all HSE sequences (61%) from the "outside" to the "inside" patient zone were due to 'self-contact'. Current hand hygiene guidelines often fail to address HCW self-contact as an indication for hand hygiene [17]. Hence, such HSE are usually ignored by observers. Second, much variation exists in whether HCWs perceive their professional apparel as a potential source of bacteria, leading to variations in hand hygiene [24]. Additionally, as described by Sax & Clack, relying on automatic, unconscious behaviors fuelled by "mental models" for routine tasks is inherent to the nature of human beings, allowing mental resources to be spared for more complex tasks [11]. This suggests that people often are unaware of what exactly their hands do while they are focused on the main task goal [11]. The average of 1.48 exposures per minute to a HCW's own body is consistent with previous findings [25, 26]. However, with only 4.87 exposures per hour to "HCW Face", our results differed from studies who found that face contact occurred up to 15–23 times per hour among students during 2-h lectures [26] or during office-type work [25]. Finally, glove use was frequent, representing one fifth of all HSE. Gloves represent mobile surfaces that transport microorganisms like bare hands. Further research could explore the nature of HSE during glove use to inform best practice for glove indications.

The "first-person view" of a head-mounted action camera provides the advantage of an unobstructed view of both hands and the surfaces they touch following the healthcare worker [27] even when leaving the immediate care area, neither of which can be guaranteed with a fixed-position camera. From anecdotal reports by the participants, their awareness of wearing a camera and their activity being registered waned quickly, suggesting a minor Hawthorne effect, yet this remains to be studied systematically. Contrary to concerns about video recording in acute care settings, we found that once healthcare workers, patients, and their relatives were informed of the study goals, objections to filming were rare. Video observation of hand hygiene behavior has been used before [28–31] but never from a first-person view and never to record HSEs.

Our approach has limitations. The analysis is limited to a small sample of healthcare workers in three ICUs and in consequence not representative for care in general. We do not expect, however, the main findings of frequent HSE to be categorically different. Furthermore, while the sequential analysis we report here considers only pairs of two consecutive HSE leading up to "colonization" or "infection" events, it is important to recognize that HSE occur in long sequential chains. The exact benefit of hand hygiene at any of these moments has not been considered in our current calculation, nor in the WHO 'Five moments' concept. In this line of thought, our approach might serve as basis for more advanced future transmission risk modelling. Our definition of a *colonization event* deviated from 'Moment 1' of the WHO hand hygiene concept by including any object within the patient zone, not only the patient. We did this intentionally to identify the transmission trajectories most likely leading to contamination of high-touch surfaces near the patient and ultimately, the patient. On a technical note, the specific software is expensive and its use requires expertise. Video coding is more time-consuming than live observation. Hence, before introducing this instrument into day-to-day practice beyond research, simplification and automation is a desirable next development step. Finally, the videos were coded by a single coder (MS) and supervised by a second person (LC) due to feasibility. The possibility to pause and rewind the video likely minimized the risk of miscoding.

In conclusion, our approach produced a valid video and coding instrument for analysis of detailed HSE trajectories. Using a head-mounted action camera and a comprehensive coding system, we could show for the first time in a fast-paced, real clinical setting how frequently healthcare workers' hands touch surfaces, corroborating the fast spread of microorganisms in healthcare settings. Further development and use of this method may contribute to the design of more efficient preventive strategies.

Conclusions

Using a new head-mounted action camera and a systematic coding tool, we could show for the first time how healthcare workers' hands touch surfaces in a real-world clinical setting. This human factors approach to task analysis demonstrated the hand trajectories via which microorganisms can spread in healthcare and revealed that hand hygiene adherence is lower than usually reported by traditional on-site observations. This new instrument may assist in designing more efficient preventive strategies on an individual and systems level.

Acknowledgements
We would like to warmly thank the healthcare workers and patients who had the courage and kindness to contribute to this research.

Funding
This research was partially funded by the Swiss Science Foundation grant 32003B_149474.

Authors' contributions
All authors contributed to the design, conduct of the study, the analysis of the data, and the writing of the manuscript. All authors read and approved the final manuscript.

Ethics approval and consent to participate
Due to the quality improvement scope of this study, the Ethics Review Board of the Canton of Zurich formally waived the need for ethics review. Signed consent was sought of patients or their relatives in accordance with the University Hospital Zurich regulations for videotaping and photography. Participants gave their oral consent after an in-depth explanation of the study goals and proceedings and could opt out at any time. Data were rendered anonymous in the coding database.

Consent for publication
Not applicable

Competing interests
The authors declare that they have no competing interests.

References
1. Harbarth S, Sax H, Gastmeier P. The preventable proportion of nosocomial infections: an overview of published reports. J Hosp Infect. 2003;54:258–266; quiz 321.
2. Graves N, Weinhold D, Tong E, Birrell F, Doidge S, Ramritu P, et al. Effect of healthcare-acquired infection on length of hospital stay and cost. Infect Control Hosp Epidemiol. 2007;28:280–92. DOI: 10.1086/512642.
3. Umscheid CA, Mitchell MD, Doshi JA, Agarwal R, Williams K, Brennan PJ. Estimating the proportion of healthcare-associated infections that are reasonably preventable and the related mortality and costs. Infect Control Hosp Epidemiol. 2011;32:101–14. DOI: 10.1086/657912.
4. Antimicrobial resistance. Geneva: World Health Organization; 2014. Available from: http://apps.who.int/iris/bitstream/10665/112642/1/9789241564748_eng.pdf. Accessed 19 Oct 2017.
5. Boyce JM, Pittet D, Committee HICPA, Force HSAIHHT. Guideline for hand hygiene in health-care settings. Recommendations of the healthcare infection control practices advisory committee and the HICPAC/SHEA/APIC/IDSA hand hygiene task force. Society for Healthcare Epidemiology of America/Association for Professionals in infection control/Infectious Diseases Society of America. MMWR Recomm Rep. 2002;51:1–45, quiz CE1-4.
6. Pittet D, Allegranzi B, Sax H, Dharan S, Pessoa-Silva CL, Donaldson L, et al. Evidence-based model for hand transmission during patient care and the role of improved practices. Lancet Infect Dis. 2006;6:641–52. DOI: 10.1016/S1473-3099(06)70600-4.
7. Clack L, Schmutz J, Manser T, Sax H. Infectious risk moments: a novel, human factors-informed approach to infection prevention. Infect Control Hosp Epidemiol. 2014;35:1051–5. DOI: 10.1086/677166.
8. Thomas Y, Boquete-Suter P, Koch D, Pittet D, Kaiser L. Survival of influenza virus on human fingers. Clin Microbiol Infect. 2014;20:O58–64. DOI: 10.1111/1469-0691.12324.
9. L'Huillier AG, Tapparel C, Turin L, Boquete-Suter P, Thomas Y, Kaiser L. Survival of rhinoviruses on human fingers. Clin Microbiol Infect. 2015;21: 381–5. DOI: 10.1016/j.cmi.2014.12.002.
10. Sax H, Allegranzi B, Uçkay I, Larson E, Boyce J, Pittet D. My five moments for hand hygiene': a user-centred design approach to understand, train, monitor and report hand hygiene. J Hosp Infect. 2007;67:9–21. 10.1016/j.jhin.2007.06.004.
11. Sax H, Clack L. Mental models: a basic concept for human factors design in infection prevention. J Hosp Infect. 2015;89:335–9. 10.1016/j.jhin.2014.12.008.
12. Boyce JM. Hand hygiene compliance monitoring: current perspectives from the USA. J Hosp Infect. 2008;70(Suppl 1):2–7. DOI: 10.1016/S0195-6701(08)60003-1.
13. Braun BI, Kusek L, Larson E. Measuring adherence to hand hygiene guidelines: a field survey for examples of effective practices. Am J Infect Control. 2009;37:282–8. DOI: 10.1016/j.ajic.2008.09.002.
14. Organization. WH. WHO guidelines for hand hygiene in health care. Geneva, Switzerland: World Health Organization; 2009.
15. Sax H, Allegranzi B, Chraïti MN, Boyce J, Larson E, Pittet D. The World Health Organization hand hygiene observation method. Am J Infect Control. 2009; 37:827–34. DOI: 10.1016/j.ajic.2009.07.003.
16. Ward MA, Schweizer ML, Polgreen PM, Gupta K, Reisinger HS, Perencevich EN. Automated and electronically assisted hand hygiene monitoring systems: a systematic review. Am J Infect Control. 2014;42:472–8. DOI: 10.1016/j.ajic.2014.01.002.
17. WHO guidelines on hand hygiene in health care. Geneva: World Health Organization; 2009. Available from: http://apps.who.int/iris/bitstream/10665/44102/1/9789241597906_eng.pdf. Accessed 19 Oct 2017.
18. Pires D, Soule H, Bellissimo-Rodrigues F, Gayet-Ageron A, Pittet D. Hand hygiene with alcohol-based hand rub: how long is long enough? Infect Control Hosp Epidemiol. 2017;38:547–52. DOI: 10.1017/ice.2017.25.
19. Stanton NA. Hierarchical task analysis: developments, applications, and extensions. Appl Ergon. 2006;37:55–79. DOI: 10.1016/j.apergo.2005.06.003.
20. Clack L, Sax H. Annals for hospitalists inpatient notes - human factors engineering and inpatient care-new ways to solve old problems. Ann Intern Med. 2017;166:HO2–3. DOI: 10.7326/M17-0544.
21. Clack L, Sax H. Human factors design. In: Pittet D, Boyce J, Allegranzi B, editors. Hand hygiene - a handbook for medical professionals. Hospital medicine: current concepts. Chichester, UK: John Wiley & Sons, Inc.; 2017. p. 185–8.
22. Longtin Y, Schneider A, Tschopp C, Renzi G, Gayet-Ageron A, Schrenzel J, et al. Contamination of stethoscopes and physicians' hands after a physical examination. Mayo Clin Proc. 2014;89:291–9. DOI: 10.1016/j.mayocp.2013.11.016.
23. Gurses AP, Seidl KL, Vaidya V, Bochicchio G, Harris AD, Hebden J, et al. Systems ambiguity and guideline compliance: a qualitative study of how intensive care units follow evidence-based guidelines to reduce healthcare-associated infections. Qual Saf Health Care. 2008;17:351–9. DOI: 10.1136/qshc.2006.021709.
24. Whitby M, Pessoa-Silva CL, McLaws ML, Allegranzi B, Sax H, Larson E, et al. Behavioural considerations for hand hygiene practices: the basic building blocks. J Hosp Infect. 2007;65:1–8. DOI: 10.1016/j.jhin.2006.09.026.
25. Nicas M, Best D. A study quantifying the hand-to-face contact rate and its potential application to predicting respiratory tract infection. J Occup Environ Hyg. 2008;5:347–52. DOI: 10.1080/15459620802003896.
26. Kwok YL, Gralton J, McLaws ML. Face touching: a frequent habit that has implications for hand hygiene. Am J Infect Control. 2015;43:112–4. DOI: 10.1016/j.ajic.2014.10.015.
27. Nair AG, Kamal S, Dave TV, Mishra K, Reddy HS, Della Rocca D, et al. Surgeon point-of-view recording: using a high-definition head-mounted video camera in the operating room. Indian J Ophthalmol. 2015;63:771–4. DOI: 10.4103/0301-4738.171506.
28. Swoboda SM, Earsing K, Strauss K, Lane S, Lipsett PA. Electronic monitoring and voice prompts improve hand hygiene and decrease nosocomial infections in an intermediate care unit. Crit Care Med. 2004;32:358–63. DOI: 10.1097/01.CCM.0000108866.48795.0F.

29. Sahud AG, Bhanot N, Radhakrishnan A, Bajwa R, Manyam H, Post JC. An electronic hand hygiene surveillance device: a pilot study exploring surrogate markers for hand hygiene compliance. Infect Control Hosp Epidemiol. 2010;31:634–9. DOI: 10.1086/652527.
30. Armellino D, Hussain E, Schilling ME, Senicola W, Eichorn A, Dlugacz Y, et al. Using high-technology to enforce low-technology safety measures: the use of third-party remote video auditing and real-time feedback in healthcare. Clin Infect Dis. 2012;54:1–7. DOI: 10.1093/cid/cir773.
31. Palmore TN, Henderson DK. Big brother is washing...Video surveillance for hand hygiene adherence, through the lenses of efficacy and privacy. Clin Infect Dis. 2012;54:8–9. DOI: 10.1093/cid/cir781.

9

An in vitro comparison of standard cleaning to a continuous passive disinfection cap for the decontamination of needle-free connectors

Anna L. Casey[*], Tarja J. Karpanen, Peter Nightingale and Tom S. J. Elliott

Abstract

Background: The optimal decontamination method for needle-free connectors is still unresolved. The objective of this study was to determine if a continuous passive disinfection cap is as effective as standard cleaning for the microbial decontamination of injection ports of two types of needle-free connectors.

Methods: The injection ports of needle-free connectors were inoculated with *Staphylococcus aureus* and allowed to dry. Disinfection caps containing 70% (*v/v*) isopropyl alcohol (IPA) were attached to the connectors for one, three or 7 days and were compared with needle-free connectors cleaned with 2% (*w/v*) chlorhexidine gluconate (CHG) in 70% (*v/v*) IPA. The number of *S. aureus* remaining on the injection ports was evaluated. Median $\log_{10}$ reductions and 95% confidence interval (CI) were calculated and data analyzed using the Mann-Whitney test.

Results: The application of the disinfection cap resulted in a significantly higher reduction in *S. aureus* than the 2% (*w/v*) CHG in 70% (*v/v*) IPA wipe, achieving a > 5 $\log_{10}$ reduction in CFU at each time point.

Conclusions: The disinfection caps resulted in a significantly higher reduction in *S.aureus* on the injection ports when compared to the use of a 2% (*w/v*) CHG in 70% (*v/v*) IPA wipe. This offers an explanation for the lower rates of central-line associated bloodstream infection (CLABSI) associated with the use of disinfection caps reported in clinical studies.

Keywords: Disinfection cap, Wipe, Needle-free connectors, Isopropyl alcohol, Chlorhexidine

Background

There have been varying reports on the rates of bloodstream infection (BSI) associated with needle-free connectors including an increase in incidence following a change from split-septum connectors to mechanical connectors [1]. The Centers for Disease Control and prevention (CDC) has subsequently recommended that when needleless systems are used, a split-septum valve may be preferred over some mechanical valves [2]. Furthermore, The Society for Healthcare Epidemiology of America (SHEA) and the Infectious Diseases Society of America (IDSA) advised that positive-pressure needleless connectors with mechanical valves should not be used before a thorough assessment of risks, benefits, and education regarding proper use [3]. The FDA requested that manufacturers of positive-displacement devices should conduct post-market surveillance to demonstrate that their devices were not associated with an increased risk of BSI compared to other types of device. A SHEA/IDSA practice update subsequently stated that the optimal needle-free connector design for the prevention of infection was still unresolved and an assessment of risks, benefits and education was again recommended [4].

Many factors have been attributed to the level of infection risk associated with needle-free connectors and includes the efficacy of disinfection of the injection ports [5]. It has also been suggested that surface disinfection

* Correspondence: anna.casey@uhb.nhs.uk
University Hospitals Birmingham NHS Foundation Trust, Birmingham B15 2TH, UK

of needle-free connectors is not intuitive which may lead to non-compliance [5].

Caps which attach to injection ports of needle-free connectors incorporating disinfectants have been developed. Menyhay and Maki described such a device containing 2% chlorhexidine gluconate (CHG) in 70% isopropyl alcohol (IPA) in 2006 [6]. The caps act as passive disinfection devices which are designed to ensure that needle-free connectors are always clean.

Several clinical studies have evaluated the use of these passive disinfection devices, all of which demonstrate benefits including significant reductions in the rates of hub microbial colonisation [7], and central-line associated bloodstream infections (CLABSI) [8–12].

Whilst these studies represent the clinical scenario whereby adherence to decontaminating the needle-free connector may not always be optimal, they do not investigate the efficacy of a defined cleaning method compared to passive disinfection caps under optimal, controlled conditions.

The aim of the study was to determine under controlled laboratory conditions whether a commercially available continuous passive disinfection cap which contains 70% (*v/v*) IPA was as effective for microbial decontamination of two different needle-free connectors when compared to defined standard cleaning with a 2% (*w/v*) CHG in 70% (*v/v*) IPA wipe.

Methods
Needle-free connectors and cleaning devices
The needle-free connectors used in this study were a neutral displacement connector - MicroClave™ (ICU Medical) and a positive-displacement connector - CareSite™ (BBraun). Curos® caps containing 70% (*v/v*) IPA (3 M Healthcare) were compared to 2% (*w/v*) CHG in 70% (*v/v*) IPA wipes (Sani-cloth CHG 2%, PDI) for decontamination of the needle-free connectors.

Contamination of needle-free connectors
An overnight culture of *Staphylococcus aureus* National Collection of Type Cultures (NCTC) 6538 on tryptic soy agar (Oxoid) was used to prepare a 1×10^8 CFU/mL suspension in tryptone sodium chloride (1 g/L tryptone [Oxoid], 8.5 g/L NaCl [Sigma-Aldrich] in distilled water) containing 3 g/L bovine albumin faction V [VWR International] and 3 ml/L defibrinated sheep blood [TCS Biosciences] in accordance with BS EN 16615:2015 [13].

Following one activation of each connector, the external injection port of each sterile needle-free connector were inoculated with a 50 µL suspension containing at least 5×10^6 CFU of *S. aureus* and allowed to air dry for 4 h at 20 °C. Whilst the high inoculum of *S.aureus* used in this study would not be expected in the clinical scenario, it permitted the identification of any differences present between the

two decontamination methods, was also representative of European standard antiseptic test conditions [13], and simulated a worst-case scenario in the clinical situation.

Evaluation of the variability in wiping technique by different operators
Needle-free connectors were cleaned for 15 s (through 180° 15 times) with a 2% (*w/v*) CHG in 70% (*v/v*) IPA wipe and allowed to dry for 30 s (this method was completed independently by two different experienced operators). A total of 54 of each type of needle-free connnector were studied (27 of each needle-free connector by each operator).

Evaluation of the prolonged effect of the decontamination procedures
Disinfection caps were attached to the needlefree-connectors for 1, 3 or 7 days and were compared with needle-free connectors cleaned with a 2% (*w/v*) CHG in 70% (*v/v*) IPA wipe. All the needle-free connectors were subsequently left at 20 °C in air for 1, 3 or 7 days. A total of 54 of each needle-free connector were studied per time point following each decontamination procedure. An identical number of control needle-free connectors which were contaminated as above and which were not decontaminated were also similarly studied and acted as positive controls for each sampling point.

Evaluation of the effect of a pre- and post-device activation wipe
Following contamination with *S. aureus*, 54 of each type of needle-free connector were cleaned as above for 15 s with a 2% (*w/v*) CHG in 70% (*v/v*) IPA wipe and allowed to dry for 30 s. These were then incubated for 7 days at 20 °C and then cleaned again with a 2% (*w/v*) CHG in 70% (*v/v*) IPA wipe prior to microbiological sampling.

Microbiological sampling of needle-free connectors
Needle-free connectors were immersed into bijous containing 1 mL of neutralizing solution consisting of 30 g/L Tween 80, 30 g/L saponin, 3 g/L lecithin, 1 g/L L-histidine, 5 g/L sodium thiosulphate in tryptone sodium chloride (all VWR International). Nullification of antimicrobial activity and non-microbial toxicity was verified prior to commencement of the study (unpublished data). The bijous were then sonicated for 10 min at 50 Hz. The entire volume of neutralizing solution was inoculated (in addition to dilutions from positive control connectors) onto chromogenic *S. aureus* plates (ChromID *S. aureus* [Biomerieux]) in duplicate.

Sample size calculation and statistical analysis
The aim of the study sample size was to demonstrate that each decontamination method achieved a 5 $\log_{10}$ reduction in the number of *S. aureus* (or 99.999% reduction).

Based on preliminary work, it was concluded that 54 of each type of needle-free connector in each scenario should give at least a 90% chance of achieving a 5 $\log_{10}$ reduction in CFU. Median $\log_{10}$ reductions and 95% confidence interval (CI) were calculated and data analyzed using the Mann-Whitney test. The level of significance was < 0.05.

Results

CFU counts on positive control needle-free connectors
The minimum CFU count on the controls (the needle-free connectors which were not decontaminated after inoculation with *S. aureus*) during the study was 5.17 $\log_{10}$ CFU for MicroClave™ and 5.49 $\log_{10}$ CFU for CareSite™ therefore total kill (TK) always represented a $\geq$ 5.17 or $\geq$ 5.49 $\log_{10}$ CFU reduction, respectively.

Evaluation of the variability in wiping technique by different operators
There was no significant difference between the two operators in terms of $\log_{10}$ CFU reduction of *S. aureus* following 15 s decontamination with a 2% (*w/v*) CHG in 70% (*v/v*) IPA wipe and drying for 30 s for both the MicroClave™ (4. 69, 95% CI = 3.56–5.29 vs 4.61, 95% CI = 3.99–5.21, *P* = 0. 73) and CareSite™ (5.10, 95% CI = 4.11-TK vs 5.10, 95% CI = 3.04-TK, *P* = 0.32). Furthermore, there was no difference in the overall $\log_{10}$ CFU reduction between the two different types of needle-free connectors (*P* = 0.18 for Micro-Clave™ and *P* = 0.70 for CareSite™).

Evaluation of the decontamination procedures on *S. aureus* counts.
The median and 95% CI $\log_{10}$ CFU reduction in *S. aureus* after decontamination for 15 s with a 2% (*w/v*) CHG in 70% (*v/v*) IPA wipe followed by incubation at room temperature for 1, 3 or 7 days or after application of the disinfection cap for 1, 3 or 7 days is shown in Table 1. The application of the disinfection cap resulted in a significantly higher $\log_{10}$ CFU reduction of the *S. aureus* than the 2% (*w/v*) CHG in 70% (*v/v*) IPA wipe, achieving a > 5 $\log_{10}$ reduction in CFU at each time point. Furthermore, there was no difference in the $\log_{10}$ CFU reduction of *S. aureus* between the two different types of needle-free connectors with any decontamination regime at any time-point.

Evaluation of the effect of a pre- and post-device activation wipe
Decontamination of both types of needle-free device with a 2% (*w/v*) CHG in 70% (*v/v*) IPA wipe both following inoculation with *S. aureus* and following each subsequent incubation period resulted in a higher $\log_{10}$ CFU reduction as compared to only cleaning following contamination for MicroClave™ only (*P* = 0.009). However, in line with the above findings, the disinfection cap still resulted in a significantly higher $\log_{10}$ CFU reduction (Table 1) as compared to the two decontaminations with 2% (*w/v*) CHG in 70% IPA (*v/v*) wipes for both needle-free connectors (MicroClave™ *P* = 0.041, CareSite™ *P* < 0. 0001, median [95% CI] = TK [TK-TK] for both types of connector).

Discussion
This study demonstrated that under controlled laboratory conditions a disinfection cap containing 70% (*v/v*) IPA was more effective at reducing microbial contamination of contaminated injection ports of needle-free connectors when compared to cleaning with 2% (*w/v*) CHG in 70% (*v/v*) IPA wipes even for 15 s. Indeed, the study demonstrated that the caps were associated with a significantly higher $\log_{10}$ CFU reduction than a 2% (*w/v*) CHG in 70% (*v/v*) IPA wipe at 1, 3 and 7 days and a

Table 1 Median (95%CI) $\log_{10}$ reductions of CFU of *Staphylococcus aureus* on two types of needle-free connectors injection ports after 1, 3 and 7 days following two decontamination methods

Day	Decontamination method	Connector studied: MicroClave®	Comparison of wipe vs disinfection cap (*P* value)	Connector studied: CareSite®	Comparison of wipe vs disinfection cap (*P* value)	Comparison of MicroClave® vs CareSite® (*P* value)
1	2% (*w/v*) CHG in 70% (*v/v*) IPA wipe	> 6.45[a] (4.97-TK)	< 0.0001[b]	TK (4.29-TK)	< 0.0001[b]	0.49
	Disinfection cap	TK (TK-TK)		TK (TK-TK)		0.75
3	2% (*w/v*) CHG in 70% (*v/v*) IPA wipe	4.66 (4.34–4.95)	< 0.0001[b]	4.77 (4.39–5.68)	< 0.0001[b]	0.98
	Disinfection cap	TK (TK-TK)		TK (TK-TK)		0.057
7	2% (*w/v*) CHG in 70% (*v/v*) IPA wipe	TK (TK-TK)	< 0.0001[b]	TK (5.20-TK)	< 0.0001[b]	0.15
	Disinfection cap	TK (TK-TK)		TK (TK-TK)		1.00

[a]the median was half-way between the values of 6.45 and total kill (TK)
[b]The reductions were greater for the disinfection cap

two-clean regime used at 7 days. This was the case for both types of needle-free connectors tested during this study, demonstrating the efficacy across more than one specific device. Indeed, no differences in $\log_{10}$ CFU reductions between these devices were observed. The reasons for this difference in efficacy of the cap versus wipe is unresolved but may reflect the continuous antimicrobial activity of the decontamination offered by the caps rather than the relatively short time following the wipes. Another confounding factor is compliance to decontamination of needle-free connectors in clinical practice. Adherence to recommended decontamination procedures by healthcare workers prior to access of needle-free connectors has been reported to be as low as 10% [14], whereas with the use of caps compliance has been high [8–10]. Indeed, the enhanced efficacy of the caps has also been reflected in decreased rates of CLABSI with increasing cap compliance [11, 15].

It is therefore conceivable that not only the improved antimicrobial activity of the caps versus wipes together with high levels of compliance with disinfection caps may both in part account for the lower rates of CLABSI associated with their use reported in previous clinical studies.

It could also be concluded that given the significant $\log_{10}$ CFU reductions observed with the 2% (w/v) CHG in 70% (v/v) IPA wipe in this study, there is no requirement for the additional efficacy of the disinfection cap. However, if compliance with the use of wipes is low, the disinfection caps could prove a useful tool. Furthermore, since there is concern surrounding potential chlorhexidine- and cross-resistance to antibiotics [15, 16], the use of a decontamination regime in the absence of chlorhexidine (such as the disinfection cap used in this study) may be appealing.

A potential limitation of this current study is that the selected single decontamination of the injection ports with a wipe may not be representative of the frequency with which this would occur in the clinical scenario. Similarly, if the disinfection caps were employed in the inpatient clinical scenario they would be accessed and replaced more frequently. This would be the case in clinical areas where IV devices are frequently accessed such as in critical care. However, the selected decontamination regimen used in this current study is representative of the outpatient scenario where central venous catheters may be accessed just once a week during clinic visits. We therefore considered that the comparison of the two decontamination regimes in this study to be representative of this latter clinical scenario. A further advantage of this experimental approach was it allowed the longevity of the antimicrobial activity of the cap to be evaluated.

Besides reports of overcoming compliance issues and decreased rates of CLABSI there are several other documented advantages associated with the use of disinfection caps. These include time savings [17], healthcare worker preference [17], a reduction in contamination of blood cultures [9], and cost savings [8, 9, 11].

All these advantages present a persuasive argument to utilise these devices in clinical practice.

Conclusion

The results of this study support the SHEA/IDSA practice special approach recommendation for preventing CLABSI to 'use an antiseptic-containing hub/connector cap/port protector to cover connectors (quality of evidence: I)' [4].

Abbreviations

BSI: Bloodstream infection; CDC: Centers for Disease Control and Prevention; CFU: Colony forming unit; CHG: Chlorhexidine gluconate; CI: Confidence interval; CLABSI: Central line-associated bloodstream infection; FDA: Food and Drug Administration; IDSA: Infectious Diseases Society of America; IPA: Isopropyl alcohol; NCTC: National Collection of Type Cultures; SHEA: Society for Healthcare Epidemiology of America; TK: Total kill; v/v: Volume/volume; w/v: Weight/volume

Acknowledgements

We would like to thank Karen Burgess for her assistance in the laboratory.

Funding

Funding for this study was provided by 3 M. 3 M was not involved in the collection, analysis, and interpretation of data and the preparation, submission, and review of this manuscript.

Authors' contributions

ALC, TK were involved in the design, execution and analysis of the study and writing the associated manuscript. TE and PN were involved in the design and analysis of the study and writing the manuscript. All authors read and approved the final manuscript.

Consent for publication

Not applicable

Competing interests

TSJE and ALC have received honoraria from BD for attendance at advisory board meetings and presentations at symposia. TSJE and TJK have received honoraria from 3 M for attendance at advisory board meetings and presentations at symposia. PN has no conflicts to declare. This work was presented in part as a poster at the 5th World Congress on Vascular Access, June 20-22 2018, Copenhagen, Denmark.

References

1. Jarvis WR, Murphy C, Hall KK, et al. Healthcare-associated bloodstream infections associated with negative- or positive-pressure or displacement mechanical valve needleless connectors. Clin Infect Dis. 2009;49:1821–7.
2. O'Grady NP, Alexander M, Burns LA, et al. Guidelines for the prevention of intravascular catheter-related infections. Clin Infect Dis. 2011;52(9):e162–93.

3. Marschall J, Mermel LA, Classen D, et al. Strategies to prevent central line-associated bloodstream infections in acute care hospitals. Infect Control Hosp Epidemiol. 2008;29(Suppl 1):S22–30.

4. Marschall J, Mermel LA, Fakih M, et al. Strategies to prevent central line-associated bloodstream infections in acute care hospitals: 2014 update. Infect Control Hosp Epidemiol. 2014;35(7):753–71.

5. Moureau NL, Flynn J. Disinfection of needleless connector hubs: clinical evidence systematic review. Nurs Res Pract 2015;2015:article 796762.

6. Menyhay SZ, Maki DG. Disinfection of needleless catheter connectors and access ports with alcohol may not prevent microbial entry: the promise of a novel antiseptic-barrier cap. Infect Control Hosp Epidemiol 2006;27(1):23–27.

7. Gutiérrez Nicolás F, Nazco Casariego GJ, Viña Romero MM, Gonzalaz Garcia J, Ramos Diaz R, Perez Perez JA. Reducing the degree of colonisation of venous access catheters by continuous passive disinfection. Eur J Hosp Pharm. 2016;23:131–3.

8. Merrill KC, Sumner S, Linford L, Taylor C, Macintosh C. Impact of universal disinfectant cap implementation on central-line associated bloodstream infections. Am J Infect Control. 2014;40(12):1274–7.

9. Sweet MA, Cumpston A, Briggs F, Craig M, Hamadani M. Impact of alcohol-impregnated port protectors and needleless neutral pressure connectors on central line associated bloodstream infections and contamination of blood cultures in an inpatient oncology unit. Am J Infect Control. 2012;40(10):931–4.

10. Ramirez C, Lee AM, Welch K. Central venous catheter protective connector caps reduce intraluminal catheter-related infection. The. J Assoc Vasc Access. 2012;17(4):210–3.

11. Stango C, Runyan D, Stern J, Macri I, Vacca M. A successful approach to reducing bloodstream infections based on a disinfection device for intravenous needleless connector hubs. J Infus Nurs. 2014;37(6):462–5.

12. Wright MO, Tropp J, Schora DM, et al. Continuous passive disinfection of catheter hubs prevents contamination and bloodstream infection. Am J Infect Control. 2013;41:33–8.

13. BS EN 16615:2015. Chemical disinfectants and antiseptics – quantitative test method for the evaluation of bactericidal and yeasticidal activity on non-porous surfaces with mechanical action employing wipes in the medical area (4- field test) – Test method and requirements (phase 2, step 2). Available from BSI, London.

14. Lee J. Disinfection cap makes critical difference in central line bundle for reducing CLABSIs. In: Proceedings of the APIC annual conference, vol 39. Fort Lauderdale; 2013. p. E64.

15. Kampf G. Acquired resistance to chlorhexidine – is it time to establish an 'antiseptic stewardship' initiative? J Hosp Infect. 2016;94:213–27.

16. Vali L, Davies SE, Lai LLG, Dave J, Amyes SGB. Frequency of biocide resistance genes, antibiotic resistance and the effect of chlorhexidine exposure on clinical methicillin-resistant Staphylococcus aureus isolates. J Antimicrob Chemother. 2008;61:524–32.

17. Cameron-Watson C. Port protectors in clinical practice: an audit. British J Nursing. 2016;25(8):S25–31.

10

Antibacterial efficacy of local plants and their contribution to public health in rural Ethiopia

Gutema Taressa Tura, Wondwossen Birke Eshete and Gudina Terefe Tucho[*]

Abstract

Background: Proper hand hygiene with soap and detergents prevents the transmission of many infectious diseases. However, commercial detergents are less likely to be accessible or affordable to poor people in remote rural areas. These people traditionally use some plant parts as a detergent even though their antibacterial activity has not been yet investigated. Therefore, this study aims to determine the antibacterial activities of some of the plants against bacteria isolated from humans.

Methods: Plants selected for this study are *Phytolacca dodecandra fruits*, *Rumex nepalensis* leaves, *Grewia ferruginea* bark and leaves. The samples of these plants were collected from rural areas of Jimma town based on their ethno-botanical survey and information on their local use. Acetone was used as a solvent to extract the bioactive constituents of the plants. The antibacterial activities of the plants were evaluated against reference strains and bacteria isolated from humans using disc diffusion and macro dilution methods.

Results: The plant extracts have shown varying antimicrobial activities against the bacterial species tested. Susceptibility testing shows zones of inhibition ranging from 8.0 ± 1.0 mm to 20.7 ± 5.5 mm. The MIC and MBC of the plants against the bacterial species tested were 3.13 and 12.5 mg/ml respectively. These variations are attributed to different concentrations of the bioactive constituents of the extracts like saponins, tannins, flavonoids and terpenoids.

Conclusion: The studied plants can contribute to achieve better personal hygiene since they are effective against different bacterial agents and are freely available in rural areas.

Keywords: Plants, Phytochemical, Hand hygiene, Antibacterial, Antimicrobial resistance, Public health

Background

Soap has been used for personal hygiene for many centuries. The effectiveness of soap to clean dirt is based on its detergent properties. However, soaps containing antiseptic agents in addition to detergents are available since the 19th century [1, 2]. In particular, hands perform several activities through which they come into contact with contaminated objects. Hands will be routes for disease transmission if proper hand hygiene is not performed. In fact many infectious diseases are easily transmitted through hand contacts from the immediate environment [3, 4]. Many of the diseases in developing countries are related to fecal-oral transmission attributed to insufficient personal hygiene [5]. Hand hygiene is the simplest, most cost effective and easily applicable measure that can reduce the risk of spread of infectious diseases [6–8]. Nevertheless, the effectiveness of hand hygiene depends on the habit of using soap during washing [7, 9]. However, better microbial removal and hygiene might be more achieved when antimicrobial detergents are used instead of plain soap and water [1, 7].

There are many effective antimicrobial cleaning products available to provide better cleaning services. In particular, alcohol based cleaning agents are effective against gram negative and gram positive bacteria despite some limitations related to short time residual effects [10, 11]. Nevertheless, most effective commercial antimicrobial agents are

* Correspondence: guditerefe@gmail.com; gudina.terefe@ju.edu.et
Department of Environmental health Sciences and Technology, Jimma University, Jimma, Ethiopia

less likely accessible or affordable to poor people living in remote rural areas of developing countries to meet the goal of hand hygiene [12]. Alternatively, different plants with antimicrobial properties can replace expensive commercial antimicrobial products [13, 14]. Most plant products are effective including against harmful resistant micro-organisms [15].

People in rural areas have a rich tradition of using different parts of plants for personal hygiene. For instance, *Phytolacca dodecandra (P. dodecandra)* fruits, *Rumex nepalensis (R. nepalensis)* leaves and *Grewia ferruginea (G. ferruginea)* leaves and bark are some of the most commonly used plants in different rural areas of Ethiopia for cleaning purposes (i.e. bathing, washing clothes etc.). There are a lot of effective different plants used for personal hygiene in different parts of the world [16–19]. Several medicinal plants have been studied for their antibacterial activities against different pathogenic bacteria species [20–22]. Many of them were also found to be effective against resistant microbial strains [16, 23]. However, the antibacterial activities of plants used for personal hygiene have not been yet determined. These plants can be cost effective alternatives to modern detergents if their antibacterial activities are determined and promoted. Studying their antibacterial activity is not only to promote them as alternatives but also to preserve indigenous knowledge about the use of local plants for personal hygiene [24]. Therefore, this study aims to evaluate the antibacterial activities of some plants used for personal hygiene against bacterial colonizing the skin. The results can be vital in the promotion of low cost and effective cleaning materials in rural areas and in preserving indigenous knowledge about plants used for personal hygiene.

Methods
Plant sample collection and preparation
Different parts of healthy test plants of *P. dodecandra* (local name "Andoode") fruits, *R. nepalensis* (local name

"Timiji") leaves, *G. ferruginea* (local name "Dhoqonu") leaves and bark were collected from rural areas within the Jimma zone. The selection of the test plants was based on ethno-botanical surveys and relevant information of traditional use of the plants as detergents [21, 25]. The parts of the plants considered for sampling are frequently used for cleaning purposes.

The collected samples were washed under running clean tap water to eliminate adhering dust and any foreign particles and shaded to dry at room temperature for about 7–14 days. The dried samples were grinded with a mechanical grinder, sieved with a 2.5 mm sieve size and stored at 4 °C until considered for extraction [26]. The bioactive constituents of the plants were extracted with acetone. Acetone was selected as a solvent based on its low toxicity, easiness of extraction and easy evaporation [27]. The extraction was performed by dissolving 200 g of each plant's powder in 700 ml of acetone, shaken at constant speed of 300 rpm (HY-5A Maneuver style vibrator shaker) and filtered with Whatman No.1 filter paper. The contents were then dried and weighed for their extract yields and stored at 4 °C for microbial assay. The percentage extract yields of the plants were calculated as: Percentage extract yield $(\%) = \frac{\text{Weight of dried extract}}{\text{Weight of dried powder}} \times 100$ (Table 1).

Phytochemical screening
The phytochemical screenings of the plants were made based on qualitative methods used in other studies [28–30]. Saponins, tannins, flavonoids and terpenoids were bioactive compounds considered for identification based on their antimicrobial activities [31–35]. The concentration of the constituents was determined based on their relative color strength; the deeper the color the stronger the concentration of the constituents in the extracts.

Table 1 Ethno-botanical and relevant information of the plants

Name			Parts used	Traditional use	Picture of the plant part
Scientific	Family	Local			
Phytolacca dodecandra	Phytolaccaceae	Andoodee (Indodi)	Fruit	Used for washing of clothes, hands and body	
Rumex nepalensis	Polygonaceae	Timijii (Tult)	Leaf	Used for washing of hands and hair	
Grewia ferruginea	Tiliaceae	Dhoqonu (Lenkoata)	Leaf	Used for washing hair	
Grewia ferruginea	Tiliaceae	Dhoqonu (Lenkoata)	Bark	Used for washing hair	

Identification of Saponins was made by using a foam test by adding 5 ml of distilled water to 0.5 g of the extracts, shaken vigorously and observed for its frothing. Again three drops of olive oil were added and shaken vigorously for the formation of emulsions indicating the presence of saponins. The test for identification of tannins was done by mixing 0.5 g of the extracts with distilled water and heating on a water bath until the extracts were fully dissolved. The formation of a dark green color indicates the presence of tannins upon addition of 0.1% ferric chloride. Identification of the presence of flavonoids was made by adding 0.2 g of the extracts to 2 ml of 2% solution of NaOH. An intense yellow color was formed which turned colorless upon addition of few drops of diluted HCl indicating the presence of flavonoids. Finally, identification of terpenoids was made by mixing 0.2 g of the extracts with 2 ml of chloroform ($CHCl_3$) and 3 ml of concentrated sulfuric acid (H_2SO_4) whereby the formation of a layer with a reddish-brown color interface indicates the presence of terpenoids.

Isolation and identification of bacteria species
Isolation and susceptibility testing of the bacterial species were done by using standardized procedures [36–38]. Isolation of the test bacteria was done by using sterile cotton swabs soaked in 0.85% sterile saline solution. The samples were taken from palms, fingers and fingernails of the left and right hands of individuals working in hospital and food handling activities and preserved at 4 °C in saline solution.

Prior to culturing, MacConkey agar, Mannitol salt agar, Xylose Lysine Desoxycholate agar (XLD agar) and selenite F broth were prepared according to the instruction of the manufacturer and the operating standard procedures [38, 39]. Subsequently, the swab samples were soaked in saline solution, vigorously shaken and 0.2 ml of the solution was cultured on the media and incubated in an inverted position at 37 °C for 24 h. The media containing inoculum was then observed for the formation of distinct isolated colonies for further sub-culturing. Colonies for sub-culture were considered based on the colony morphology of culture positive samples. Accordingly, Lactose fermenting colonies (LFCs) and non-lactose fermenting colonies (NLFCs) were characterized by pink color and pale color respectively on MacConkey agar. Small colonies surrounded by yellow zones or colonies changed the color of Mannitol Salt Agar (MSA) to yellow and white creamy colonies were also identified. Following gram staining, different biochemical and enzymatic reaction tests were done to identify bacteria into species. Therefore, we used oxidase, catalase, Klinger iron agar (KIA), lysine iron agar (LIA), Indole, Motility, Citrate, Urease, Triple sugar iron Agar (TSIA) and TSIA tests.

Due to resource constraints, classification of bacteria was done using the following basic biochemical approach [4, 38, 40]. Accordingly, the identification of *Salmonella* species was made by culturing the colony on Xylose Lysine Desoxycholate agar media enriched with a Selenite broth; thus colonies with a black center were identified as *Salmonella* species. Identification of *E.coli* was made by using MacConkey salt agar and fermentation of lactose with the formation of flat dry pink of irregular colonies. Identification of *S.aureus* was made by using Mannitol salt agar with the subsequent formation of yellow/golden colored colonies. *P. aeruginosa* identification was made by using nutrient agar and MacConkey agar. Colonies with large and irregular opaque bluish-green pigment on nutrient agar and non-lactose fermentation with colorless colonies on MacConkey agar were identified as *P. aeruginosa*. These species of bacteria are responsible for many communicable diseases in developing countries. In addition, most of them are resistant to ordinary antibacterial agents and are considered for the current antibacterial activity testing.

E. coli (ATCC 25922), P. aeruginosa (DSMZ 1117), S. typhimurium (ATCC 13311) and S. aureus (ATCC 25923), all American Type Culture Collections were obtained from the Microbiology lab of Jimma University as reference bacteria strains for a quality control.

Antibacterial activity testing
Inoculums for antibacterial testing were prepared by transferring pure bacteria strains grown on nutrient agar media to 5 ml sterile physiological saline solution (0.85% NaCl w/v). The suspended turbidity was adjusted to 0.5 McFarland standards corresponding to 1.5×10^8 CFU/ml [41]. The antibacterial activity testing of the plants was done by using a disc diffusion method [37]. The standardized suspension of bacterial strains of 1.5×10^8 CFU/ml was prepared and diffused on the Mueller Hinton agar (MHA) media with sterile swabs. Sterile filter paper discs of 6 mm diameter were impregnated with a 200 mg concentration of the plant extracts dissolved in 1 ml of DMSO, then placed on swabbed agar and incubated at 37° C for 24 h. The diameters of zones of inhibition were measured in millimeters using a ruler and the average of triplicate results were presented. A positive and negative control was done by 1% phenol solution and DMSO (without plant extracts) respectively.

Determining MIC and MBC of the plants
The Minimum Inhibitory Concentration (MIC) and Minimum Bactericidal Concentration (MBC) of the plants were determined based on standard procedures and cited literatures [42–44]. Accordingly, a stock solution with the concentration of the plant extracts of

200 mg in 1 ml of DMSO was diluted using a two-fold serial dilution. This provides the series of test concentrations of 100, 50, 25, 12.5, 6.25 and 3.13 mg/ml respectively. The plant's antibacterial activity testing was done by incubating each concentration of the extract with inoculum containing 0.1 ml of microbial cell at 37 °C for 24 h [45, 46]. The smallest concentration that inhibited the growth of the test bacteria was considered as MIC of the plants. The MBC of the plants was determined by transferring inoculums from MIC tubes to freshly prepared nutrient agar, incubated for 24 h at 37 °C with different concentrations of the extracts [23]. The smallest concentration of the extracts with no visible bacterial growth after incubation was taken as MBC.

Results
The extract yields of the plants and their phytochemical constituents
The method used for the extraction achieved varying extract yields ranging from 6.40 g to 15.47 g (Table 2). The highest percent extract yield was obtained from *P. dodecandra* fruits (7.74%) and the lowest (3.2%) was from *G. ferruginea* bark. Variations were also observed in the concentration of the phytochemical constituents of the plant parts and species. Phytochemical constituents are bioactive compounds with many antibacterial activities. Accordingly, all the evaluated plant species contain saponins, tannins and flavonoids in varying concentrations. However, terpenoids were not found in *P. dodecandra* fruits and *R. nepalensis* leaves (Table 3).

Antibacterial activities of the plants
The antibacterial activities of the plants are shown in Table 4. The data shows huge antibacterial activity variation among different plant species and parts. The extracts of the plants achieved varying zones of inhibition against both isolate and reference (standard) bacteria species. The highest zone of inhibition (20.7 ± 5.5 mm) was achieved with *R. nepalensis* leaves extract against reference *Salmonella* strain (*S. typhimerium*). The zones of inhibition of *P. dodecandra* fruits, and *G. ferruginea* leaves and bark against different bacterial species range from 9.0 ± 1.0 to 16.7 ± 1.2 mm (Mean ± SD). However, all of them achieved a relatively smaller zone of inhibition against isolated bacteria than their reference counterparts. The MIC and the MBC of the studied plants are shown in Fig.1. Their MIC

ranges from 3.13 mg/ml to 50 mg/ml while their MBC are between 6.25 mg/ml and 100 mg/ml. This implies that a higher concentration is needed for killing bacteria than for inhibiting their growth. The *G. ferruginea* leaves and bark extract showed the lowest MIC and MBC against *Salmonella* species while *R. nepalensis* similarly showed the lowest values against *E. coli*. Relatively, larger MIC and MBC were obtained with the extract of *G. ferruginea* and *R. nepalensis* against *S. aureus* and *P. aeruginosa*.

Discussion
Evaluation of the antibacterial activities of the plants
Among modern methods of extraction, maceration is effective in extracting bioactive compounds at room temperature [47]. These compounds contain broad spectrum antibacterial agents acting against different species of bacteria [34, 35, 48, 49]. Different plant species contain different concentrations of bioactive compounds (Table 3). The variation in antibacterial activity against both test and reference bacteria is found to be attributable to variation in bioactive constituents of the plants. The variation was also significant even within the same plant when evaluated against different bacteria species. The antibacterial activity of *R. nepalensis* against *Salmonella* species (*S. typhimurium*) and *P. aeruginosa* is a good example. This plant showed the highest inhibition against *Salmonella* species and no inhibition against *P. aeruginosa*. The variation can be attributed to the high concentration of tannins and the lack of terpenoids in this plant. Nevertheless, most plant extracts achieved smaller zones of inhibition against test bacteria than reference bacterial species due to probability of antibacterial resistance with isolate species. However, all the evaluated plant extracts possess antimicrobial activity with high susceptibility pattern of low MIC and MBC. Their low MIC and MBC indicates their high efficacy against nonresistant and resistant bacteria species [50]. In particular, plants with a high concentration of flavonoids (i.e. *P. dodecandra and G. ferruginea*) have shown better antibacterial activity against isolate bacterial species than the remaining test plant species and parts. Literature reported flavonoids as bioactive compounds with high antimicrobial activities against resistant strains [51, 52].

The bioactive constituents have different mechanism of action against bacterial cells. Tannins and Flavonoids act on bacterial cells through the formation of a complex

Table 2 The extract yields of the plants

S.No.	Plant parts	Weight of powder (gram)	Weight of extract (gram)	Percent extract yield (%)
1	*P.dodecandra fruit*	200	15.47	7.74
2	*R.nepalensis leaves*	200	7.10	3.55
3	*G.ferruginea bark*	200	6.40	3.20
4	*G.ferruginea leaves*	200	11.14	5.57

Table 3 Phythochemical constituents of the plants

S. No.	Phytochemical components	P.dodecandra fruit	R.nepalensis leaf	G.ferruginea bark	G.ferruginea leaf
1	Saponins	++	+	+++	+++
2	Tannins	++	+++	++	+
3	Flavonoids	+++	+	+++	++
4	Terpenoids	–	–	++	+++

Key: = absent; + = present in small amount; ++ = Present in moderate amount; +++ = present in high amount

with cell walls, binding to proteins, disruption of membranes and inhibition of enzymes. Antibacterial effects of saponins are achieved through inactivation of extracellular medium and membranes of the bacterial cell [13]. Saponins-rich extracts are less active against *S. aureus* compared to gram negative bacteria like *E.coli* and *P. aeruginosa* [53]. Studies indicated that most pathogenic bacteria such as *S.aureus* and *E.coli* isolated from the hands of health workers are resistant to many antimicrobial agents [54, 55]. However, the plants evaluated in the current study showed moderate to highest antibacterial activities against these organisms probably due to availability of bioactive compounds in high concentration. In particular, plants containing tannins, flavonoids and saponins are effective against resistant bacterial species [16]. This shows the effectiveness of the studied plants against various bacterial species.

Contribution of the plants to rural sanitation and public health

Most people living in rural areas of developing countries do not have sufficient income to afford the costs of modern antibacterial detergents. Moreover, most of them do not have sufficient awareness of the use of antibacterial detergents as a first line of defense against many communicable diseases [9, 56]. In addition, most of them do not have access to basic sanitation and clean water supply. Lack of access to basic sanitation and clean water can be solved by building the system providing the services. However, fecal-oral contamination and transmission of related diseases are inevitable if good hand hygiene is not practiced [57]. In areas where

commercial detergents are not available or affordable the studied plants can be used as an alternative. These plants are available in most rural areas throughout the year to use without any costs. Moreover, research shows that *S. aureus*, *E. coli* and *P. aeruginosa* species are resistant to most antibacterial agents [27]. However, all the test plants in the current study have shown antibacterial activity against these organisms with varying concentrations. This implies the possibility to use the ingredients of the plants in the formulation of commercial antibacterial detergents. However, the current study was not designed to provide its efficacy against resistant bacteria in a short contact time. Therefore, further investigation is needed to determine their efficacy with a short contact time. Nevertheless, the results are robust in promoting plant materials for hand hygiene in remote rural areas where commercial detergents are not available or not affordable to the poor.

Conclusion

The current study evaluated the antibacterial activities of three plant species traditionally used as detergents in rural areas of Ethiopia. All the test plant species have shown moderate to high antibacterial activity against the test bacteria species. *P.dodecandra* fruit and *G.ferruginea* bark and leaves have shown zones of inhibition ranging from 8 to 11 mm against *E. coli*, *S. aureus*, *P. aeruginosa* and *Salmonella* species. *R. nepalensis* also has shown zones of inhibition ranging from 9 to 12 mm against all test bacterial species except *P. aeruginosa*. In addition, all of them achieved better antibacterial activity with the smallest concentration of the extracts (i.e. lowest MIC

Table 4 Zone of inhibition (mean ± SD, n = 3) of the plants extracts in mm

Extracts	Bacteria strains							
	E.coli		S. aureus		P. aeruginosa		Salmonella spp.	
	Isolate	Ref.	Isolate	Ref.	Isolate	Ref.	Isolate	Ref.
P.dodecandra fruits	9.7 ± 0.6	11.3 ± 1.5	10.3 ± 2.1	12.3 ± 2.3	9.3 ± 2.5	12.0 ± 1.0	11.0 ± 1.0	16.3 ± 0.6
G. ferruginea leaf	10.0 ± 1.0	12 ± 0.0	9.7 ± 0.6	11.7 ± 0.6	9.0 ± 1.0	10.7 ± 1.5	11.0 ± 1.0	14.3 ± 0.6
G. ferruginea bark	8.0 ± 1.0	12.0 ± 2.6	9.0 ± 1.0	11.3 ± 2.9	9.7 ± 2.5	10.3 ± 1.2	9.3 ± 0.6	16.7 ± 1.2
R. nepalensis leaf	9.0 ± 1.0	10.3 ± 0.6	9.0 ± 1.0	12.0 ± 3.5	NI	NI	10.0 ± 1.0	20.7 ± 5.5
Phenol	7.3 ± 0.6	8.7 ± 1.5	8.0 ± 1.0	8.7 ± 1.2	7.7 ± 0.6	8.0 ± 1.7	5.0 ± 4.4	5.0 ± 4.4
DMSO	0	0	0	0	0	0	0	0

Key: ± SD = Standard Deviation, Ref. = Reference bacteria strain, NI = No Zone of inhibition, n = number of replicates

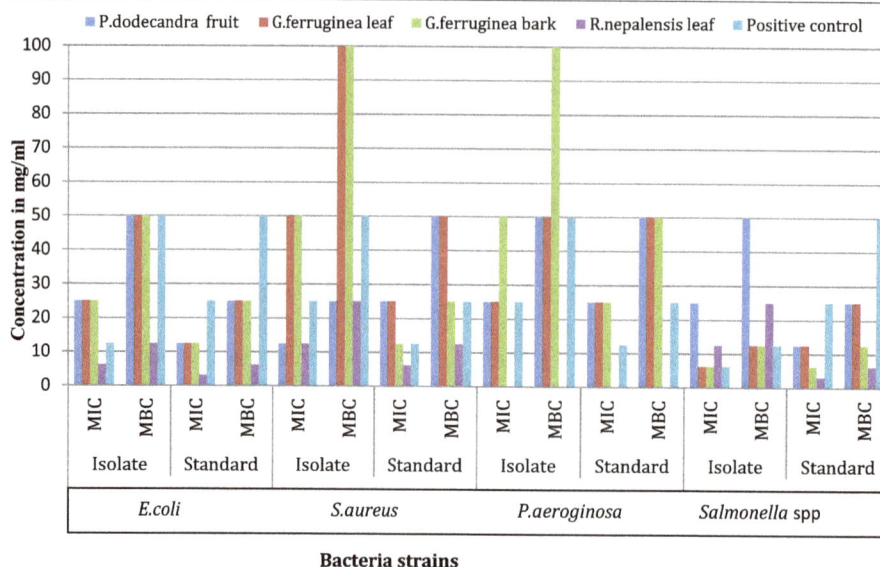

Fig. 1 MIC and MBC of the test plants and the positive control against different bacterial species

and MBC). The difference in antibacterial activity of the plants can be attributed to varying availability of the bioactive constituents. However, all of them contain effective bioactive constituents such as tannins, flavonoids and saponins in varying concentration. These constituents are effective against different bacterial species including resistant strains. Therefore, all the test plants are strong enough to replace commercial detergents and achieve good personal hygiene in rural areas where the accessibility or affordability of commercial detergents are limited or absent. These plants are abundantly available in rural areas to be a promising source of commercial antimicrobial agent production if further investigation is considered.

Abbreviations
DMSO: Dimethylsulfoxide; KIA: Klinger iron agar; LFCs: Lactose Fermenting Colonies; LIA: Lysine iron agar; MBC: Minimum Bactericidal Concentration; MHA: Mueller Hinton Agar; MIC: Minimum Inhibitory Concentration; NLFC: Non-lactose fermenting colonies; XLD: Xylose Lysine Desoxycholate

Acknowledgements
"Not applicable" in this section.

Funding
This study was supported by Jimma University College of public health and medical sciences research and post graduate office.

Authors' contributions
GTT (Gutema), designed the study, collected the data, did the experiment, analyzed the data, and wrote the first draft of the manuscript. GTT (Gudina) participated in the design of the study, supervised the whole process, reviewed and modified the draft of the manuscript. WBE (Wondwossen) participated in the study, supervision and review of manuscript. All authors read and approved the final manuscript.

Consent for publication
"Not applicable" in this section.

Competing interests
The authors declare that they have no competing interests.

References
1. Boyce JM, Pittet D. Guideline for hand hygiene in health-care settings: recommendations of the healthcare infection control practices advisory committee and the hicpac/shea/apic/idsa hand hygiene task force. Am J Infect Control. 2002;30(8):S1–S46.
2. Wolf R, et al. Soaps, shampoos, and detergents. Clin Dermatol. 2001; 19(4):393–7.
3. Simonne, A., Hand hygiene and hand sanitizers, in Department of Family, Youth and Community Sciences, Institute of Food and Agricultural Sciences (IFAS).2016, University of Florida.
4. Tambekar D, et al. Prevention of transmission of infectious disease: studies on hand hygiene in health-care among students. Cont J Biomed Sci. 2007;1: 6–10.
5. Tambekar DH, Shirsat SD. Hand washing: a cornerstone to prevent the transmission of Diarrhoeal infection. Asian J Med Sci. 2009;1(3):100–3.
6. Cossu A, et al. Assessment of sanitation efficacy against Escherichia Coli O157: H7 by rapid measurement of intracellular oxidative stress, membrane damage or glucose active uptake. Food Control. 2017;71:293–300.
7. Burton M, et al. The effect of handwashing with water or soap on bacterial contamination of hands. Int J Environ Res Public Health. 2011;8(1):97–104.
8. Curtis V, Cairncross S. Effect of washing hands with soap on diarrhoea risk in the community: a systematic review. Lancet Infect Dis. 2003;3(5):275–81.
9. Biran A, et al. The effect of a soap promotion and hygiene education campaign on handwashing behaviour in rural India: a cluster randomised trial. Tropical Med Int Health. 2009;14(10):1303–14.
10. Barnes, S., D. Concepcion, and G. Felizardo, Guide to the Elimination of Infections in Hemodialysis. Washington.–APIC.–2010.–78 p, 2010.
11. Larson E, et al. Skin reactions related to hand hygiene and selection of hand hygiene products. Am J Infect Control. 2006;34(10):627–35.
12. Revelas A. Acute gastroenteritis among children in the developing world: review. South Afr J Epidemiol Infect. 2012;27(4):156–62.
13. Cowan MM. Plant products as antimicrobial agents. Clin Microbiol Rev. 1999;12(4):564–82.
14. Handali S, et al. Formulation and evaluation of an antibacterial cream from Oxalis Corniculata aqueous extract. Jundishapur J Microbiol. 2011;4(4):255–60.
15. Wallace RJ. Antimicrobial properties of plant secondary metabolites. Proc Nutr Soc. 2004;63(04):621–9.
16. Ahmad I, Beg AZ. Antimicrobial and phytochemical studies on 45 Indian medicinal plants against multi-drug resistant human pathogens. J Ethnopharmacol. 2001;74(2):113–23.

17. Asafu Maradufu JKO, Sang BC, Khang'ati JE. Using Senecio lyratipartitus extract after anal ablution - Various documents on results from research grant. Baraton: University of Eastern Africa; 2013.

18. Vyas P. Antimicrobial activity of ayurvedic hand sanitizers. Int J Pharm & Bio Arch. 2011;2(2):1–5.

19. Wani NS, et al. Formulation and evaluation of herbal sanitizer. Int J PharmTech Res. 2013;5(1):40–3.

20. Geyid A, et al. Screening of some medicinal plants of Ethiopia for their anti-microbial properties and chemical profiles. J Ethnopharmacol. 2005; 97(3):421–7.

21. Suleman S, Alemu T. A survey on utilization of ethnomedicinal plants in Nekemte town, east Wellega (Oromia), Ethiopia. J Herbs, Spices Med Plants. 2012;18(1):34–57.

22. Tadeg H, et al. Antimicrobial activities of some selected traditional Ethiopian medicinal plants used in the treatment of skin disorders. J Ethnopharmacol. 2005;100(1):168–75.

23. Aliyu A, et al. Activity of plant extracts used in northern Nigerian traditional medicine against methicillin-resistant Staphylococcus Aureus (MRSA). Nigerian J Pharm Sci. 2008;7(1):1–8.

24. Mehta, P. and K. Bhatt, Traditional soap and detergent yielding plants of Uttaranchal. 2007.

25. Kumbi ET. Use and conservation of traditional medicinal plants by indigenous people in gimbi woreda, western wellega, ethiopia. Addis Ababa: Addis Ababa University; 2010.

26. Cannell RJ. How to approach the isolation of a natural product, in Natural Products Isolation: Springer; 1998. p. 1–51.

27. Tiwari P, et al. Phytochemical screening and extraction: a review. Internationale Pharmaceutica Sciencia. 2011;1(1):98–106.

28. Joshi B, et al. Phytochemical extraction and antimicrobial properties of different medicinal plants: Ocimum Sanctum (Tulsi), Eugenia Caryophyllata (clove), Achyranthes Bidentata (Datiwan) and Azadirachta Indica (Neem). Journal of Microbiology and Antimicrobials. 2011;3(1):1–7.

29. Longanga Otshudi A. A. Vercruysse, and A. Foriers, Contribution to the ethnobotanical, phytochemical and pharmacological studies of traditionally used medicinal plants in the treatment of dysentery and diarrhoea in Lomela area, Democratic Republic of Congo (DRC). J Ethnopharmacol. 2000; 71(3):411–23.

30. Yadav R, Agarwala M. Phytochemical analysis of some medicinal plants. Journal of phytology. 2011;3(12):1–5.

31. Joshi RK. Chemical constituents and antibacterial property of the essential oil of the roots of Cyathocline purpurea. J Ethnopharmacol. 2013;145(2):621–5.

32. Al-Snafi AE. Chemical constituents and pharmacological effects of Citrullus Colocynthis-a review. IOSR Journal Of Pharmacy. 2016;6(3):57–67.

33. Ezema BE, Odoemelam EI, Agbo MO. Phytochemical and antibiotic evaluation of the methanol extract of Loranthus Micranthus Linn parasitic on kola Accuminate. International Journal of PharmTech Research. 2016;9(2):176–81.

34. Boğa M, et al. Phytochemical profile and some biological activities of three Centaurea species from Turkey. Trop J Pharm Res. 2016;15(9):1865–75.

35. Kalaiselvi V, Binu TV, Radha SR. Preliminary phytochemical analysis of the various leaf extracts of Mimusops Elengi L. South Indian J Biol Sci. 2016;2(1):24–9.

36. Coyle, M.B., Manual of antimicrobial susceptibility testing. 2005: American Society for Microbiology.

37. Jorgensen, J.H. and J.D. Turnidge, Susceptibility test methods: dilution and disk diffusion methods, in Manual of Clinical Microbiology, Eleventh Edition. 2015, American Society of Microbiology. p. 1253–1273.

38. CLSI, ed. Performance Standards for Antimicrobial Susceptibility Testing 26th Edition. ed. P.C.a.L.S.I. CLSI supplement M100S. Wayne. 2016, Clinical and Laboratory Standards Institute.

39. Atlas RM. Handbook of microbiological media, fourth edition, vol. 1-1953: CRC Press; 2010.

40. Cheesbrough M. District laboratory practice in tropical countries: Cambridge university press; 2006.

41. Kiehlbauch JA, et al. Use of the National Committee for clinical laboratory standards guidelines for disk diffusion susceptibility testing in New York state laboratories. J Clin Microbiol. 2000;38(9):3341–8.

42. CLSI, Methods for dilution antimicrobial susceptibility tests f or bacteria that grow aerobically; approved St andard—ninth edition. CLSI document M07-A9. Wayne, PA:, 2012, Clinical and Laboratory Standards Institute.

43. Sule I, Agbabiaka T. Antibacterial effect of some plant extracts on selected Enterobacteriaceae. Ethnobotanical leaflets. 2008;2008(1):137.

44. Makut M, et al. Phytochemical screening and antimicrobial activity of the ethanolic and methanolic extracts of the leaf and bark of Khaya Senegalensis. Afr J Biotechnol. 2008;7(9);1216–9.

45. Das K, Tiwari R, Shrivastava D. Techniques for evaluation of medicinal plant products as antimicrobial agents: current methods and future trends. J Medicinal Plants Res. 2010;4(2):104–11.

46. Jagessar R, Mohamed A, Gomes G. An evaluation of the antibacterial and antifungal activity of leaf extracts of Momordica Charantia against Candida Albicans, Staphylococcus Aureus and Escherichia Coli. Nature and Science. 2008;6(1):1–14.

47. Gupta A, Naraniwal M, Kothari V. Modern extraction methods for preparation of bioactive plant extracts. International Journal of Applied and Natural Sciences (IJANS). 2012;1(1):8–26.

48. Ichim E, Marutescu L, Popa M, Cristea S. Antimicrobial efficacy of some plant extracts on bacterial ring rot pathogen, Clavibacter michiganensis ssp. sepedonicus. The EuroBiotech Journal. 2017;1(1):93–6.

49. Mohan Ch M, Smitha PV. Phytochemical composition and antimicrobial activity of three plant preparations used in folk medicine and their synergistic properties. J Herbs, Spices & Med Plants. 2011;17(4):339–50.

50. Njume C, Jide AA, Ndip RN. Aqueous and organic solvent-extracts of selected south African medicinal plants possess antimicrobial activity against drug-resistant strains of helicobacter pylori: inhibitory and bactericidal potential. Int J Mol Sci. 2011;12:5652–65.

51. Kumari I. Antibacterial activity of bud extract of Euphorbia Hirta L. against gram-positive bacteria Staphylococcus Aureus. Indian Journal of Applied Research. 2017;6(10);307–08.

52. Cushnie TT, Lamb AJ. Antimicrobial activity of flavonoids. Int J Antimicrob Agents. 2005;26(5):343–56.

53. Maatalah MB, et al. Antimicrobial activity of the alkaloids and saponin extracts of anabasis articulata. J Biotechnol Pharm Res. 2012;3(3):54–7.

54. Aiello AE, et al. A comparison of the bacteria found on the hands of 'homemakers' and neonatal intensive care unit nurses. J Hosp Infect. 2003; 54(4):310–5.

55. Chauhan, V., In vitro assessment of indigenous herbal and commercial antiseptic soaps for their antimicrobial activity, 2006, M. Sc. Dissertation in Biotechnology, Department of Biotechnology and Environmental Sciences, Thapar Institute of Engineering & Technology, Deemed University, Patiala, India.

56. Biran A, et al. Effect of a behaviour-change intervention on handwashing with soap in India (SuperAmma): a cluster-randomised trial. Lancet Glob Health. 2014;2(3):e145–54.

57. Pittet D, Allegranzi B, Boyce J. The World Health Organization guidelines on hand hygiene in health care and their consensus recommendations. Infect Control Hosp Epidemiol. 2009;30(07):611–22.

Intervening with healthcare workers' hand hygiene compliance, knowledge, and perception in a limited-resource hospital in Indonesia

Dewi Santosaningsih[1,2,3], Dewi Erikawati[1], Sanarto Santoso[1], Noorhamdani Noorhamdani[1,2], Irene Ratridewi[2], Didi Candradikusuma[2], Iin N. Chozin[2], Thomas E. C. J. Huwae[2], Gwen van der Donk[3], Eva van Boven[3], Anne F. Voor in 't holt[3], Henri A. Verbrugh[3] and Juliëtte A. Severin[3*]

Abstract

Background: Hand hygiene is recognized as an important measure to prevent healthcare-associated infections. Hand hygiene adherence among healthcare workers is associated with their knowledge and perception. This study aimed to evaluate the effect of three different educational programs on improving hand hygiene compliance, knowledge, and perception among healthcare workers in a tertiary care hospital in Indonesia.

Methods: The study was performed from May to October 2014 and divided into a pre-intervention, intervention, and post-intervention phase. This cluster randomized controlled trial allocated the implementation of three interventions to the departments, including role model training-pediatrics, active presentation-surgery, a combination of role model training and active presentation-internal medicine, and a control group-obstetrics-gynecology. Both direct observation and knowledge-perception survey of hand hygiene were performed using WHO tools.

Results: Hand hygiene compliance was observed during 2,766 hand hygiene opportunities, and knowledge-perception was assessed among 196 participants in the pre-intervention and 88 in the post-intervention period. After intervention, the hand hygiene compliance rate improved significantly in pediatrics (24.1% to 43.7%; $P < 0.001$), internal medicine (5.2% to 18.5%; $P < 0.001$), and obstetrics-gynecology (10.1% to 20.5%; $P < 0.001$). The nurses' incorrect use of hand rub while wearing gloves increased as well ($P < 0.001$). The average knowledge score improved from 5.6 (SD = 2.1) to 6.2 (SD = 1.9) ($P < 0.05$). In the perception survey, "strong smell of hand alcohol" as a reason for non-compliance increased significantly in the departments with intervention (10.1% to 22.9%; $P = 0.021$).

Conclusion: The educational programs improved the hand hygiene compliance and knowledge among healthcare workers in two out of three intervention departments in a limited-resource hospital in Indonesia. Role model training had the most impact in this setting. However, adjustments to the strategy are necessary to further improve hand hygiene.

Keywords: Hand hygiene, Healthcare-associated infections, Indonesia

* Correspondence: j.severin@erasmusmc.nl
[3]Department of Medical Microbiology and Infectious Diseases, Erasmus University Medical Center, 's-Gravendijkwal 230, Rotterdam 3015 CE, The Netherlands

Background

Healthcare-associated infections (HAIs) are known to be a threat in healthcare facilities, affecting morbidity, mortality, and length of stay of patients, and increase costs worldwide [1–5]. One of the most important measures to control the transmission of pathogens that may cause HAIs is hand hygiene [6, 7]. In 2005, the World Health Organization (WHO) launched the Clean Care is Safer Care campaign to encourage Member States to advocate hand hygiene. To support local improvement, a range of tools was published that were based on a multi-modal strategy with the following five components: system change, training and education, evaluation and feedback, reminders in the workplace, and institutional safety climate [1, 8]. Although the WHO guidelines and tools were designed in a way that would be of use in any setting regardless of the resources available and the cultural background, it was recognized that adaptation according to local needs, resources, and settings would be necessary [6]. Especially in developing countries, hand hygiene improvement requires a different approach than in developed countries [9]. In Indonesia, a low-middle income country, many efforts have been made over the past decade to improve the overall quality of healthcare including a national hospital accreditation program that incorporates infection control components. However, hospitals are still facing problems that typically occur in a developing country, such as overcrowding of wards and shortage of certain supplies [10, 11]. It is unknown which of the elements of the WHO multi-modal approach would have the greatest impact on the improvement of hand hygiene in such a setting [8]. Additionally, there is also only limited data on hand hygiene barriers [12]. This kind of information is necessary to redesign the approach into a suitable and feasible program for Indonesia and similar countries. This study aimed to assess the healthcare workers' (HCWs') hand hygiene compliance, knowledge, and perception in a limited-resource hospital in Indonesia before and after the implementation of three different educational programs.

Methods

Setting

The study was performed in Dr. Saiful Anwar hospital, a 902-bed tertiary care hospital, in Malang, Indonesia. In this hospital, there are four classes of care, including VIP (very important person), class I, II and III related to the room and care facilities. In this study, four departments including pediatrics, surgery, internal medicine, and obstetrics-gynecology (obst-gyn) were involved with characteristics as presented in Table 1. The alcohol-based hand rub that is used in the hospital is produced by the hospital pharmacist according to the WHO formulation II[6]. A hand rub container was attached to the footboard of each bed and next to each entrance door.

The Dr. Saiful Anwar hospital has an infection prevention control team that consists of eight infection prevention control nurses (IPCN), each representing a specific ward (internal medicine, surgery, obst-gyn, pediatrics, intensive care unit, VIP unit, emergency unit, and operation room unit). These nurses work part time as an infection control practitioner and part time as a nurse providing patient care in the wards. The IPCN coordinate a larger team of 48 infection prevention control-linked nurses (IPCLN) who are selected among senior nurses from the different wards. IPCN and IPCLN were recruited based on Pedoman Pencegahan dan Pengendalian Infeksi di Rumah Sakit dan Fasilitas Pelayanan Kesehatan Lainnya (Guideline of Infection Prevention and Control for Hospitals and other Healthcare Services) published by Ministry of Health of the Republic of Indonesia, 2008. Before the start of the study and partly during the study period, the hospital was preparing for a national hospital accreditation. Therefore, the hand hygiene procedure, according to the existing guideline, had been introduced to HCW by the IPCN and IPCLN in collaboration with the hospital accreditation team. In addition, posters presenting the hand hygiene procedures had been posted in the workplaces. Nevertheless, observations of the hand hygiene compliance had not been conducted by the infection prevention control team until the present study started.

Table 1 Characteristics of participating wards

Dept.	Type of ward involved	Facilities	Number of patients per room	Ratio nurse: patients	Type of intervention
IM	General ward: 4 rooms	Class I[a] (1 room)	1	1:5	Active presentations and role model training
		Class II[b] (1 room)	7–8	1:8	
		Class III[c] (2 rooms)	30	1:8	
SUR	Acute surgery unit: 1 room	Class III[c]	30	1:4	Active presentations
	General ward: 1 room	Class II[b]	7–8	1:6	
OBG	General ward: 2 rooms	Class III[c]	30	1:5	No intervention (control group)
PED	High care unit: 1 room	Class II[b]	14	1:2	Role model training
	Neonatology ward: 6 rooms	Class II[b]	7	1:5	

Abbreviations: *Dept.* Department, *IM* internal medicine, *SUR* surgery, *OBG* obstetrics-gynecology, *PED* pediatrics
[a]Patients have to share the bathroom with another patient; [b]patients share a bathroom together; [c]only one bathroom per room

Design

The design of the study was a pilot cluster randomized controlled trial, with a total duration of 24 weeks. The study was divided into three phases: pre-intervention (May to June 2014; 8 weeks), intervention (July to August 2014; 8 weeks), and post-intervention (September to October 2014; 8 weeks). The interventions consisted of three different educational programs: (1) active presentations; (2) role model training; (3) a combination of active presentations and role model training. By drawing lots, the four departments were randomly assigned to either one of the three educational interventions or to no intervention (Table 1). Active presentations to the HCW were held on at least three different occasions per ward to ensure that all HCW could participate and focused on the threat of HAIs and hand hygiene procedures [6]. In the intervention with role model training, IPCLN, as role models, received training about the hand hygiene educational program focusing on hand hygiene training techniques, including active presentations, discussions, practicing the hand hygiene procedure and the observation method. The theoretical part of HAIs and their prevention through high hand hygiene compliance was also presented to IPCLN. Therefore, they were able to motivate other HCW to better adhere to the hand hygiene procedures in the ward. The combination of active presentations and role model training was executed separately from the other interventions.

The main outcome and secondary outcome of the study was the hand hygiene compliance among HCW, including doctors, nurses, and students (either nursing students or medical students), and knowledge-perception regarding HAIs and hand hygiene among HCW obtained by a survey in the pre-intervention phase compared to the post-intervention phase, respectively. The direct observation method was applied to establish hand hygiene compliance rates, because this is considered the gold standard [13]. The observations were carried out several times a week during differing time slots, but not during the weekend. Every moment of observation lasted about 30 to 60 min. The outcomes of these observations were presented as percentages of compliance representing the fraction of the number of times when hand hygiene should have taken place correctly, and the number of times it had actually taken place correctly. The hand hygiene compliance observation sheet as well as knowledge and perception questionnaires were based on the WHO tools [6]. The knowledge survey consisted of three single item and three multiple item (i.e., more than one answer) questions on the following topics: transmission of microorganisms, source of HAIs, and hand hygiene indications. A correct answer was awarded with one point, with a maximum score of 12 points for 12 correct answers. A wrong answer led to one score deduction for multiple item questions,

and a score of zero for a wrong answer to a single item question. The perception survey consisted of 12 yes/no questions, 13 of a 4-Likert-items scale questions (the last two points of the scale were considered as positive perception), and 3 open-ended questions, and included: intention to adhere to hand hygiene, risk of cross-transmission and HAIs related to non-compliance, social norms concerning hand hygiene, and hand hygiene methods, indications, importance, promotion, and compliance barriers. In addition, the three open-ended questions concerned the perception of HCW on the risk of patients acquiring HAIs, the hand hygiene compliance rate that should be achieved, and self-reporting of the hand hygiene compliance level.

When the HCW were providing patient care in the wards and filling out the surveys, two observers concurrently recorded their clothing regarding jewelry on the arms or fingers, long sleeves, and nail polish.

The study was approved by the medical ethics committee (No 129/EC/KEPK-JK/05/2012). Informed consent was not obtained, since it involved little risk of harm for the participants and the study was regarded as a hospital infection control program. Anonymity of HCW was guaranteed in the knowledge and perception survey.

Statistical analysis

The overall compliance to hand hygiene with confidence intervals (95%CI) was calculated using the standard normal distribution. To assess differences in compliance and each of the WHO five moments of hand hygiene at the different departments between pre- and post-intervention, the Pearson Chi-Square statistic or the Fisher's exact test was used when applicable. If the compliance in pre- and post-intervention at the departments with intervention (i.e., pediatrics, surgery and internal medicine) was significantly different from the department without intervention (i.e., obst-gyn), the Pearson Chi-Square statistic was used followed by the Mantel-Haenszel statistic. In addition, knowledge and perception improvement were analyzed using the independent T-test and the Chi-Square test, respectively. Backward multiple logistic regression analysis was performed to determine factors associated with hand hygiene compliance and included department, class, room type, nurse-to-patient ratio, moment of hand hygiene, and HCWs' professions before and after intervention. A P value of < 0.05 was considered statistically significant and all analyses were performed using IBM SPSS version 21 (SPSS Inc., Chicago, IL, USA).

Results

Compliance to hand hygiene

During the study period, 2,766 potential hand hygiene opportunities were observed at the 4 participating departments. The overall compliance to hand hygiene was 19.5% (95%CI: 18.0 to 20.9). After intervention, the hand hygiene compliance rate increased both in the departments with intervention (i.e., pediatrics, internal medicine, and surgery) and in the department without intervention (i.e., obst-gyn) from 16.1% to 27.1% and from 10.1% to 20.5%, respectively. Departments pediatrics, internal medicine and obst-gyn improved significantly when comparing pre-intervention to post-intervention ($P < 0.001$). However, the intervention did not significantly improve hand hygiene compliance in the surgery department ($P = 0.05$). When considering the different types of HCW, hand hygiene compliance of doctors and nurses improved significantly post-intervention ($P < 0.001$), but not among students ($P = 0.840$). For the 538 opportunities with good hand hygiene compliance, it was observed that HCW used hand rub at 379 (70.6%) opportunities, whereas at 159 (29.6%) opportunities they washed their hands. We did not find a significant increase in the use of hand rub in the departments with intervention (Table 2). For the 2,228 opportunities with non-compliance, we found that HCW used hand rub while wearing gloves (GA) at 74 (3.3%) opportunities, wore gloves when it was not necessary at 157 (7.0%) opportunities, and did not perform hand hygiene at all at 1,997 (89.6%) opportunities. When comparing pre-intervention and post-intervention phases, the nurses who did not perform hand hygiene at all and wore gloves when it was not necessary decreased significantly ($P = 0.024$ and $P = 0.046$, respectively), however their use of hand rub while wearing gloves increased ($P < 0.001$). Similarly, the students who wore gloves when it was not necessary decreased but the use of hand rub while wearing gloves increased significantly ($P < 0.001$) (Table 3). With regard to clothing among nurses in the pre-intervention phase, 17% of the nurses wore jewelry, 31% of the nurses had long sleeves and 33% wore both jewelry and had long sleeves. Thus, a total of 81% did not wear appropriate clothing.

Based on the five moments of hand hygiene recommended by the WHO, the highest compliance was to moment 4 (27.4%) (i.e., after touching a patient). The lowest compliance was to moment 5 (12.2%) (i.e., after touching patient surroundings). Table 4 shows compliance considering the five moments pre-intervention and post-intervention at the four participating departments.

Hand hygiene compliance pre-intervention compared to post-intervention

Independent of phase (i.e., pre-intervention and post-intervention), we observed a statistically significant difference between compliance at departments obst-gyn and surgery ($P < 0.001$), and between obst-gyn and pediatrics ($P < 0.001$). When adding phase as a confounding factor, the relationships remained significant ($P = 0.001$ and $P < 0.001$, respectively). Independent of

phase (i.e., pre-intervention and post-intervention), we did not observe a statistically significant difference between compliance at departments obst-gyn and internal medicine ($P = 0.207$). When adding phase as confounding factor, the relationship remained non-significant ($P = 0.069$).

Factors associated with hand hygiene compliance

Multivariate analysis showed that when comparing the pre- and post-intervention phase, the pediatric and surgery department was significantly associated with hand hygiene compliance improvement among HCW (odds ratio [OR] 4.078 and 1.963; 95%CI 1.513-10.994 and 1.178-3.270, respectively). Other factors associated with the hand hygiene compliance at the different departments were general adult room (OR 1.710; 95%CI 1.002-2.918), class III room facilities (OR 1.993; 95%CI 1.168-3.400), WHO moment of before touching a patient and after touching a patient (OR 1.442; 95%CI 1.057-1.968 and OR 2.333; 95%CI 1.850-2.943, respectively). Professional categories being either a doctor or a nurse was also associated with hand hygiene compliance improvement in the post-intervention phase (OR 1.366; 95%CI 1.012-1.843 or OR 1.279; 95%CI 1.019-1.604) (Table 5).

Knowledge and perception

A total of 284 HCW participated in the knowledge and perception survey regarding hand hygiene and HAIs in the pre- (total $n = 196$; internal medicine, 56; surgery, 33; obst-gyn, 47, and pediatrics, 60) and post-intervention phase (total $n = 88$; internal medicine, 33; surgery, 18; obst-gyn, 15; pediatrics, 22). Overall, the average score was 5.8 (SD = 2.1), the median score was 6 and the mode score was 7/12, whereas the minimum and maximum score were 1/12 and 11/12, respectively. After interventions, the average of knowledge score improved from 5.6 (SD = 2.1) to 6.2 (SD = 1.9) ($P < 0.05$). We classified the knowledge score to be low level (0-5) and high level (6-12) and noted a significant increase in the proportion of high level scores in the pediatrics department ($P < 0.05$) after the intervention. There was not a significant change identified in other departments (Table 2). Also, we did not find a significant increase in the proportion of high level scores among doctors, nurses, and students in the four departments. The results of the perception survey on intention to adhere to hand hygiene, risk of cross-transmission and HAIs related to non-compliance, social norms concerning hand hygiene, hand hygiene indications, methods and promotion are presented in Table 6. In the departments with intervention, positive perception was demonstrated by 69.1 to 98.7% of HCW in the pre-intervention phase and 67.1 to 98.6% of HCW in the post-intervention phase to all perception items. The survey in the department without an intervention showed that 63.8% to 100% of HCW in the pre-intervention phase and

Table 2 Compliance and knowledge of hand hygiene in pre- and post-intervention

Department[a] HCW	Compliance rate[b] Overall % (95%CI)	Pre-intervention (%)	Post-intervention (%)	P value	Score	Proportion of HCW based on Knowledge score group Pre-intervention (%)	Post-intervention (%)	P value
PED	32.4 (28.6–36.2)	80/332 (24.1)	107/245 (43.7)	<0.001	0 – 5	30/60[d] (50.0)	5/22 (22.7)	0.043
HR		53/80 (66.2)	70/107 (65.4)	1.000	6 – 12	30/60[d] (50.0)	17/22 (77.3)	
HW		27/80 (33.8)	37/107 (34.6)					
Doctor		21/84 (25.0)	55/117 (47.0)	0.002	0 – 5	8/17 (47.1)	0/2 (0)	0.322
					6 – 12	9/17 (52.9)	2/2 (100)	
Nurse		23/105 (21.9)	45/87 (51.7)	<0.001	0 – 5	13/23 (56.5)	5/18 (27.8)	0.063
					6 – 12	10/23 (43.5)	13/18 (72.2)	
Student		36/143 (25.2)	7/41 (17.1)	0.280[c]	0 – 5	8/17 (47.1)	0/2 (0)	0.322
					6 – 12	9/17 (52.9)	2/2 (100)	
IM	12.3 (10.0–14.6)	19/364 (5.2)	74/399 (18.5)	<0.001	0 – 5	28/56 (50.0)	11/33 (33.3)	0.184
HR		11/19 (57.9)	42/74 (56.8)	1.000	6 – 12	28/56 (50.0)	22/33 (66.7)	
HW		8/19 (42.1)	32/74 (43.2)					
Doctor		3/40 (7.5)	10/37 (27.0)	0.032	0 – 5	5/13 (38.5)	NA	NA
					6 – 12	8/13 (61.5)	NA	
Nurse		6/180 (3.3)	55/295 (18.6)	<0.001	0 – 5	11/26 (42.3)	8/24 (33.3)	0.570
					6 – 12	15/26 (57.7)	16/24 (66.7)	
Student		11/144 (7.6)	9/67 (13.4)	0.181	0 – 5	9/12 (75.0)	2/5 (40.0)	0.280
					6 – 12	3/12 (25.0)	3/5 (60.0)	
SUR	21.3 (18.3–24.3)	83/440 (18.9)	73/293 (24.9)	0.05	0 – 5	16/33[e] (48.5)	10/18 (55.6)	0.771
HR		69/83 (83.1)	64/73 (87.7)	0.501	6 – 12	17/33[e] (51.5)	8/18 (44.4)	
HW		14/83 (16.9)	9/73 (12.3)					
Doctor		7/57 (12.3)	8/30 (26.7)	0.091	0 – 5	4/8 (50.0)	NA	NA
					6 – 12	4/8 (50.0)	NA	
Nurse		31/238 (13.0)	46/118 (39.0)	<0.001	0 – 5	7/12 (58.3)	6/7 (85.7)	0.333
					6 – 12	5/12 (41.7)	1/7 (14.3)	
Student		45/145 (31.0)	19/145 (13.1)	<0.001[c]	0 – 5	2/8 (25.0)	4/11 (36.4)	1.000
					6 – 12	6/8 (75.0)	7/11 (63.6)	
OBG	14.6 (12.0–17.2)	40/395 (10.1)	61/298 (20.5)	<0.001	0 – 5	20/47[f] (42.6)	3/15[g] (20.0)	0.138
HR		32/40 (80.0)	38/61 (62.3)	0.078	6 – 12	27/47[f] (57.4)	12/15[g] (80.0)	
HW		8/40 (20.0)	23/61 (37.7)					
Doctor		0/18 (0)	3/12 (25.0)	0.054	0 – 5	5/10 (50.0)	NA	NA
					6 – 12	5/10 (50.0)	NA	
Nurse		24/173 (13.9)	30/157 (19.1)	0.199	0 – 5	2/12 (16.7)	1/7 (14.3)	1.000
					6 – 12	10/12 (83.3)	6/7 (85.7)	
Student		16/204 (7.8)	28/129 (21.7)	<0.001	0 – 5	10/21 (47.6)	2/7 (28.6)	0.662
					6 – 12	11/21 (52.4)	5/7 (71.4)	

Abbreviations: *IM* internal medicine, *SUR* surgery, *OBG* obstetrics-gynecology, *PED* pediatrics, *HCW* healthcare workers, *HR* handrubbing, *HW* handwashing, *NA* not available

[a]Departments of Pediatrics, Surgery and Internal Medicine with intervention, Department of Obstetrics-gynecology without intervention; [b]the percentage of correct hand hygiene actions undertaken on moments when hand hygiene was considered necessary according to the WHO "five moments"; [c]Significantly worse instead of significantly better; [d]3 HCWs did not mention the profession in the questionnaire; [e]5 HCWs did not mention the profession in the questionnaire; [f]4 HCWs did not mention the profession in the questionnaire; [g]1 HCW did not mention the profession in the questionnaire; score range 0-5 = 0-42% correct; score range 6-12 = 50%-100% correct

80 to 100% of HCW in the post-intervention phase answered with positive response. There was no significant improvement of the hand hygiene perception before and after the interventions. However, "strong smell of hand-alcohol" as a reason not to perform hand hygiene increased significantly in the departments with intervention. The

Table 3 Behavior of HCW at moments of non-compliance ($n = 2{,}228$ out of $n = 2{,}766$ observed moments)

Behavior	Phase	Total	HCW					
			Doctors (%)	P value	Nurses (%)	P value	Students (%)	P value
GA	Pre	4/1308 (0.3)	0/168 (0)	NA	1/612 (0.2)	<0.001	3/528 (0.6)	<0.001
	Post	70/920 (7.6)	0/120 (0)		41/481 (8.5)		29/319 (9.1)	
Gloves[a]	Pre	114/1308 (8.7)	1/168 (0.6)	1.000	67/612 (10.9)	0.046	46/528 (8.7)	<0.001
	Post	43/920 (4.7)	0/120 (0)		35/481 (7.3)		8/319 (2.5)	
No HH	Pre	1190/1308 (90.9)	167/168 (99.4)	1.000	544/612 (88.9)	0.024	479/528 (90.7)	0.292
	Post	807/920 (87.7)	120/120 (100.0)		405/481 (84.2)		282/319 (88.4)	

Abbreviations: *HCW* healthcare workers, *HH* hand hygiene, *GA* gloves and alcohol (using an alcohol based hand rub while wearing gloves), *Pre* pre-intervention, *Post* post-intervention
[a]Wearing gloves when it was not necessary

Table 4 Compliance to the five different WHO moments of hand hygiene pre-intervention and post intervention

WHO moment	Total (%)	Compliance (%)		P value
		Pre-intervention	Post-intervention	
1: Before	86/438 (19.6)	57/267 (21.3)	29/171 (17.0)	0.259
Pediatrics		30/89 (33.7)	9/39 (23.1)	0.298
Internal medicine		6/64 (9.4)	7/87 (8.0)	0.774
Surgery		7/67 (10.4)	11/22 (50.0)	<0.001
Obstetrics-gynecology		14/47 (29.8)	2/23 (8.7)	0.069
2: Before	16/123 (13.0)	7/87 (8.0)	9/36 (25.0)	0.017
Pediatrics		4/20 (20.0)	4/8 (50.0)	0.172
Internal medicine		0/31 (0)	2/14 (14.3)	0.092
Surgery		2/20 (10.0)	2/4 (50.0)	0.115
Obstetrics-gynecology		1/16 (6.3)	1/10 (10.0)	1.000
3: After	3/12 (25.0)	2/9 (22.2)	1/3 (33.3)	1.000
Pediatrics		0/4 (0)	1/1 (100)	0.200
Internal medicine		0/1 (0)	0/0 (0)	NA
Surgery		1/3 (33.3)	0/0 (0)	NA
Obstetrics-gynecology		1/1 (100)	0/2 (0)	0.333
4: After	299/1093 (27.4)	112/544 (20.6)	187/549 (34.1)	<0.001
Pediatrics		40/133 (30.1)	79/119 (66.4)	<0.001
Internal medicine		12/96 (12.5)	38/139 (27.3)	0.006
Surgery		42/178 (23.6)	42/180 (23.3)	0.953
Obstetrics-gynecology		18/137 (13.1)	28/78 (35.9)	<0.001
5: After	134/1100 (12.2)	45/624 (7.2)	89/476 (18.7)	<0.001
Pediatrics		6/86 (7.0)	14/45 (31.1)	<0.001
Internal medicine		2/172 (1.2)	27/159 (17.0)	<0.001
Surgery		31/172 (18.0)	18/87 (20.7)	0.605
Obstetrics-gynecology		6/194 (3.1)	30/185 (16.2)	<0.001

Abbreviations: *WHO* World Health Organization
1 = before touching a patient; 2 = before a procedure; 3 = after a procedure or body fluid exposure risk; 4 = after touching a patient; 5 = after touching a patient's surroundings

Table 5 Multivariate analysis of the factors associated with hand hygiene compliance in the pre-and post-intervention phase

Factors	Univariate		P value	Multivariate		P value
	Number of HH compliance (%)			OR	95% CI	
	PI (n = 223)	PoI (n = 315)				
Department:			<0.001			
Obst-gyn	40 (17.9)	61 (19.4)		1		
Internal medicine	20 (9.0)	74 (23.5)		-	-	NS
Pediatric	80 (35.9)	107 (34.0)		4.078	1.513–10.994	0.005
Surgery	83 (37.2)	73 (23.2)		1.963	1.178–3.270	0.010
Class of room facilities:			<0.001			
Class I	1 (0.4)	20 (6.3)		1	-	NS
Class II	108 (48.4)	175 (55.6)		-	1.168–3.400	0.011
Class III	114 (51.1)	120 (38.1)		1.993		
Room type:			<0.001			
Neonatology	50 (22.4)	72 (22.9)		-	-	NS
General ward	92 (41.3)	192 (61.0)		1.710	1.002–2.918	0.049
High/acute care unit	81 (36.3)	51 (16.2)		1		
Ratio nurse: patients:						NS
1:2	30 (13.5)	35 (11.1)	0.015			
1:4–6	174 (78.0)	226 (71.7)				
1:8	19 (8.5)	54 (17.1)				
Moment of HH:			<0.001			
Moment 1	57 (25.6)	29 (9.2)		1.442	1.057–1.968	0.021
Moment 2	7 (3.1)	9 (2.9)		-		NS
Moment 3	2 (0.9)	1 (0.3)		-		NS
Moment 4	112 (50.2)	187 (59.4)		2.333	1.850–2.943	<0.001
Moment 5	45 (20.2)	89 (28.3)		1		
HCW categories:			<0.001	-		
Doctor	31 (13.9)	76 (24.1)		1.366	1.012–1.843	0.042
Nurse	84 (37.7)	176 (55.9)		1.279	1.019–1.604	0.034
Student	108 (48.4)	63 (20.0)		1		

Abbreviations: HH hand hygiene, *PI* pre-intervention, *PoI* post-intervention, *HCW* healthcare workers
Moment 1: before touching a patient; Moment 2: before a procedure; Moment 3: after a procedure or body fluid exposure risk; Moment 4: after touching a patient; Moment 5: after touching a patient's surroundings

perception of HCW in the departments with intervention regarding the average percentage of hospitalized patients who will develop a HAI increased significantly from 49.7 to 58.6% ($P < 0.05$) in the post-intervention phase. In addition, the self-reporting of hand hygiene compliance rate decreased from 85.5% to 75.1% ($P < 0.001$). We did not find any significant difference in the perception survey in the department without intervention between pre- and post-intervention (Table 6).

Discussion

We report the first cluster randomized controlled trial evaluating the effect of three different educational programs on HCWs' hand hygiene compliance and knowledge-perception in a limited-resource hospital in Indonesia. Particularly in our hospital, educational programs on hand hygiene were not applied regularly. Therefore, the educational programs used in this study were introduced in our hospital for the first time. In the departments with an intervention of role model training (i.e., pediatrics and internal medicine), the hand hygiene compliance improved, but only pediatrics department with the sole intervention of role model training was significantly better than the control group. The hand hygiene compliance improvement co-occurred with a statistically significant improvement of the knowledge score. Therefore, we conclude that role model training has the most impact on improving hand hygiene

Table 6 Perception associated with HAIs and hand hygiene adherence among HCW between departments

Perception	No. of HCW (%)					
	Departments with intervention		P value	Department without intervention		P value
	Pre (n = 149)	Post (n = 73)		Pre (n = 47)	Post (n = 15)	
Formal training on HH within 3 years[a]	107 (71.8)	51 (70.8)	0.875	30 (63.8)	13 (86.7)	0.118
Intention to adhere to HH[a]	137 (91.9)	70 (95.9)	0.396	45 (95.7)	15 (100.0)	1.000
The impact of a HAIs on a patient's clinical outcome[b]	115 (77.2)	64 (87.7)	0.119	41 (87.2)	14 (93.3)	0.759
Effectiveness of HH in preventing HAIs[b]	140 (94.0)	65 (89.0)	0.220	41 (87.2)	12 (80.0)	0.674
Importance of HH in the ward among all patient safety issues[b]	136 (91.3)	63 (86.3)	0.480	40 (85.1)	14 (93.3)	0.676
Performing HH as WHO recommended method[b]	126 (84.6)	62 (84.9)	0.944	45 (95.7)	13 (86.7)	0.244
Importance that the head of department attach to the HH behavior[b]	121 (81.2)	61 (83.6)	0.292	41 (87.2)	13 (86.7)	1.000
Importance that the colleagues attach to the HH behavior[b]	103 (69.1)	56 (76.7)	0.147	37 (78.7)	13 (86.7)	0.713
Importance that the patients attach to the HH behavior[b]	109 (73.2)	49 (67.1)	0.557	37 (78.7)	12 (80.0)	1.000
Effort to perform HH as WHO recommended method[b]	135 (90.6)	68 (93.2)	0.768	42 (89.4)	14 (93.3)	0.824
Reasons for HCW not to perform HH on a moment that it is expected[a]:						
a) Too much time	12 (8.2)	2 (2.8)	0.151	3 (6.5)	0	1.000
b) Not enough facilities	27 (19.0)	15 (21.1)	0.718	6 (13.6)	2 (13.3)	1.000
c) Skin dry or irritated	26 (18.6)	16 (22.5)	0.584	10 (21.7)	2 (14.3)	0.713
d) Hand-alcohol is not effective for hand hygiene	26 (18.2)	12 (16.9)	1.000	6 (13.3)	1 (6.7)	0.668
e) Strong smell of hand-alcohol	14 (10.1)	16 (22.9)	0.021	7 (15.2)	1 (7.1)	0.667
f) The hand-alcohol substance is not convenient (sticky)	25 (17.9)	13 (19.4)	0.848	7 (15.9)	5 (33.3)	0.263
g) The hand becomes sweaty	27 (19.6)	9 (13.4)	0.331	7 (15.9)	0	0.178
h) Feeling dirty hand after using hand-alcohol	11 (8.1)	4 (6.0)	0.777	6 (14.0)	1 (7.1)	0.669
Hand hygiene procedure as WHO guideline[a]:						
a) Information about five moments for HH is known well	129 (86.6)	67 (91.8)	0.369	45 (95.7)	15 (100.0)	1.000
b) Information about six steps of HH is known well	146 (98.0)	68 (93.2)	0.134	46 (97.9)	15 (100.0)	1.000
c) Know when to apply HH	143 (96.0)	69 (94.5)	0.838	46 (97.0)	15 (100.0)	1.000
d) Know how to apply HH	147 (98.7)	72 (98.6)	0.221	47 (100.0)	15 (100.0)	-
e) Enough reminders in the ward	121 (81.2)	59 (80.8)	0.998	43 (91.5)	13 (86.7)	0.626

Perception	%					
	(95% CI)					
	Departments with intervention		P	Department without intervention		P
	Pre	Post		Pre	Post	
Average percentage of hospitalized patients who will develop a HAIs	49.7 (44.9–54.5)	58.6 (52.8–64.4)	0.026	57.7 (51.6–63.8)	64.0 (51.3–76.7)	0.320
Average percentage of situations HCW perform HH when required	69.3 (65.2–73.3)	68.1 (63.4–72.8)	0.736	75.3 (70.0–80.6)	76.3 (62.8–89.9)	0.860
Percentage of situations requiring HH do the HCW actually perform HH, either by handrubbing or handwashing (self-reporting)	85.5 (82.6–88.4)	75.1 (70.5–79.7)	<0.001	81.8 (76.8–86.7)	85.3 (78.8–91.8)	0.425

Abbreviations: HAIs healthcare-associated infections, HH hand hygiene, HCW healthcare workers
[a]"yes" response; [b]high/very high response

compliance in this setting. Erasmus et al. and other studies have also pointed out the importance of role models [14–16]. However, it is possible that the factor of positive role models is even more important in societies where job seniority plays a great role, such as in Indonesia.

The improvement in the pediatrics department might also be associated with fewer activities related to hand hygiene opportunities in patient care ($n = 577$) compared to internal medicine ($n = 763$), surgery ($n = 733$), and obst-gyn ($n = 693$). Pittet et al. reported the inverse relationship of activity level in the ward with hand hygiene compliance rate [17, 18]. The low activity level might also be associated with the improvement of hand hygiene adherence in general in wards and in rooms with class III type facilities. Overall, however, the hand hygiene compliance rate was low. Compared to Pakistan, also a low-middle income country [1], overall hand hygiene compliance rate in our study was lower. On the other hand, the HCW assured that they performed hand hygiene very well based on the perception survey (85.5% and 75.1% in the pre- and post-intervention phase, respectively). Therefore, the HCW may not change behavior [12]. Additionally, only good knowledge about the hand hygiene procedure did not lead to the high hand hygiene compliance among HCW. Other factors including awareness, action control, facilitation, social influence, attitude, self-efficacy, and intention might also be associated with the adherence to hand hygiene procedure. However, further investigation is needed [2].

Although hand hygiene compliance improved after intervention, we noted higher compliance rates after a procedure or body fluid exposure risk (although for only a low number of observed opportunities) and after touching a patient than before performing patient care. The lowest adherence was at the moment after touching a patients' surroundings. Therefore, the reason to perform hand hygiene was more to protect the HCW themselves than patients [1, 17, 19, 20]. In addition, effectiveness of hand hygiene to prevent HAIs was hampered by inappropriate clothing such as hand-accessories and long sleeves by most HCW, so transmission of pathogens was unavoidable.

Based on healthcare profession, hand hygiene adherence improved among doctors and nurses in general, although it was not significant in the surgery department. The hand hygiene performance among students did not improve significantly, and even decreased in the surgery and pediatrics departments. This might be associated with the weekly rotation of students' traineeships in our hospital leading to missing education programs, the attitudes of mentors and role models, curriculum enforcement, beliefs, and the use of gloves [21]. In such situations, students may transmit the pathogens causing HAIs from patient to patient [22].

Our data showed that wearing gloves regardless of the recommendation for gloves during patient care (i.e., wearing gloves when writing in the patient medical record) hampered HCWs' hand hygiene adherence. WHO observed such misuse of gloves not only in limited-resource hospitals, but also in hospitals where gloves are widely available [6]. After intervention, wearing gloves without indication decreased but shifted to handrubbing while using gloves during patient care. Then, HCW did not change gloves between patients or between contacts of different sites on the same patient. Nurses declared that glove decontamination resulted from a limited examination gloves supply in our hospital (750 pairs per room in Class III). However, WHO does not recommend glove decontamination [6] because of material damage, which can endanger the protective function of gloves. Similar problems were encountered by the WHO in Ebola-affected countries, where gloves were frequently disinfected with chlorine solutions [23].

This study has some limitations. Firstly, the preparation of national hospital accreditation was held in the same period as this study, which may have influenced the knowledge and perception on hand hygiene among HCW. In addition, the HCW were busy preparing the accreditation, so participation in the knowledge and perception survey after intervention was limited. Secondly, the HCW may have changed behavior during hand hygiene observation because of their awareness of the observer (Hawthorn effect) [24, 25]. This could also be an additional explanation for the significant improvement in hand hygiene compliance in the control department. Thirdly, the study was performed in a tertiary academic hospital that included medical students and nursing students, in the delivery of patient care. Modification of the hand hygiene educational program is suggested when it is applied in either secondary or non-academic hospitals according to the hospital resources.

Conclusions

In summary, role model training as part of a multi-model strategy has the most impact on knowledge and perception regarding hand hygiene and HAIs among HCW, and improves the hand hygiene compliance in a limited-resource hospital in Indonesia. However, we showed that the hand hygiene compliance rate remained rather low, therefore, the multi-modal hand hygiene strategy should be re-customized considering local resources, administrative support, and education/training focused on the barriers of non-established practice [1, 6, 26, 27].

Abbreviations

CI: Confidence interval; GA: Gloves and alcohol handrub usage; HAIs: Healthcare-associated infections; HCW: Healthcare workers; HH: Hand hygiene; HR: Handrubbing; HW: Handwashing; IM: Internal medicine; IPCLN: Infection prevention control-linked nurses; IPCN: Infection prevention control nurses; NA: Not available; OBG: Obstetrics-gynecology; OR: Odds ratio; PED: Pediatrics; PI: Pre-intervention; PoI: Post-intervention; SD: Standard deviation; SUR: Surgery; VIP: Very important person; WHO: World Health Organization

Acknowledgments

We thank the dean of the Faculty of Medicine, Brawijaya University, Malang, Indonesia and the director of the Dr. Saiful Anwar hospital, Malang, Indonesia who facilitated our work in this teaching hospital. We also thank Irwan Subekti, Tjutjuk Hardiyanto, Anis Chabibah as infection prevention control nurses as well as Muhammad Yasin and Arina Dita as infection prevention control-linked nurses who were involved in the distribution and collection of questionnaires among HCW, and supported the hand hygiene education program in this study.

Intervening with healthcare workers' hand hygiene compliance, knowledge, and perception...

89

Funding
No financial support in this study.

Authors' contributions
All authors participated in conception and study design other than additional contributions. SS and NN contributed with substantive intellectual expertise in this study. DE, IR, DC, INC, TECJH, GvdD, and EvB were involved in data collection as well as preliminary data analysis and interpretation. DS, AFV, JAS, and HAV contributed to final data analysis and interpretation in addition to writing and finalizing the manuscript. All authors read and approved the final manuscript.

Competing interest
The authors declare that they have no competing interests.

Consent for publication
Was not obtained, since it involved little risk of harm for the participants and the study was regarded as a hospital infection control program. Anonymity of HCW was guaranteed in the knowledge and perception survey.

Author details
[1]Department of Microbiology, Faculty of Medicine, Brawijaya University/Dr. Saiful Anwar Hospital, Malang, Indonesia. [2]Infection Prevention and Control Committee, Dr. Saiful Anwar Hospital, Malang, Indonesia. [3]Department of Medical Microbiology and Infectious Diseases, Erasmus University Medical Center, 's-Gravendijkwal 230, Rotterdam 3015 CE, The Netherlands.

References
1. Allegranzi B, Gayet-Ageron A, Damani N, Bengaly L, McLaws M-L, Moro M-L, Memish Z, Urroz O, Richet H, Storr J, Donaldson L, Pittet D. Global Implementation of WHO's multimodal strategy for Improvement of hand-hygiene: a quasi-experimental study. Lancet Infect Dis. 2013;13:843–51.
2. Huis A, van Achterberg T, de Bruin M, Grol R, Schoonhoven L, Hulscher M. A systematic review of hand hygiene improvement strategies: a behavioral approach. Implement Sci. 2012;7:1–14.
3. Gurley ES, Zaman RU, Sultana R, Bell M, Fry AM, Srinivasan A, Rahman M, Rahman MW, Hossain MJ, Luby SP. Rates of hospital acquired respiratory ilness in Bangladesh Tertiarty Care Hospitals: results from a low-cost pilot surveillance strategy. Clin Infect Dis. 2010;50:1084–90.
4. Duerink DO, Roeshadi D, Wahjono H, Lestari ES, Hadi U, Wille JC, De Jong RM, Nagelkerke NJ, Van den Broek PJ, Study Group 'Antimicrobial Resistance in Indonesia Prevalence and Prevention' Amrin. Surveillance of Healthcare-Associated Infections in Indonesian hospitals. J Hosp Infect. 2006;62:219–29.
5. Murni IM, Duke T, Kinney S, Daley AJ, Soenarto Y. Reducing hospital-acquired infections and improving the rational use of antibiotics in a developing country: an effectiveness study. Arch Dis Child. 2014;0:1–6.
6. World Health Organization. WHO Guidelines on Hand Hygiene in Health Care. France: WHO press; 2009.
7. Asadollahi M, Bostanabad MA, Jebraili M, Mahallei M, Rasooli AS, Abdolalipour M. Nurses' knowledge regarding hand hygiene and its individual and organizational predictors. J Caring Sci. 2015;4:45–53.
8. World Health Organization. Guide to implementation: a guide to the implementation of the WHO multimodal hand hygiene improvement strategy. 2009. http://apps.who.int/iris/bitstream/10665/70030/1/WHO_IER_PSP_2009.02_eng.pdf. Accessed 9 Feb 2017.
9. Jumaa PA. Hand hygiene: simplex and complex. Int J Infect Dis. 2005;9:3–14.
10. Peabody JW, Taguiwalo MM, Robalino DA, Frenk J. Improving the quality of care in developing countries. In: Jamison DT, Breman JG, Measham AR, editors. Disease control priorities in developing countries. 2nd ed. New York: Oxford University Press; 2006. p. 1293–307.
11. Nejad SB, Allegranzi B, Syed SB, Ellis B, Pittet D. Healthcare-associated infection in Africa: a systematic review. Bull World Health Organ. 2011;89:757–65.
12. Duerink DO, Hadi U, Lestari ES, Roeshadi D, Wahyono H, Nagelkerke NJD, Van der Meulen RG, Van den Broek PJ. A tool to assess knowledge, attitude and behavior of Indonesian healthcare workers regarding infection control. Acta Med Indones. 2013;45:206–15.
13. Boyce JM. Update on hand hygiene. Am J Infect Control. 2013;41:S94 6.
14. Erasmus V, Brouwer W, van Beeck EF, Oenema A, Daha TJ, Richardus JH, Vos MC, Brug J. A qualitative exploration of reasons for poor hand hygiene among hospital workers: lack of positive role models and of convincing evidence that hand hygiene prevents cross transmission. Infect Control Hosp Epidemiol. 2009;30:415–9.
15. Lee SS, Park SJ, Chung MJ, Lee JH, Kang HJ, Lee JA, Kim YK. Improved hand hygiene compliance is associated with the change of perception toward hand hygiene among medical personnel. J Infect Chemother. 2014;46:165–71.
16. Buffet-Bataillon S, Leray E, Poisson M, Michelet C, Bonnaure-Mallet M, Cormier M. Influence of job seniority, hand hygiene education, and patient to nurse ratio on hand disinfection compliance. J Hosp Infect. 2010;76:32–5.
17. Pittet D. Improving adherence to hand hygiene practice: a multidisciplinary approach. Emerg Infect Dis. 2001;7:234–40.
18. Pittet D. Compliance with hand disinfection and its impact on hospital acquired infections. J Hosp Infect. 2001;48 (Supplement A):S40–6.
19. Teker B, Ogutlu A, Gozdas HT, Ruayercan S, Hacialioglu G, Karabay O. Factors affecting hand hygiene adherence at a private hospital in Turkey. Eurasian J Med. 2015;47:208–12.
20. Randle J, Arthur A, Vaughan N. Twenty-four-hour observational study of hospital hand hygiene compliance. J Hosp Infect. 2010;76:252–5.
21. al Kadi A, Salati SA. Hand hygiene practices among medical students. Interdiscip Perspect Infect Dis. 2012; doi:10.1155/2012/679129.
22. Reem H, Kharraz R, Alshanqity A, AlFawaz D, Eshaq AM, Abu-Zaid A. Hand Hygiene: knowledge and attitudes of fourth-year clerkship medical students at Alfaisal University, College of Medicine, Riyadh, Saudi Arabia. Cureus. 2015;7:e310.
23. Hopman J, Kubilay Z, Allen T, Edrees H, Pittet D, Allegranzi B. Efficacy of chlorine solution used for hand hygiene and gloves disinfection in Ebola settings: a systematic review. Antimicrob Resist Infect Control. 2015;4 Suppl 1:O13.
24. Srigley JA, Furness CD, Baker GR, Gardom M. Quantification of the Hawthorn effect in hand hygiene compliance monitoring using an electronic monitoring system: a retrospective cohort study. BMJ Qual Saf. 2014;23:974–80.
25. Rosenthal VD, McCormick RD, Guzman S, Villamayor C, Orellano PW. Effect of education and performance feedback on handwashing; The benefit of administrative support in Argentian hospitals. Am J Infect Control. 2003;31:85–92.
26. Pittet D, Hugonnet S, Harbarth S, et al. Effectiveness of a hospital-wide programme to improve compliance with hand hygiene. Lancet. 2000;356:1307–12.
27. Allegranzi B, Pittet D. Role of hand hygiene in healthcare-associated infection prevention. J Hosp Infect. 2009;73:305–15.

12

Temporal relationship between antibiotic use and respiratory virus activities in the Republic of Korea

Sukhyun Ryu[1,2], Sojung Kim[3], Bryan I. Kim[2], Eili Y. Klein[4,5], Young Kyung Yoon[6] and Byung Chul Chun[2,7*]

Abstract

Background: Inappropriate use of antibiotics increases resistance and reduces their effectiveness. Despite evidence-based guidelines, antibiotics are still commonly used to treat infections likely caused by respiratory viruses. In this study, we examined the temporal relationships between antibiotic usage and respiratory infections in the Republic of Korea.

Methods: The number of monthly antibiotic prescriptions and the incidence of acute respiratory tract infections between 2010 and 2015 at all primary care clinics were obtained from the Korean Health Insurance Review and Assessment Service. The monthly detection rates of respiratory viruses, including adenovirus, respiratory syncytial virus, influenza virus, human coronavirus, and human rhinovirus, were collected from Korea Centers for Disease Control and Prevention. Cross-correlation analysis was conducted to quantify the temporal relationship between antibiotic use and respiratory virus activities as well as respiratory infections in primary clinics.

Results: The monthly use of different classes of antibiotic, including penicillins, other beta-lactam antibacterials, macrolides and quinolones, was significantly correlated with influenza virus activity. These correlations peaked at the 0-month lag with cross-correlation coefficients of 0.45 ($p < 0.01$), 0.46 ($p < 0.01$), 0.40 ($p < 0.01$), and 0.35 (< 0.01), respectively. Furthermore, a significant correlation was found between acute bronchitis and antibiotics, including penicillin (0.73, $p < 0.01$), macrolides (0.74, $p < 0.01$), and quinolones (0.45, $p < 0.01$), at the 0-month lag.

Conclusions: Our findings suggest that there is a significant temporal relationship between influenza virus activity and antibiotic use in primary clinics. This relationship indicates that interventions aimed at reducing influenza cases in addition to effort to discourage the prescription of antibiotics by physicians may help to decrease unnecessary antibiotic consumption.

Keywords: Antibiotic use, Influenza, Respiratory virus, Korea, Time-series analysis

Background

Overuse and inappropriate use of antibiotics drive the emergence and spread of antimicrobial resistance [1, 2]. In the Republic of Korea, the number of antibiotic prescriptions is relatively higher (31.7 defined daily dose [DDD] per 1000 inhabitants per day) than in other member countries of the Organization for Economic Co-operation and Development (mean, 23.7 DDD per 1000 inhabitants per day) [3]. In Korea, the majority of antibiotics (ca. 90%) are prescribed in primary care and mainly for acute respiratory tract infections (ARTIs; ca. 57%) [4]. ARTIs are mainly viral in origin, are generally self-limiting, and do not require antibiotics [5, 6]. Secondary bacterial pneumonia is the most important clinical complication of respiratory viral infections. However, previous studies have shown that antibiotics do not improve outcomes for patients with ARTIs [7–10].

To prevent overuse and inappropriate use of antibiotics, it is essential to identify and understand antibiotic prescribing patterns and determining factors, however, little

* Correspondence: chun@korea.ac.kr
[2]Department of Epidemiology and Health Informatics, Graduate School of Public Health, Korea University, Seoul, Republic of Korea
[7]Department of Preventive Medicine, Korea University College of Medicine, Seoul, Republic of Korea

is known about antibiotic prescribing patterns in the Republic of Korea. The purpose of this study was to describe antibiotic prescription patterns in primary care clinics over a 6-year period and to identify its temporal relationship with respiratory viruses and ARTIs.

Methods
Antibiotic use data
The National Health Insurance covers 98% of the total Korean population, providing near- complete coverage of all antibiotic prescriptions in the Republic of Korea. Reimbursement data from over 80,000 healthcare service providers in Korea were collected from the Korean Health Insurance Review and Assessment Service (KHIRA). The data covers 46 million patients annually, approximately 90% of the population of the Republic of Korea, and includes patients' diagnoses (recorded using the *International Classification of Diseases, Clinical Modification, 10th Revision* [ICD-10-CM]), and prescription drugs [11, 12]. We collected monthly antibiotic prescription data from primary care clinics between January 2010 and December 2015 in accordance with the Anatomic Therapeutic Chemical Classification System (J01A: tetracyclines; J01C: beta-lactam antibacterials, penicillins; J01D: other beta-lactam antibacterials [cephalosporins, monobactams, and carbapenems]; J01F:macrolides, lincosamides, and streptogramins; J01G: aminoglycosides; J01MA: fluoroquinolones). Prescription data were converted to DDD per 1000 inhabitants per day (DID), the assumed average maintenance dose per day for a prescribed medication. Population data were obtained from census data provided by Korean Statistical Information Service.

Respiratory virus surveillance data
The number of acute respiratory virus diagnoses was collected from the Korea Influenza and Respiratory Virus Surveillance System (KINRESS) from the Korea Centers for Disease Control and Prevention. KINRESS collects nasopharyngeal specimens from patients with acute respiratory symptoms, including cough, rhinorrhea, and sore throat, from sentinel primary care clinics. This weekly laboratory-based surveillance system has been in operation since 2009 to measure respiratory virus activity at the community level, including adenovirus (ADV), influenza virus (IFV; A, B), human coronavirus (hCoV; 229E, OC43, NL63), human rhinovirus (hRV), and respiratory syncytial virus (RSV; A, B). Laboratory confirmation of respiratory pathogens was performed using multiplex polymerase chain reaction (PCR) or real-time reverse transcription PCR [13, 14].

Incidence of acute respiratory tract infections
We obtained the monthly number of ARTI diagnoses between 2010 and 2015 from the KHIRA database using ICD-10-CM codes. All patients diagnosed with an ARTI, regardless of age or gender, were included. ARTIs were defined as acute bronchitis and acute upper respiratory tract infection. In addition, we included acute tonsillitis and pneumonia as comparators as they are more likely to require antibiotics than other ARTIs [15]. Incidence was calculated by dividing the number of ARTI diagnoses by the population of the Republic of Korea during the study period.

Statistical analysis
We used regression analysis to describe the trends of antibiotic use, respiratory virus activity, and the incidence of ARTIs, including acute bronchitis, overall.

To identify the temporal relationship between antibiotic prescriptions and respiratory virus activity and the incidence of ARTIs, we performed a cross-correlation function test. This cross-correlation test is widely used in identifying the time lags of onetime series (respiratory virus) with the possible predictors of another time series (antibiotic use) [16, 17].

The Box-Jenkins method was applied to fit time-series data to seasonal autoregressive moving average models [18, 19]. Stationary time series was evaluated using the augmented Dickey-Fuller test to determine whether differencing is required to rule out spurious correlations. The Akaike information criterion test, the portmanteau test, and a normality check of the residuals were conducted to identify the best model fit. Cross-correlation analysis using the residuals from each time-series model was used to evaluate the temporal relationship between the antibiotic prescription rate and respiratory virus detection as well as the incidence of ARTIs.

The statistical package R, version 3.2.4 (R Foundation for Statistical Computing, Vienna, Austria) was used for all statistical analysis. All p-values were 2-sided and considered significant at $p < 0.05$.

Results
Antibiotic use
The average DID of the total antibiotic prescriptions during the study period was 26.2 (range, 20.3-31.2). For primary clinics, the prescribing rate was 25.2 (range, 20.6-31. 2) DID in 2010 and 26.9 (range, 20.4-30.1) in 2015 with a tendency to increase ($p < 0.01$) (Fig. 1a).

The most commonly used classes of antibiotic were penicillin (DID range, 7.1-12.7; mean, 10.1), other beta-lactams antibacterials (DID range, 6.3-9.0; mean, 7.7), macrolides (DID range, 2.4-5.5; mean, 3.9), fluoroquinolones (DID

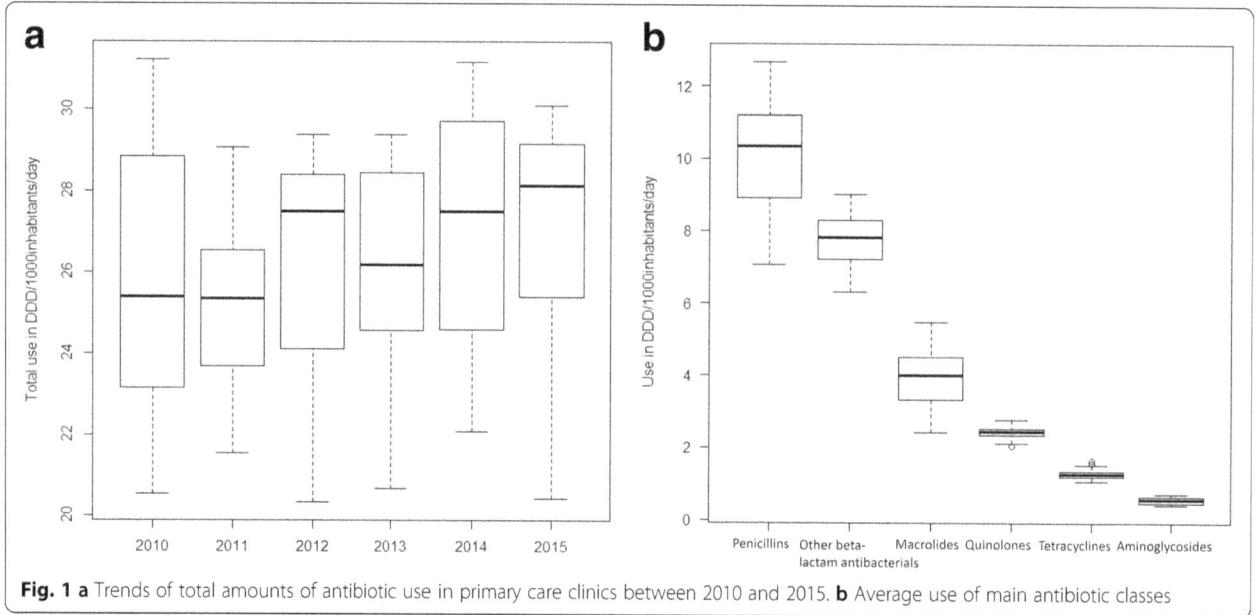

Fig. 1 a Trends of total amounts of antibiotic use in primary care clinics between 2010 and 2015. **b** Average use of main antibiotic classes

range, 2.0-2.8; mean, 2.4), tetracyclines (DID range, 1.1-1.6; mean, 1.3), and aminoglycosides (DID range, 0.4-0.7; mean, 0.6) (Fig. 1b).

Acute respiratory virus activities

Mean annual detection rates of respiratory viruses fluctuated highly in 2011 and 2012, but was largely stable in the other years, though estimated ranges were relatively large. In 2010, 47% (range, 27-72%) of isolates had a virus, while only 39% (range, 21-62%) were detected in 2015 (Fig. 2a).

The most commonly detected respiratory viruses were hRV (range, 2-35%; median, 16%), IFV (range, 0-62%;

median, 2%), ADV (range, 2-28%; median, 6%), RSV (range, 0-24; median, 2%), and hCoV (range, 0-19%; median, 2%) (Fig. 2b).

Incidence of acute respiratory tract infections

The annual incidence of acute bronchitis increased significantly from 3836 (range, 1964-5665; mean, 3836) per 100,000 individuals in 2010 to 4612 (range, 2440-6034; mean, 4612) per 100,000 individuals in 2015 ($p < 0.01$) (Fig. 3a). The average incidences of acute bronchitis, acute tonsillitis, acute upper respiratory tract infections, and pneumonia were 4334, 1864,

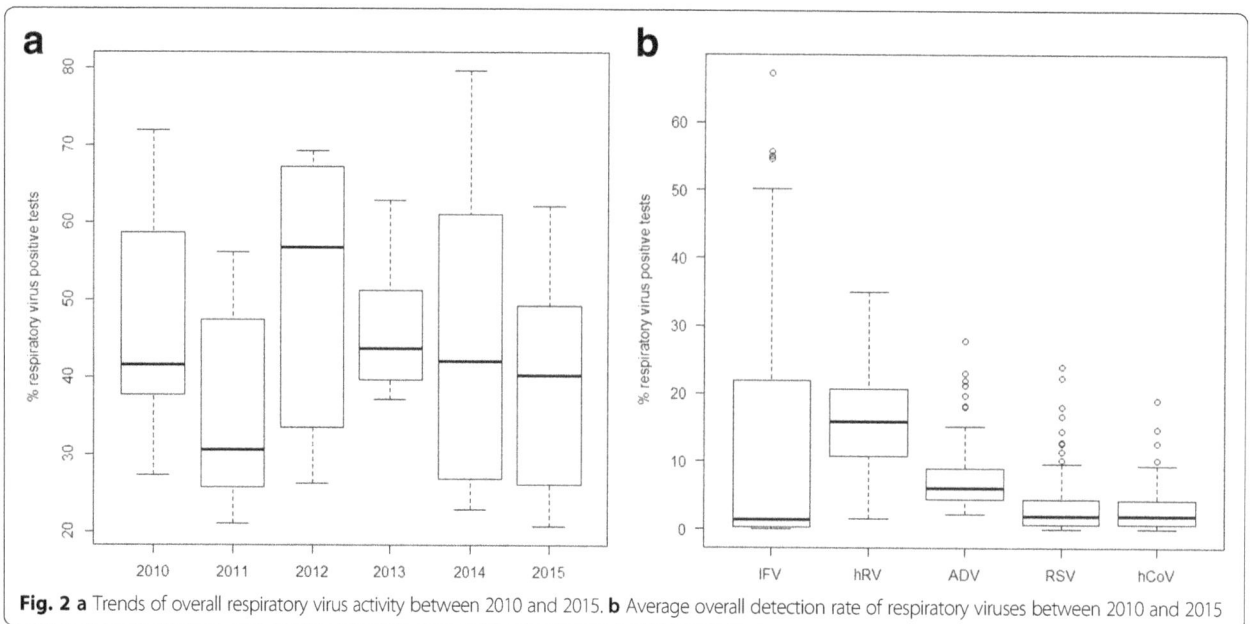

Fig. 2 a Trends of overall respiratory virus activity between 2010 and 2015. **b** Average overall detection rate of respiratory viruses between 2010 and 2015

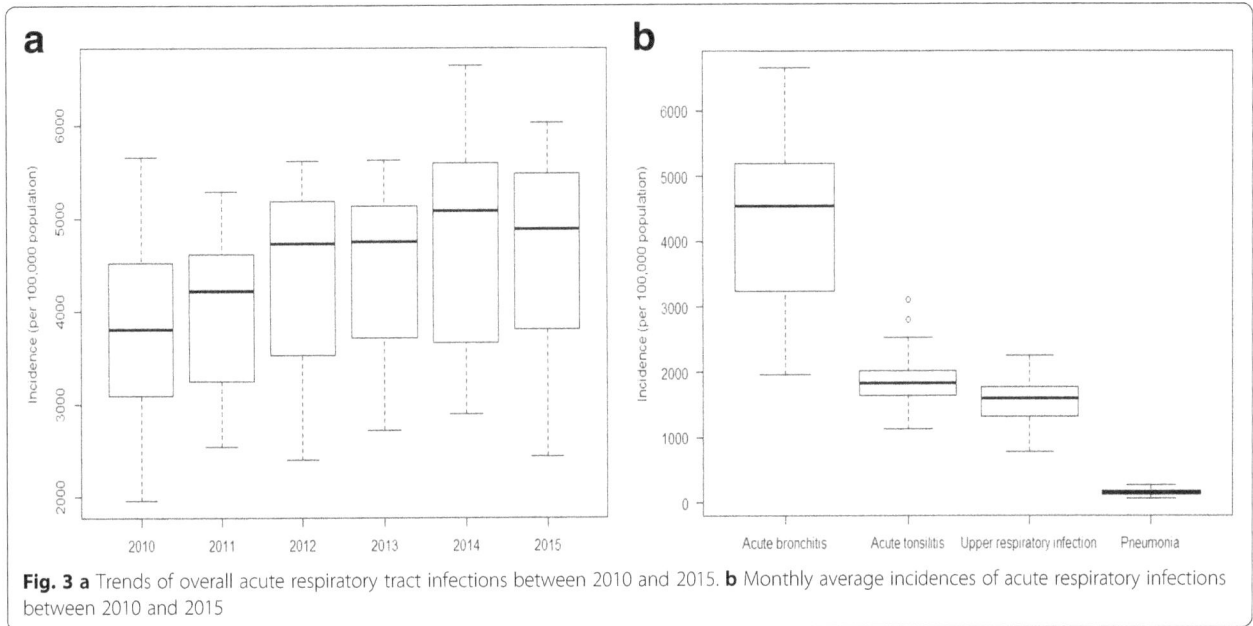

Fig. 3 a Trends of overall acute respiratory tract infections between 2010 and 2015. **b** Monthly average incidences of acute respiratory infections between 2010 and 2015

1526, and 153 per 100,000 individuals, respectively (Fig. 3 (b)).

Correlation analysis of antibiotic use with respiratory virus detection and incidence of respiratory infections

Monthly time series of antibiotic use, respiratory virus detection, and incidence of ARTIs are presented in Fig. 4. Seasonal antibiotic use clearly followed a similar oscillatory pattern to influenza virus detection. Antibiotic use also had a similar seasonal pattern as the incidences of acute bronchitis, acute upper respiratory tract infections, and acute tonsillitis.

The total monthly rate of antibiotic prescriptions was highly cross-correlated with the monthly detection rate of influenza virus (cross-correlation coefficient 0.47, $p < 0.01$). In bivariate analyses, antibiotic use rates for the 4 most commonly used antibiotics (penicillins, other beta-lactam antibacterials, macrolides, and fluoroquinolones) were significantly cross-correlated with influenza virus detection at the 0-month lag with cross-correlation coefficients of 0.45 ($p < 0.01$), 0.46 ($p < 0.01$), 0.40 ($p < 0.01$), and 0.35 (< 0.01), respectively (Table 1). However, no cross-correlation was found between antibiotic classes with lower-use rates (< 2 DID) and the influenza virus detection rate. There was significant cross-correlation between hRV and tetracycline with a 2-month lag (cross-correlation coefficient 0.24, $p = 0.04$).

For ARTIs, the correlation coefficiencts of antibiotic use and the incidence of acute bronchitis were 0.73 ($p < 0.01$) for penicillins, 0.69 ($p < 0.01$) for other beta-lactam antibacterials, 0.74 ($p < 0.01$) for macrolides and 0.45 ($p < 0.01$) for fluoroquinolones (Table 2). Acute upper respiratory infection was significantly correlated

with penicillins (0.33, $p < 0.01$), other beta-lactam antibacterials (0.32, $p < 0.01$), macrolides (0.24, $p = 0.04$), and fluoroquinolones (0.31, $p < 0.01$) without a lag. Again, no cross-correlation was found between classes of antibiotics with lower-use rates (< 2 DID) and ARTIs.

For comparators that were more likely to require antibiotics than ARTIs, pneumonia was significantly correlated with penicillins (0.36, $p < 0.01$), macrolides (0.53, $p < 0.01$), aminoglycosides (0.38, $p < 0.01$), and other beta-lactam antibacterials (0.25, $p < 0.03$) without a lag. Furthermore, acute tonsillitis was significantly correlated with penicillin (0.69. $p < 0.01$), other beta-lactam antibacterials (0.68, $p < 0.01$), macrolides (0.59, $p < 0.01$), and fluoroquinolones (0.35, $p < 0.01$) without a lag.

Discussion

Our study is the first to identify the temporal relationship between the number of monthly antibiotic prescriptions and the detection rates of respiratory viruses and ARTIs in the Republic of Korea. Our results suggest that seasonal variation in the numbers of commonly prescribed antibiotics (penicillins, other beta-lactam antibacterials, macrolides, and fluoroquinolones) was significantly associated with the change in the activity of influenza in the community. Seasonal variation of antibiotic prescriptions has been documented in the United States [17, 20], Canada [21], and Europe [22]. Furthermore, it has also been shown that the incidence of influenza is highly correlated with the seasonal pattern of antibiotic prescriptions and that changes in testing can affect prescription rates of antibiotics [23–26]. These previous findings support our results that the seasonality of antibiotic use is significantly associated with influenza virus activity in the country.

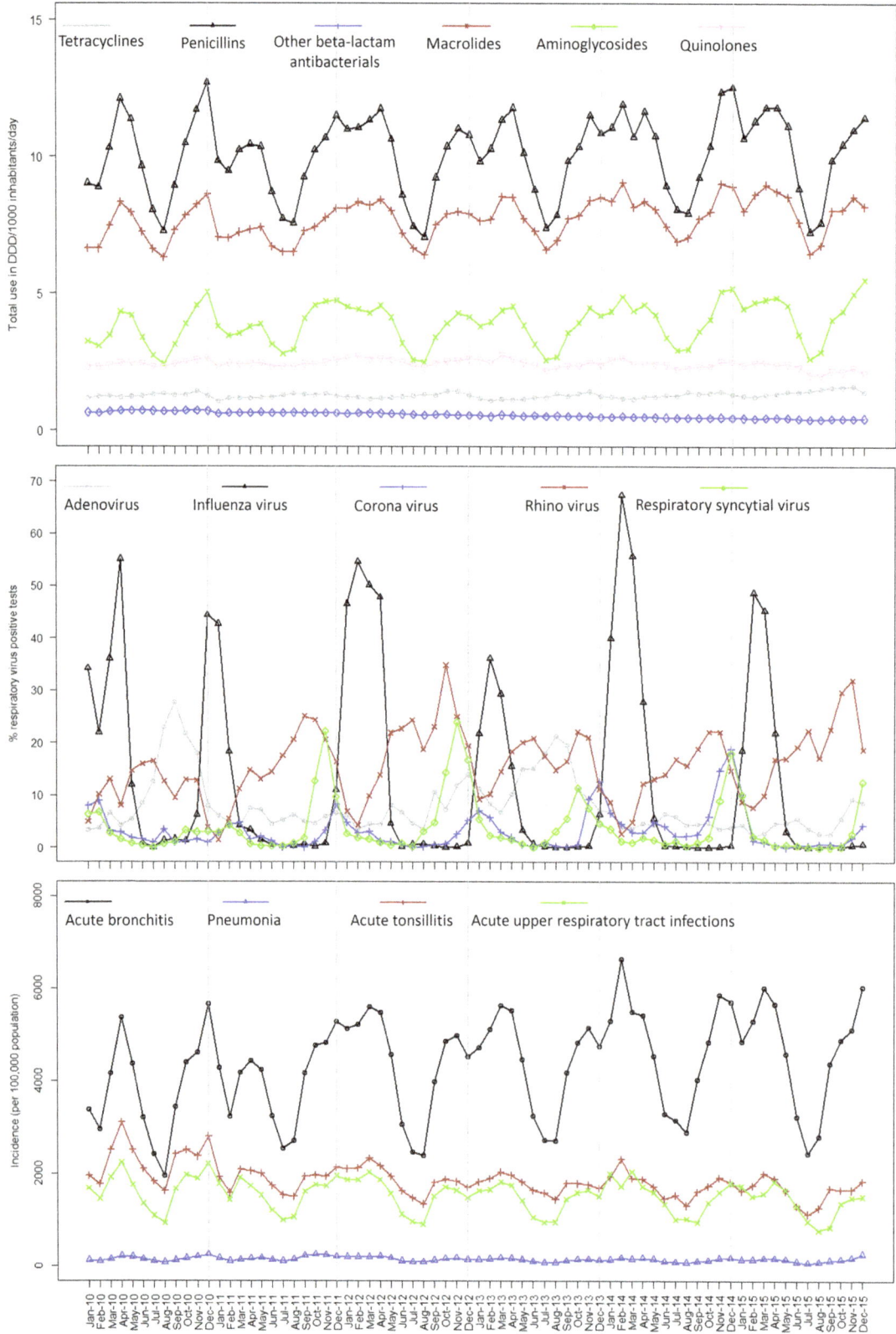

Fig. 4 Descriptive trends of antibiotic use, respiratory virus activities, and the incidence of acute respiratory disease

Table 1 Cross-correlation coefficients between antibiotic use and respiratory viruses (2010-2015)

Antibiotics	RSV	IFV	hCoV	hRV	ADV
Tetracyclines	−0.14 $p = 0.24$ 0-month lag	0.05 $p = 0.67$ 7-month lag	−0.09 $p = 0.43$ − 3-month lag	0.24 $p = 0.04$ 2-month lag	− 0.07 $p = 0.55$ 0-month lag
Penicillins	− 0.01 $p = 0.98$ 10-month lag	0.45 $p < 0.01$ 0-month lag	0.06 $p = 0.64$ 2-month lag	−0.13 $p = 0.29$ 2-month lag	− 0.09 $p = 0.44$ 6-month lag
Other beta-lactam antibacterials	−0.02 $p = 0.90$ 1-month lag	0.46 $p < 0.01$ 0-month lag	0.02 $p = 0.85$ 1-month lag	−0.14 $p = 0.24$ 2-month lag	−0.11 $p = 0.34$ 0-month lag
Macrolides	0.12 $p = 0.31$ 10-month lag	0.40 $p < 0.01$ 0-month lag	−0.06 $p = 0.60$ 1-month lag	−0.08 $p = 0.50$ 8-month lag	− 0.16 $p = 0.18$ 9-month lag
Aminoglycosides	−0.03 $p = 0.79$ 10-month lag	0.15 $p = 0.20$ 0-month lag	0.11 $p = 0.36$ 1-month lag	0.10 $p = 0.39$ 0-month lag	−0.11 $p = 0.37$ 5-month lag
Fluoroquinolones	−0.02 $p = 0.84$ 3-month lag	0.35 $p < 0.01$ 0-month lag	−0.03 $p = 0.83$ 2-month lag	−0.04 $p = 0.76$ 2-month lag	− 0.16 $p = 0.19$ 6-month lag

Abbreviations: *ADV* adenovirus, *hCoV* human coronavirus, *hRV* human rhinovirus, *IFV* Influenza virus, *RSV* respiratory syncytial virus

Aside from the correlation between hRV and tetracycline, other viruses were not significantly correlated with antibiotic use. This may be due to the low numbers of antibiotic use against hRV.

Regarding the cross-correlation between influenza virus activity and the incidence of pneumonia, no significant temporal relationship was found within a 1-month lag (β = 0.23, p = 0.05). This is likely because of the low incidence of pneumonia (153 cases per 100,000 persons). This is not surprising as pneumonia is an uncommon diagnosis in the outpatient setting compared to acute bronchitis (4334 cases per 100,000 persons). Pneumonia is a quite severe infection and often requires hospitalization for confirmation. Thus, many acute bronchitis prescriptions might reflect uncertainty on the clinician part as to whether the patient may have pneumonia, and are prescribing out of an abundance of caution despite the potential downside consequences of unnecessary antibiotic use.

Regarding the relationship between influenza virus activity and the incidence of acute tonsillitis, a significant cross-correlation was found (β = 0.29, p = 0.01) at the 0-month lag. This result is consistent with previous literature documenting the most common cause of tonsillitis is viral infection including influenza virus [27]. Conservative management is the main treatment option for patients with tonsillitis except in the case of streptococcal infections (detection rate in Korea: 8.3%) [27]. Our results demonstrated that antibiotic use was significantly correlated with acute tonsillitis with a larger magnitude than influenza virus activity. This correlation likely

Table 2 Cross-correlation coefficients between antibiotic use and acute respiratory tract infections (2010-2015)

Antibiotics	Acute bronchitis	Acute tonsillitis	Acute upper respiratory infection	Pneumonia
Tetracyclines	0.44 $p = 0.66$ 0-month lag	0.11 $p = 0.34$ 0-month lag	0.03 $p = 0.97$ −10-month lag	−0.01 $p = 0.90$ 0-month lag
Penicillins	0.73 $p < 0.01$ 0-month lag	0.69 $p < 0.01$ 0-month lag	0.33 $p < 0.01$ 0-month lag	0.36 $p < 0.01$ 0-month lag
Other beta-lactam antibacterials	0.69 $p < 0.01$ 0-month lag	0.68 $p < 0.01$ 0-month lag	0.32 $p < 0.01$ 0-month lag	0.25 $p = 0.03$ 0-month lag
Macrolides	0.74 $p < 0.01$ 0-month lag	0.59 $p < 0.01$ 0-month lag	0.24 $p = 0.04$ 0-month lag	0.53 $p < 0.01$ 0-month lag
Aminoglycosides	0.14 $p = 0.28$ 0-month lag	0.20 $p = 0.09$ −3-month lag	−0.04 $p = 0.75$ 0-month lag	0.38 $p < 0.01$ 0-month lag
Fluoroquinolones	0.45 $p < 0.01$ 0-month lag	0.35 $p < 0.01$ 0-month lag	0.31 $p < 0.01$ 0-month lag	0.23 $p = 0.05$ 0-month lag

results from the physician's anxiety over the potential risk of developing secondary bacterial infections. Antibiotics prescribed for respiratory viruses are positively associated with poor quality prescribing [24, 28]. Patient satisfaction has been shown to be a major driver as well. Even patients who received a delayed antibiotic prescription were less likely to be satisfied with treatment than those who immediately received a prescription, even if the treatment outcomes were not different [29, 30]. This underlying situation may have contributed to the high rates of antibiotic use for diagnoses that generally do not require antibiotics.

Our results further suggest that antibiotic use could be lowered by reducing influenza transmission or through education campaigns aimed at the public and physicians to discourage inappropriate prescribing of antibiotics, particularly during influenza season [31]. Moreover, increasing vaccine coverage, which covers only approximately 43% of the Korean population, may reduce unnecessary antibiotic use [32]. Improved point-of-care tests for detecting influenza virus may also be likely to reduce antibiotic use [25, 26].

Our findings are subject to several limitations. First, our study is ecological and utilizes population-level data and thus may not represent associations at the individual level. Nonetheless, the significant relationship between the overuse of antibiotics and influenza virus circulation was also observed in a previous cohort study [33]. Second, since enterovirus (mean detection rate: 3.1%) has not been assessed in the KINRESS since 2011 and the mean detection rates of other respiratory viruses, such as human metapneumovirus (hMPV), human bocavirus (hBoV), and human parainfluenza virus (hPIV) were relatively low (hMPV: 1.28%, hBoV: 1.6%, hPIV: 4.0%), these viruses were not considered in this study. Third, we used primary care clinic-based sentinel surveillance data for respiratory virus detection. These data could underestimate the strength of virus activity; however, the pattern of influenza virus activity was similar to the pattern of influenza-like-illness in the country. Fourth, the number of samples collected was not consistent year on year due to the variation of respiratory virus activity (yearly mean number of samples collected is 12,938). Fifth, ARTIs may include other infectious diseases requiring antibiotic treatment, such as bacterial pneumonia.

Conclusions

Our study identified a strong temporal association between antibiotic use, and influenza virus activity, and the incidence of ARTIs. We detected a significant correlation between antibiotic use of common antibiotics (penicillins, other beta-lactam antibacterials, macrolides, and fluoroqui-

nolones) and influenza virus activity as well as the incidence of acute bronchitis and acute upper respiratory tract infections. Our results indicate that interventions aimed at reducing influenza infections and discouraging the use of antibiotics by physicians and the public may help to decrease antibiotic consumption. Additional studies, including precise evaluations of the Korean Influenza National Immunization Program, on antibiotic prescription patterns, may identify additional opportunities to reduce antibiotic prescriptions.

Abbreviations
ADV: Adenovirus; ARTIs: Acute respiratory tract infections; DDD: Defined daily dose; DID: Defined daily dose per 1000 inhabitants per day; hBoV: Human bocavirus; hCoV: Human coronavirus; hMPV: Human metapneumovirus; hPIV: Human parainfluenza virus; hRV: Human rhinovirus; ICD-10-CM: International Classification of Diseases, Clinical Modification, Tenth Revision; IFV: Influenza virus; KHIRA: Korean Health Insurance Review and Assessment Service; KINRESS: Korea Influenza and Respiratory Virus Surveillance System; RSV: Respiratory syncytial virus

Acknowledgments
This work was conducted in partial fulfillment of the doctoral thesis requirement of the Graduate School of Public Health, Korea University, Seoul, Korea.

Funding
This work was supported by the Research Institute for Healthcare Policy, KMA in 2016.

Authors' contributions
RS was responsible for the design of the study and RS, KS, and KBI collected and analyzed the data. RS, KEI, and CBC prepared the initial and revised draft of the manuscript. RS, KEI, YKY, and CBC were responsible for validation, analysis and interpretation of the data. All authors contributed to the final version of the manuscript. All authors read and approved the final manuscript.

Competing interests
The authors declare that they have no competing interests.

Author details
[1]Division of Infectious Disease Control, Gyeonggi Provincial Government, Suwon, Republic of Korea. [2]Department of Epidemiology and Health Informatics, Graduate School of Public Health, Korea University, Seoul, Republic of Korea. [3]Department of Insurance Benefit, National Health Insurance Service, Seoul, Republic of Korea. [4]Center for Disease Dynamics, Economics & Policy, Washington D.C., USA. [5]Department of Emergency Medicine, Johns Hopkins University, Baltimore, USA. [6]Division of Infectious Diseases, Department of Internal Medicine, Korea University College of Medicine, Seoul, Republic of Korea. [7]Department of Preventive Medicine, Korea University College of Medicine, Seoul, Republic of Korea.

References
1. World Health Organization. Antimicrobial resistance: global report on surveillance. Geneva: WHO Press, World Health Organization; 2014.
2. Boucher HW, Talbot GH, Bradley JS, Edwards JE, Gilbert D, Rice LB. Bad bugs, no drugs: no ESKAPE! An update from the infectious disease Society of America. Clin Infect Dis. 2009;48:1–2.

3. Organization for Economic Co-operation and Development (OECD). Antimicrobial resistance: OECD; 2016. http://www.oecd.org/els/health-systems/antimicrobial-resistance.htm. Accessed 10 Apr 2017

4. Health Insurance Review and Assessment (HIRA). In-depth analysis and evaluation of drug use. Seoul: HIRA; 2015.

5. Smith S, Fahey T, Smucny J, Becker L. Antibiotics for acute bronchitis. Cochrane Database Syst Rev. 2012;4:CD000245.

6. Ebell MH, Radke T. Antibiotic use for viral acute respiratory tract infections remains common. Am J Manag Care. 2015;21:e567–75.

7. Evans AT, Hussain S, Durairaj L, Sadowski LS, Charles-Damte M, Wang Y. Azithromycin for acute bronchitis: a randomized, double-blind, controlled trial. Lancet. 2002;35:1648–54.

8. Little P, Stuart B, Moore M. Amoxicillin for acute lower-respiratory tract infection in primary care when pneumonia is not suspected: a 12-country, randomized, placebo-controlled trial. Lancet Infect Dis. 2013;13:123–9.

9. Llor C, Moragas A, Bayona C, Morros R, Pera H, Plana-Ripoll O, et al. Efficacy of anti-inflammatory or antibiotic treatment in patients with non-complicated acute bronchitis and discoloured sputum: randomised placebo controlled trial. BMJ. 2013;347:f5762.

10. Ganestam F, Lundborg CS, Grabowska K, Cars O, Linde A. Weekly antibiotic prescribing and influenza activity in Sweden: a study throughout five influenza seasons. Scand J Infect Dis. 2003;35:836–42.

11. Kim L, Kim KA, Kim S. A guide for the utilization of health insurance review and assessment service national patient sample. Epidemiol Health. 2014;36:e2014008.

12. Health Insurance Review and Assessment. Healthcare Bigdata Hub. http://opendata.hira.or.kr. Accessed 10 Mar 2017.

13. Park JS, Jung HD, Jung HM, Kim SS, Kim CK. Prevalence of respiratory viruses in patients with acute respiratory infections in Korea. J Allergy Clin Immunol. 2016;137:AB31.

14. Korea Centers for Disease Control and Prevention. Weekly surveillance reports for influenza and other respiratory viruses. Chengju. http://www.cdc.go.kr/CDC/info/CdcKrInfo0502.jsp?menuIds=HOME001-MNU1154-MNU0005-MNU0048-MNU0050. Accessed 10 Mar 2017

15. Zoorob R, Sidani MA, Fremont RD, Kihlberg C. Antibiotic use in acute upper respiratory tract infection. Am Fam Physician. 2012;11:817–22.

16. Gilca R, Fortin E, Frenette C, Longtin Y, Gourdeau M. Seasonal variation in Clostridium difficile infections are associated with influenza and respiratory syncytial virus activity independently of antibiotic prescriptions: a time series analysis in Quebec. Canada Antimicrob Agents and Chemother. 2012;56:639–46.

17. Sun L, Klein KY, Laximinarayan R. Seasonality and temporal correlation between community antibiotic use and resistance in the United States. Clin Inf Dis. 2012;7:1–8.

18. Cowperwait PSP, Metcalfe AV. Introductory time series with R. New York: Springer; 2009.

19. Box GEP, Jenkins GM, Reinsel GC. Time series analysis: forecasting and control. 3rd ed. Englewood Cliffs: Prentice Hall; 1994.

20. Suda KJ, Hicks LA, Roberts RM, Hunkler RJ, Taylor TH. Trends and seasonal variation in outpatient antibiotic prescription rates in the United States, 2006 to 2010. Antimicrob Agents Chemother. 2014;58:2763–6.

21. Cebotareco N, Bush PJ. Reducing antibiotics for colds and flu: a student-thought program. Health Educ Res. 2008;23:146–57.

22. Goossens H, Ferech M, Stichele RV, Elseviers M. Outpatient antibiotic use in Europe and association with resistance: a cross-national database study. Lancet. 2005;365:579–87.

23. Fleming DM, Ross AM, Cross KW, Kendall H. The reducing incidence of respiratory tract infection and its relation to antibiotic prescribing. Br J Gen Pract. 2003;53:778–83.

24. Polgreen PM, Yang M, Laxminarayan R, Cavanaugh JE. Respiratory fluoroquinolone use and influenza. Infect Control Hosp Epidemiol. 2011;32:706–9.

25. Belshe RB, Gruber WC. Safety, efficacy and effectiveness of cold-adapted, live, attenuated, trivalent, intranasal influenza vaccine in adults and children. Philos Trans R Soc Lond Ser B Biol Sci. 2001;356:1947–51.

26. Noyola DE, Demmler GJ. Effect of rapid diagnosis on management of influenza a infection. Pediatr Infect Dis J. 2000;19:303–7.

27. Korea Centers for Disease Control and Prevention (KCDC). Guidelines for the antibiotic use in children with acute upper respiratory tract infections. Osong: KCDC; 2016. p. 20–5.

28. Dallas A, Magin P, Morgan S, Tapley A, Henderson K, Ball J, et al. Antibiotic prescribing for respiratory infections: a cross-sectional analysis of the ReCEnT study exploring the habits of early-career doctors in primary care. Fam Pract. 2015;32:49–55.

29. Arroll B, Kenealy T, Kerse N. Do delayed prescriptions reduce antibiotic use in respiratory tract infection? A systematic review. Br J Gen Pract. 2003;53:871–7.

30. Spurling GK, Del Mar CB, Dooley L, Foxlee R, Farley R. Delayed antibiotics for respiratory infections. Cochrane Database Syst Rev. 2013;4:CD004417.

31. Sabuncu E, David J, Bernede-Bauduin C, Pepin S, Leroy M, Boelle PY, et al. Significant reduction of antibiotic use in the community after a nationwide campaign in France, 2002-2007. PLoS Med. 2009;6:e1000084.

32. Yang HJ, Cho SI. Influenza vaccination coverage among adults in Korea: 2008-2009 to 2011-2012 seasons. Int J Environ Res Public Health. 2014; 11:12162–73.

33. Nitsch-Osuch A, Gyrczuk E, Wardyn A, Zycinska K, Brydak L. Antibiotic prescription practices among children with influenza. Adv Exp Med Biol. 2016;905:25–31.

13

Infection control at an urban hospital in Manila, Philippines: a systems engineering assessment of barriers and facilitators

Kaitlin F. Mitchell[1,2], Anna K. Barker[1,2], Cybele L. Abad[3] and Nasia Safdar[2,4,5*]

Abstract

Background: Healthcare facilities in low- and middle-income countries, including the Philippines, face substantial challenges in achieving effective infection control. Early stages of interventions should include efforts to understand perceptions held by healthcare workers who participate in infection control programs.

Methods: We performed a qualitative study to examine facilitators and barriers to infection control at an 800-bed, private, tertiary hospital in Manila, Philippines. Semi-structured interviews were conducted with 22 nurses, physicians, and clinical pharmacists using a guide based on the Systems Engineering Initiative for Patient Safety (SEIPS). Major facilitators and barriers to infection control were reported for each SEIPS factor: person, organization, tasks, physical environment, and technology and tools.

Results: Primary facilitators included a robust, long-standing infection control committee, a dedicated infection control nursing staff, and innovative electronic hand hygiene surveillance technology. Barriers included suboptimal dissemination of hand hygiene compliance data, high nursing turnover, clinical time constraints, and resource limitations that restricted equipment purchasing.

Conclusions: The identified facilitators and barriers may be used to prioritize possible opportunities for infection control interventions. A systems engineering approach is useful for conducting a comprehensive work system analysis, and maximizing resources to overcome known barriers to infection control in heavily resource-constrained settings.

Keywords: Systems Engineering Initiative for Patient Safety, Philippines, Infection control, Hand hygiene, Intervention implementation

Background

No health care facility in the world is immune to the burden of hospital-acquired infections (HAIs). Those in low- and middle-income countries such as the Philippines experience especially high rates of HAIs [1, 2], perhaps due to the added challenges they face in achieving effective infection control. These challenges include a higher prevalence of multi-drug resistant organisms (MDROs), lack of HAI surveillance, antibiotic overuse and misuse, and international migration of their healthcare workforce [3–5]. Assessing and improving the quality of infection

* Correspondence: ns2@medicine.wisc.edu
[2]Division of Infectious Diseases, Department of Medicine, University of Wisconsin-Madison, Madison, WI, USA
[4]William S. Middleton Memorial Veterans Hospital, Madison, WI, USA

control policies, hand hygiene, and HAI surveillance in these settings is critical [6].

In order to develop effective interventions, it is essential to understand how the work system in a healthcare setting may impede successful implementation [7]. The Systems Engineering Initiative for Patient Safety, or SEIPS framework, is well suited for its ability to analyze the impacts of a work system on both patient and organizational outcomes [8]. The work system includes the components of person (e.g. skills, motivation, and needs), tasks (e.g. job content), tools and technologies (e.g. information technologies or medical devices), the physical environment (e.g. layout and work station design), and organizational components (e.g. patient safety culture and communication). This model has been used to improve patient safety in a variety of healthcare contexts, including both outpatient and inpatient settings [9, 10].

Although the Philippines has a high HAI burden, an understanding of the facilitators and barriers to hospital infection control in this country is lacking [1–3]. To address this gap, we used the SEIPS framework to evaluate barriers and facilitators to infection control at a private, tertiary hospital located in Manila.

Methods
Location
The study was conducted at a private, 800-bed, tertiary hospital in Manila, Philippines. The facility is one of five hospitals in the Philippines accredited by the Joint Commission International. It employs 1000 physicians and over 2000 allied medical and administrative staff, and handles both routine and complex cases in many departments. The hospital has an infection control program that was established in 1986, and at the time of our study included six dedicated infection control nursing staff. Infection control policies are implemented and reviewed by the Hospital Infection Control Executive Committee. The facility has designated medical floors for those needing airborne isolation (e.g. pulmonary tuberculosis).

Study population
We completed a total of 22 semi-structured interviews with physicians (n = 10; three male, seven female), nurses including infection control staff (n = 10; two male, eight female), and clinical pharmacists (n = 2; two female). Potential participants were selected by convenience sampling to cover a range of job types, experience levels, and clinical departments. Subjects who were available during the time investigators were conducting interviews were asked if they could participate and were identified on clinical wards by members of the research team. A few participants, including the two clinical pharmacists, were approached and recruited directly. Departments included cardiology, clinical pharmacy, gastroenterology, infection control, internal medicine, obstetrics and gynecology, oncology, pediatrics, and pulmonary medicine. Most participants worked in general wards in these departments, although two worked in the emergency department and two worked in the intensive care units (ICUs). Criteria for inclusion were formal employment by the hospital and active involvement in patient care. Status as a medical or nursing student or as a non-English speaker were criteria for exclusion, although no potential participants were excluded for these reasons.

Data collection
Interview questions were adapted for context from an interview guide our group previously used to study facilitators and barriers to infection control at a large, private hospital in Gurgaon, India [11]. The questions were based on the SEIPS framework and included questions in the categories for work systems: person, organization, task, physical environment, and technology and tools. Interviews were audio recorded and typically lasted ten to twenty minutes in length. No identifiable information was collected. Preliminary analysis was conducted throughout the study to refine the interview guide and assess theoretical saturation. No further interviews were completed once theoretical saturation was reached.

Data analysis
All interviews were transcribed. Interview transcripts were independently coded in NVivo software (Version 11, QSR International) by two individuals to identify trends, following a previously described method for line-by-line coding [12]. The two versions of coding were compared and found to have high inter-rater reliability. As a quality improvement project, this study was granted exemption from review by the UW-Madison Institutional Review Board and received expedited review and approval at the study site.

Results
Data were categorized based on the SEIPS model work system (Fig. 1 and Table 1).

Person
The multiple roles of the hospital's infection control nursing staff were regarded as having a positive impact on the infection control process. They conducted HAI surveillance through review of medical records and bedside follow-up of high-risk patients. Infection control staff monitored hand hygiene compliance by performing daily audits through direct observation on each ward, and they also reviewed video footage of provider entry and exit from patient rooms using the hospital's closed-circuit television system (Table 1, quotations 1 and 2). The infection control nurses and their duties were viewed with respect, and were regarded by other clinical staff as a vital component of the healthcare process (Table 1, quotation 3).

Another person-level factor was differing hand hygiene compliance between healthcare worker types. Both doctors and nurses reported that nurses had the highest hand hygiene compliance, while attending physicians had the lowest (Table 1, quotation 3). It was also noted that amongst the doctors, older consulting physicians tended to be the least compliant. This behavior was suggested to have a magnified impact on hand hygiene practices, as the senior physicians set "an example" for others (Table 1, quotation 5). Several doctors reported

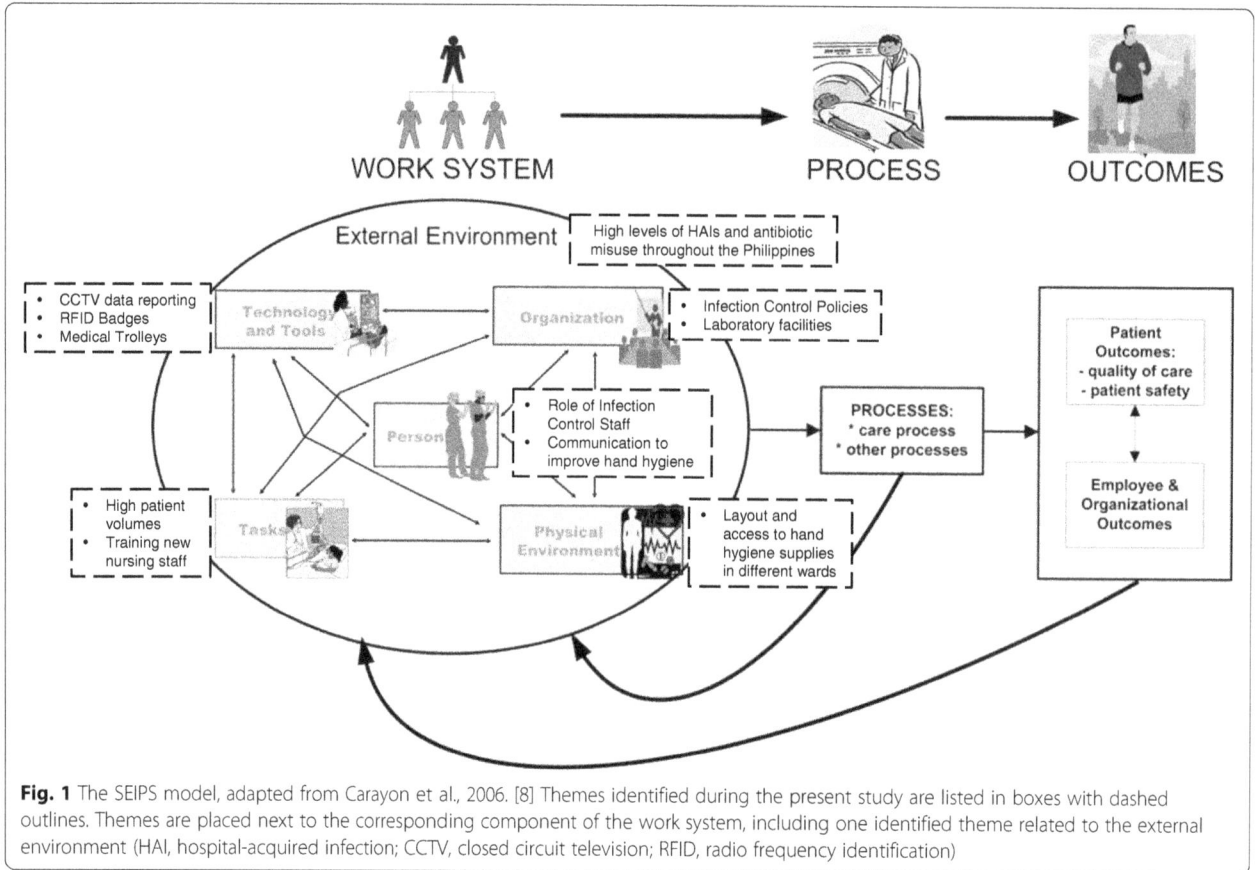

Fig. 1 The SEIPS model, adapted from Carayon et al., 2006. [8] Themes identified during the present study are listed in boxes with dashed outlines. Themes are placed next to the corresponding component of the work system, including one identified theme related to the external environment (HAI, hospital-acquired infection; CCTV, closed circuit television; RFID, radio frequency identification)

that verbal reminders, either from nurses or other physicians, would be a useful strategy to improve hand hygiene. However, it was also noted that the success of reminders would depend on the social dynamic between individual healthcare workers, as some attending physicians were more likely to be amenable to receiving feedback than others (Table 1, quotation 6).

Organization

The hospital's infection control executive committee was recognized as the organizational body that develops fundamental infection control guidelines such as those for hand hygiene, antimicrobial stewardship, and contact and other precautions. The representation of multiple departments on the committee was described as a necessary aspect of developing these guidelines (Table 1, quotation 7). These policies were monitored by the infection control staff, described above. The committee also organized promotional events and offered training for hand hygiene (Table 1, quotation 8). The committee and infection control guidelines could be called upon to resolve any disputes regarding appropriate patient care pertinent to infection control (Table 1, quotation 9). For example, they could be consulted for decisions regarding the appropriate placement of patients on the hospital's isolation ward.

The hospital has prioritized funding and staffing for laboratory facilities, which were vital for performing tests to inform patient treatment plans and infection control surveillance. The turnaround time and communication of lab results through electronic reports were described favorably (Table 1, quotation 10). Efficient laboratory testing was thought to be particularly important for detecting antibiotic-resistant infections in patients who may have been exposed in the community, or another healthcare setting, prior to admission (Table 1, quotation 11).

Task

There was considerable variation in the patient-to-provider ratios described across hospital departments, based on patient complexity and length of stay. The number of patients per nurse was estimated to be 1:1 or 2:1 in the ICUs, 5:1 or 6:1 in the obstetrics/gynecology and cancer wards, and approximately 16:1 in the cardiology ward. Several providers noted that a lack of time due to high patient volumes was a major barrier to hand hygiene compliance (Table 1, quotation 12).

Very high rates of nursing staff turnover also contributed to a high clinical workload. One nurse estimated that within the past six months, thirty out of ninety

Table 1 Representative quotations of themes identified using the SEIPS framework

SEIPS factor	Theme	Subject position and department	Quotation
Person	Role of Infection Control Staff	1: Staff Nurse, Infection Control	1: "We're doing surveillance for infection control... like gathering data for patients who have risk devices. We're also checking the environment... to make sure that infection control policies are implemented properly."
		2: Staff Nurse, Oncology	2: "The infection control people visit us... they monitor us... they check everything on a daily basis."
		3: Head Nurse, Internal Medicine	3: "[Healthcare workers are] amenable with the infection control rules... because they're for the patients."
	Communication to improve hand hygiene	4: Resident, Emergency Medicine	4: "It's the nurses who do the hand hygiene more than the doctors"
		5: Resident, Pediatrics	5: "When [the consultants] go in and we follow, we forget to wash too."
		6: Resident, Pediatrics	6: "I think it needs to be a team effort, like a constant reminder... the head nurses talk to you: 'Doctor, you need to wash your hands'. I think it's very helpful, you need to do that... But there are some doctors here who don't really become too friendly with the nurses. They really set the barrier between them."
Organization	Infection Control Policies	7: Staff Nurse, Infection Control	7: "HICEC is divided into committees... the executive committee makes the policies... we also have the nurses and staff from all different departments. Whenever we make a policy we make sure that all of [the representatives] approve."
		8: Resident, first year	8: "It's part of the infection control committee responsibilities to do regular lectures on hand hygiene."
		9: Head Nurse, Internal Medicine	9: "We can coordinate with HICEC if we have a misunderstanding with the doctors... because we have a set of admitting guidelines for what is allowed in our ward, so sometimes we just have to tell the doctors that. You can also ask HICEC [to do that]."
	Laboratory Facilities	10: Attending Physician, Gastroenterology	10: "[The lab] immediately informs us... so that we can treat right away."
		11: Resident, Pediatrics	11: "We try our best to prevent [resistant infections] here... but other doctors in other places, and the lay people, don't have any idea what antibiotic resistance means."
Tasks	High Patient Volumes	12: Resident, Emergency Medicine	12: "There are times we have to see one patient, just remove the gloves, and move onto the next patient, so there's no [time for] alcohol in between."
	Training of New Nursing Staff	13: Resident, first year	13: "[Nurses] get their training and then leave after about two to three years."
		14: Head Nurse, Emergency Medicine	14: "We teach them all the standard precautions and diseases that any nurse could encounter."
Physical Environment	Layout and Access to Hand Hygiene Supplies	15: Head Nurse, Internal Medicine	15: "The baby-friendly [obstetrics/gynecology ward] is much better with the hand hygiene because they have their own station there."
		16: Resident, Emergency Medicine	16: "The alcohol rub is more in the station, where the medications are prepared [by the nurses]... so it's not really that accessible to us."

Table 1 Representative quotations of themes identified using the SEIPS framework *(Continued)*

		17: Resident, Pediatrics	17: "I see some patients get the alcohol and place it in their room… one of the patients actually got the whole alcohol container."
		18: Resident, Emergency Medicine	18: "There are some doctors who bring their own, or at least have it hooked on to them. And then that's the time when they can do hand rubbing."
Technology and Tools	CCTV Data Reporting	19: Head Nurse, Emergency Medicine	19: "[Each person] is not being reported, the whole emergency department is being reported. It's not working I think, because when we look at the results they're not specific."
		20: Resident, Pediatrics	20: "They should call out those who don't really hand wash, and talk to them directly. Because [the providers] don't know they're being monitored, so they think they can get away with it."
	RFID Badges	21: Staff Nurse, Infection Control	21: "Every time the healthcare worker will enter the patient's room, the ID will alarm if you don't do hand hygiene."
	Medical Trolleys	22: Head Nurse, Oncology	22: "The problem here is sometimes the nurses have too many things in their arms… [they need somewhere to] place things first while they're rubbing their hands."

HICEC hospital infection control executive committee, *CCTV* closed circuit television, *RFID* radio frequency identification

nurses had left the emergency department staff. The emigration of skilled healthcare workers from the Philippines was described as common; many nurses were motivated to move for higher-paying jobs abroad, leaving vacant positions that required continual resources to fill (Table 1, quotation 13). Most newly-hired nurses began jobs at this hospital directly out of nursing school, and needed a considerable amount of on-the-job infection control training (Table 1, quotation 14).

Physical environment

Variations in the layout and quantity of hand hygiene supplies were believed to affect hand hygiene feasibility in certain departments. Alcohol-based hand rub dispensers were reported to be located outside of patient rooms, though the emergency department and ICU had additional dispensers located within patient rooms or cubicles. Sinks for handwashing were positioned at the nursing stations on most wards. However, the airborne isolation floor, emergency department isolation room, obstetrics/gynecology ward, and one select floor of private rooms had additional sinks within patient rooms. Several nurses described that the additional hand hygiene locations were an asset for those units (Table 1, quotation 15).

Multiple doctors stated that even though there were alcohol-based hand rub dispensers on every ward, these dispensers could not always be used conveniently (Table 1, quotation 16). Another barrier to the availability of hand hygiene supplies was the occasional theft of

sanitizer or whole dispensers by patients, which was reported in multiple areas including the emergency department (Table 1, quotation 17). Several providers believed that the hospital could increase hand hygiene compliance by providing personal alcohol-based hand rub dispensers to each healthcare worker (Table 1, quotation 18).

Technology and tools

This facility employed multiple technologies for hand hygiene auditing. A closed circuit television surveillance system was used to collect video footage of healthcare worker hand hygiene practices at the time of entry and exit from patient rooms. Although infection control nurses frequently reviewed the video footage, the data were not effectively communicated to clinical staff. Several doctors and nurses believed this footage was rarely or never reviewed. Others had received department-level feedback of hand hygiene compliance, but felt that reporting of compliance data to individual providers would be more helpful (Table 1, quotations 19 and 20).

Radio-frequency identification (RFID) badges utilized in the ICU were another innovative technology at this facility. These badges were detected by sensors on alcohol-based hand rub dispensers that recorded the duration and frequency of hand hygiene occurrences. The badges also provided instant reminder alarms for healthcare workers to perform hand hygiene (Table 1, quotation 21). All ICU nurses wore their own badge, allowing for individual compliance data to be tracked and reported in real-time on a television monitor prominently displayed in the ICU. However, visiting healthcare providers, including those that provided consults in the ICU, shared group RFID badges and their hand hygiene could not be monitored individually.

Medical trolleys were available on the airborne isolation ward of the hospital, and proved a useful tool for improving hand hygiene compliance for this area. The trolleys provided a place to set down medical supplies, making it easier for nurses to perform hand hygiene prior to entering the patient's room. Several nurses expressed that having medical trolleys available on all wards would help improve hand hygiene throughout the hospital (Table 1, quotation 22). However, this would require the purchasing of trolleys out of the budget for each additional unit.

Discussion

Our study design centered on the perspectives of healthcare providers to optimize future infection control interventions. Using the SEIPS model, we have framed multiple barriers and facilitators that were reported by nurses, doctors, and pharmacists at a private hospital in Manila, Philippines.

The long-established prioritization of an infection control program at this hospital is an organizational strength that is often lacking from the infrastructure of healthcare facilities in low- and middle-income countries [1, 13]. The representation of multiple departments on the program's executive committee is aligned with a World Health Organization recommendation that hospital infection control policies be developed by a multidisciplinary team [14]. This program is especially important given the high prevalence of HAIs and inappropriate usage of antibiotics throughout the Philippines [3, 15–17], which likely introduce external factors into an institutional work system where infection surveillance, laboratory testing, and disease management are otherwise very consistent (External Environment in Fig. 1). The overall purpose and processes of the infection control executive committee were well-received by healthcare providers, likely because the long-standing policies have become a normal part of the hospital's culture during the past thirty years. Previous studies support this notion, showing that institutional etiquette and social norms can influence overall compliance with infection control programs [18].

The facility's infection control nursing staff is another asset that was acknowledged to have a positive impact on patient outcomes. The six-person team at this 800-bed hospital surpasses the Centers for Disease Control recommendation of at least one full-time infection control staff for the first 100 beds, and another staff member for each additional 250 beds [19]. Infection control staff

frequently utilize one of the tool-level factors identified in our study, the closed circuit television system, for hand hygiene surveillance. However, several providers felt that reporting the results of compliance data to large groups was ineffective for improving hand hygiene at the individual level. Implementing a monitor display may prove useful, as previous video surveillance interventions have found that continuously displaying the results of hand hygiene behavior on a monitor can yield a sustained improvement in compliance rates [20, 21].

Our study found that the prominent monitor display of RFID badge data in the hospital's ICU may be an effective way to ensure individual accountability for hand hygiene compliance. One weakness of this system is the use of a shared 'guest' badges by all clinicians who visit the ICU from other departments. This could be addressed by providing regularly visiting providers with their own badges. While this type of system can provide powerful feedback to providers, implementing the badges throughout an entire institution could be cost-prohibitive [22]. Acquiring new equipment can be difficult in a resource-constrained facility, especially since increased patient charges are often the primary means of covering such costs. This was a concern among nurses in the discussion of medical trolley purchases. While trolleys are a useful tool in the airborne isolation unit, their absence in other floors is a barrier to hand hygiene compliance. Purchasing additional trolleys would likely be less costly than adding more RFID badges. Prioritizing the purchase of new trolleys at an organizational level, rather than on a ward-by-ward basis, could rapidly improve hand hygiene feasibility for healthcare workers.

The high turnover of nursing staff is also concerning, as it necessitates constant training and use of educational resources. A systematic review of nurses' motivational factors in numerous developing countries identified key factors for successful retention packages [23]. In addition to financial incentives, these packages must include ways of strengthening healthcare workers' motivation through personal recognition and career development opportunities.

Another reported barrier was the low hand hygiene compliance of attending physicians compared to nurses, a trend that is consistent with numerous institutions worldwide [24, 25]. One potential reason for this is the minimal time physicians have between patients during rounds. As several subjects suggested, providing personal portable dispensers of alcohol-based hand rub is potentially low-cost, time-saving, and would also prevent theft concerns. This type of intervention has been successful in other facilities, resulting in up to a 64% increase in hand hygiene compliance [26–28].

Implementing a verbal reminder process for hand hygiene could be another helpful practice. Several interviews suggested having the providers with the best compliance, the nurses, remind others to perform hand hygiene. This potentially nurse-driven intervention would need to account for suboptimal communication within the hierarchy of health professionals. Previous efforts to improve interprofessional collaboration have highlighted the importance of senior doctors and nurses setting an example for more junior healthcare workers, and encourage the development of shared mental models [29, 30]. This could be fostered through increasing collaborative practice, interprofessional patient rounds, or implementing a communication skills training [31]. Increasing open communication between nurses and physicians is crucial for patient safety, and interventions based on shared accountability models have had favorable impacts on hand hygiene adherence and rates of HAIs [32, 33].

Our study had several limitations. It was conducted at a single, private hospital that is considered one of the pioneers of infection control in Manila. Private hospitals comprise 60% of the roughly 1800 hospitals in the Philippines, and generally serve patients who can afford fee-for-service payments [34]. Thus, our findings may not be generalizable to smaller, community hospitals located in more rural areas of the country or to institutions that lack organizational support for infection control policies. In our institution, for example, the rate of ESBL *Klebsiella pneumoniae* based on a hospital antibiogram in 2016 for non-ICU and ICU patients was between 16 and 19% (n = 125), compared to a much higher rate of 40% (n = 8861) among 24 surveillance sites all across the Philippines. Similarly, the rate of carbapenem resistant *Acinetobacter baumanni*, though very high at 27–34% (n = 116), was still lower than the 52.1% (n = 3967) found in these surveillance hospitals [35].

The study population was limited to a small size and selected based on convenience sampling. While we sought to include participants representing a wide range of clinical experiences, our results may not reflect hospital-wide opinions regarding infection control. Other key stakeholders, such as patients, hospital management, and environmental cleaning staff may have additional perceptions and should be included in future studies.

These limitations notwithstanding, our study findings have implications for infection preventionists, hospital epidemiologists, and clinicians in resource-constrained settings. For example, the emphasis on and interest in hand hygiene compliance monitoring at our study site suggests that interventions to optimize hand hygiene might be a high priority, even in low-resource settings. Moreover, our systems approach may serve as an exemplar for other facilities seeking to prioritize infection control resources.

Previously studied infection control interventions in the Philippines have either demonstrated minimal impact, or have examined only a single disease outcome (catheter-associated urinary tract infection) [36, 37]. These studies suggest that infection control interventions in this country have the potential for success, but are also faced with the inherent difficulties of resource-limited settings. The perceived availability of resources is another challenging aspect of intervention implementation; even if resources do exist within a healthcare facility, they will not be useful if clinicians are unaware of them or do not believe they are readily available [5]. In recognition of these concerns, we incorporated the perceptions held by key stakeholders in order to prioritize areas for future intervention.

Conclusions

Discussions with healthcare providers revealed that infection control practices in a resource-limited setting were perceived positively by most. Primary facilitators in this institution included a well-established infection control unit with support from the rest of the healthcare team and hospital organization. There are several viable opportunities for future intervention to overcome the existing barriers. These include real-time feedback of hand hygiene surveillance data, provision of medical trolleys and portable alcohol-based hand rub dispensers, improvement of retention packages for nursing staff, and advancement of interprofessional communication. These measures may provide important tools for reducing HAIs in this type of resource-limited healthcare facility.

Abbreviations
CCTV: Closed circuit television; HAI: Hospital-acquired infection; HICEC: Hospital Infection Control Executive Committee; ICU: Intensive care unit; MDRO: Multi-drug resistant organism; RFID: Radio-frequency identification; SEIPS: Systems Engineering Initiative for Patient Safety

Acknowledgements
Not applicable.

Funding
AB was supported by a pre-doctoral NIH traineeship, TL1TR000429, administered by the University of Wisconsin Madison, Institute for Clinical and Translational Research, funded by NIH award UL1TR000427.

Authors' contributions
KM drafted and critically edited the manuscript and contributed to data analysis. AB contributed to study design, data collection, data analysis, and critical manuscript editing. CA and NS contributed to study design and critical manuscript editing. All authors read and approved the final manuscript.

Consent for publication

Not applicable.

Competing interests

The authors declare that they have no competing interests.

Author details

[1]Department of Population Health Sciences, University of Wisconsin-Madison, Madison, WI, USA. [2]Division of Infectious Diseases, Department of Medicine, University of Wisconsin-Madison, Madison, WI, USA. [3]Department of Medicine, Division of Infectious Diseases, The Medical City, Pasig, Philippines. [4]William S. Middleton Memorial Veterans Hospital, Madison, WI, USA. [5]Infection Control Department, University of Wisconsin-Madison, 5221 Medical Foundation Centennial Building, 1685 Highland Ave, Madison, WI 53705, USA.

References

1. Allegranzi B, Nejad SB, Combescure C, Graafmans W, Attar H, Donaldson L, Pittet D. Burden of endemic health-care-associated infection in developing countries: systematic review and meta-analysis. In Book Burden of endemic health-care-associated infection in developing countries: systematic review and meta-analysis, vol. 377. City: Elsevier; 2011. p. 228–41.
2. Navoa-Ng JA, Berba R, Galapia YA, Rosenthal VD, Villanueva VD, Tolentino MC, Genuino GA, Consunji RJ, Mantaring JB 3rd. Device-associated infections rates in adult, pediatric, and neonatal intensive care units of hospitals in the Philippines: international nosocomial infection control consortium (INICC) findings. Am J Infect Control. 2011;39:548–54.
3. The Philippine Action Plan to Combat Antimicrobial Resistance: One Health Approach. http://arsp.com.ph/wp-content/uploads/2016/07/Action-Plan-final_orig.pdf.
4. Safdar N, Sengupta S, Musuuza JS, Juthani-Mehta M, Drees M, Abbo LM, Milstone AM, Furuno JP, Varman M, Anderson DJ, et al. Status of the prevention of multidrug-resistant organisms in international settings: a survey of the Society for Healthcare Epidemiology of America research network. Infect Control Hosp Epidemiol. 2017;38(1):53–60.
5. Allegranzi B, Pittet D. Healthcare-associated infection in developing countries: simple solutions to meet complex challenges. Infect Control Hosp Epidemiol. 2007;28:1323–7.
6. Report on the burden of endemic health care-associated infection worldwide. In Book Report on the burden of endemic health care-associated infection worldwide. Geneva: World Health Organization; 2011.
7. Carroll C, Patterson M, Wood S, Booth A, Rick J, Balain S. A conceptual framework for implementation fidelity. Implement Sci. 2007;2:40.
8. Carayon P, Hundt AS, Karsh BT, Gurses AP, Alvarado CJ, Smith M, Brennan PF. Work system design for patient safety: the SEIPS model. Qual Saf Health Care. 2006;15:i50–8.
9. Yanke E, Zellmer C, Van Hoof S, Moriarty H, Carayon P, Safdar N. Understanding the current state of infection prevention to prevent Clostridium Difficile infection: a human factors and systems engineering approach. Am J Infect Control. 2015;43:241–7.
10. Carayon P, Wetterneck TB, Rivera-Rodriguez AJ, Hundt AS, Hoonakker P, Holden R, Gurses AP. Human factors systems approach to healthcare quality and patient safety. Appl Ergon. 2014;45:14–25.
11. Barker AK, Brown K, Siraj D, Ahsan M, Sengupta S, Safdar N. Barriers and facilitators to infection control at a hospital in northern India: a qualitative study. Antimicrob Resist Infect Control. 2017;6:35.
12. Corbin J, Strauss A. Basics of qualitative research: techniques and procedures for developing grounded theory. Thousand Oaks: Sage Publications; 2014.
13. Shears P. Poverty and infection in the developing world: healthcare-related infections and infection control in the tropics. J Hosp Infect. 2007;67:217–24.
14. Prevention of hospital acquired infections - A practical guide. http://whqlibdoc.who.int/hq/2002/WHO_CDS_CSR_EPH_2002.12.pdf.
15. Rosenthal VD, Maki DG, Salomao R, et al. Device-associated nosocomial infections in 55 intensive care units of 8 developing countries. Ann Intern Med. 2006;145:582–91.
16. Hardon AP. The use of modern pharmaceuticals in a Filipino village: doctors' prescription and self medication. Soc Sci Med. 1987;25:277–92.
17. Lansang MA, Lucas-Aquino R, Tupasi TE, Mina VS, Salazar LS, Juban N, Limjoco TT, Nisperos LE, Kunin CM. Purchase of antibiotics without prescription in manila, the Philippines. Inappropriate choices and doses. J Clin Epidemiol. 1990;43:61–7.
18. De Bono S, Heling G, Borg MA. Organizational culture and its implications for infection prevention and control in healthcare institutions. J Hosp Infect. 2014;86:1–6.
19. Stone PW, Dick A, Pogorzelska M, Horan TC, Furuya EY, Larson E. Staffing and structure of infection prevention and control programs. Am J Infect Control. 2009;37:351–7.
20. Armellino D, Hussain E, Schilling ME, Senicola W, Eichorn A, Dlugacz Y, Farber BF. Using high-technology to enforce low-technology safety measures: the use of third-party remote video auditing and real-time feedback in healthcare. Clin Infect Dis. 2012;54:1–7.
21. Ellingson K, Haas JP, Aiello AE, Kusek L, Maragakis LL, Olmsted RN, Perencevich E, Polgreen PM, Schweizer ML, Trexler P, et al. Strategies to prevent healthcare-associated infections through hand hygiene. Infect Control Hosp Epidemiol. 2014;35:937–60.
22. Yao W, Chu CH, Li Z. The use of RFID in healthcare: Benefits and barriers. In 2010 IEEE International Conference on RFID-Technology and Applications; 17–19 June 2010. J Med Syst. 2012;36(6):3507-25.
23. Willis-Shattuck M, Bidwell P, Thomas S, Wyness L, Blaauw D, Ditlopo P. Motivation and retention of health workers in developing countries: a systematic review. BMC Health Serv Res. 2008;8:247.
24. Erasmus V, Daha TJ, Brug H, Richardus JH, Behrendt MD, Vos MC, van Beeck EF. Systematic review of studies on compliance with hand hygiene guidelines in hospital care. Infect Control Hosp Epidemiol. 2010;31:283–94.
25. Allegranzi B, Gayet-Ageron A, Damani N, Bengaly L, McLaws M-L, Moro M-L, Memish Z, Urroz O, Richet H, Storr J, et al. Global implementation of WHO's multimodal strategy for improvement of hand hygiene: a quasi-experimental study. Lancet Infect Dis. 2013;13:843–51.
26. Malina Y, Malina Y, Iseri M, Reiner S, Hardman J, Rogers J, Vlasses F. A Portable Trackable Hand Sanitation Device Increases Hand Hygiene. American Journal of Infection Control. 2013;41:S37–8.
27. Parks CL, Schroeder KM, Galgon RE. Personal hand gel for improved hand hygiene compliance on the regional anesthesia team. J Anesth. 2015;29:899–903.
28. Koff MD, Corwin HL, Beach ML, Surgenor SD, Loftus RW. Reduction in ventilator associated pneumonia in a mixed intensive care unit after initiation of a novel hand hygiene program. J Crit Care. 2011;26:489–95.
29. Edwards PB, Rea JB, Oermann MH, Hegarty EJ, Prewitt JR, Rudd M, Silva S, Nagler A, Turner DA, DeMeo SD. Effect of peer-to-peer nurse-physician collaboration on attitudes toward the nurse-physician relationship. J Nurses Prof Dev. 2017;33:13–8.
30. Weller JM, Barrow M, Gasquoine S. Interprofessional collaboration among junior doctors and nurses in the hospital setting. Med Educ. 2011;45:478–87.
31. Gonzalo JD, Kuperman E, Lehman E, Haidet P. Bedside interprofessional rounds: perceptions of benefits and barriers by internal medicine nursing staff, attending physicians, and housestaff physicians. J Hosp Med. 2014;9:646–51.
32. Talbot TR, Johnson JG, Fergus C, Domenico JH, Schaffner W, Daniels TL, Wilson G, Slayton J, Feistritzer N, Hickson GB. Sustained improvement in hand hygiene adherence: utilizing shared accountability and financial incentives. Infect Control Hosp Epidemiol. 2013;34:1129–36.
33. Tjia J, Mazor KM, Field T, Meterko V, Spenard A, Gurwitz JH. Nurse-physician communication in the long-term care setting: perceived barriers and impact on patient safety. Journal of patient safety. 2009;5:145–52.
34. Health Service Delivery Profile: Philippines. http://www.wpro.who.int/health_services/service_delivery_profile_philippines.pdf.

35. Antimicrobial Resistance Surveillance Program 2016 Data Summary Report. http://arsp.com.ph/wp-content/uploads/2017/06/2016_annual_report_summary.pdf.

36. Navoa-Ng JA, Berba R, Rosenthal VD, Villanueva VD, Tolentino MC, Genuino GA, Consunji RJ, Mantaring JB 3rd. Impact of an international nosocomial infection control consortium multidimensional approach on catheter-associated urinary tract infections in adult intensive care units in the Philippines: international nosocomial infection control consortium (INICC) findings. J Infect Public Health. 2013;6:389–99.

37. Gill CJ, Mantaring JB, Macleod WB, Mendoza M, Mendoza S, Huskins WC, Goldmann DA, Hamer DH. Impact of enhanced infection control at 2 neonatal intensive care units in the Philippines. Clin Infect Dis. 2009;48:13–21.

14

Candidemia in a major regional tertiary referral hospital – epidemiology, practice patterns and outcomes

Jocelyn Qi-Min Teo[1], Samuel Rocky Candra[1], Shannon Jing-Yi Lee[1], Shannon Yu-Hng Chia[1,6], Hui Leck[1], Ai-Ling Tan[2], Hui-Peng Neo[1], Kenneth Wei-Liang Leow[1], Yiying Cai[1,3], Rachel Pui-Lai Ee[3], Tze-Peng Lim[1,4], Winnie Lee[1] and Andrea Lay-Hoon Kwa[1,3,5*]

Abstract

Background: Candidemia is a common cause of nosocomial bloodstream infections, resulting in high morbidity and mortality. This study was conducted to describe the epidemiology, species distribution, antifungal susceptibility patterns and outcomes of candidemia in a large regional tertiary referral hospital.

Methods: A retrospective surveillance study of patients with candidemia was conducted at Singapore General Hospital between July 2012 and December 2015. In addition, incidence densities and species distribution of candidemia episodes were analysed from 2008 to 2015.

Results: In the period of 2012 to 2015, 261 candidemia episodes were identified. The overall incidence was 0.14/1000 inpatient-days. *C. glabrata* (31.4%), *C. tropicalis* (29.9%), and *C. albicans* (23.8%) were most commonly isolated. The incidence of *C. glabrata* significantly increased from 2008 to 2015 (Coefficient 0.004, confidence interval 0–0.007, $p = 0.04$). Fluconazole resistance was detected primarily in *C. tropicalis* (16.7%) and *C. glabrata* (7.2%). *fks* mutations were identified in one *C. albicans* and one *C. tropicalis*. Candidemia episodes caused by *C. tropicalis* were more commonly encountered in patients with haematological malignancies ($p = 0.01$), neutropenia ($p < 0.001$) and higher SAPS II scores ($p = 0.02$), while prior exposure to echinocandins was associated with isolation of *C. parapsilosis* ($p = 0.001$). Echinocandins (73.3%) were most commonly prescribed as initial treatment. The median (range) time to initial treatment was 1 (0–9) days. The 30-day in-hospital mortality rate was 49.8%. High SAPS II score (Odds ratio, OR 1.08; 95% confidence interval, CI 1.05–1.11) and renal replacement therapy (OR 5.54; CI 2.80–10.97) were independent predictors of mortality, while drain placement (OR 0.44; CI 0.19–0.99) was protective.

Conclusions: Decreasing azole susceptibilities to *C. tropicalis* and the emergence of echinocandin resistance suggest that susceptibility patterns may no longer be sufficiently predicted by speciation in our institution. Candidemia is associated with poor outcomes. Strategies optimising antifungal therapy, especially in the critically-ill population, should be explored.

Keywords: *Candida*, Bloodstream infections, Antifungal susceptibility, *fks*, Mortality

* Correspondence: andrea.kwa.l.h@sgh.com.sg
[1]Department of Pharmacy, Singapore General Hospital, Blk 8 Level 2, Outram Road, Singapore 169608, Singapore
[3]Department of Pharmacy, National University of Singapore, 18 Science Drive 4, Singapore 117543, Singapore

Background

Candida species are the leading cause of invasive fungal infections and a common cause of hospital-acquired bloodstream infections [1]. Candidemia has a profound impact on patient outcomes and the burden has increased significantly over the years. The crude mortality is high, ranging from 30–50% [2–4]; while the attributable mortality due to candidemia varied from 15–49% [5, 6]. Increasing reports of antifungal resistance, even in newer agents such as the echinocandins, further escalate the complexity in the management of candidemia [7].

Knowledge of antifungal susceptibility patterns is imperative in the selection of early and appropriate antifungal agents for improved patient outcomes. The variable epidemiology of candidemia, contributed by the geographical and temporal variations in incidence and species distribution [4, 8–10], underscores the continuing need for local surveillance of *Candida* species distribution and susceptibility patterns.

Furthermore, the introduction of new echinocandins into Singapore such as anidulafungin in 2008 and micafungin in 2013, coupled with the exponential increase in echinocandin usage in our institution for the past 5 years, suggest that current susceptibility patterns should be reviewed. A recent study has also reported the emergence of echinocandin resistance in the Asia-Pacific region [11]. The objectives of this study were 1) to investigate the incidence, species distribution and antifungal susceptibilities of candidemia, and 2) to describe the clinical features and outcomes of candidemia in our population.

Methods

Study setting and design

A retrospective surveillance study of patients with candidemia was conducted at Singapore General Hospital (SGH) between July 2012 and December 2015. SGH is the largest acute care hospital (1800 beds) in the country, and covers a wide range of medical and surgical specialties. The hospital is the national/regional referral centre for services such as plastic surgery and burns, renal medicine, nuclear medicine, pathology and haematology. SGH accounts for approximately 25% of the total acute hospital beds in the public sector and 20% of acute beds nationwide.

All adult inpatients (at least 21 years old) with ≥ 1 positive blood culture for *Candida spp.* were included into the study. Each positive *Candida* culture must be accompanied with temporally-related clinical signs and symptoms of infection for inclusion into the study. For each patient, only the first candidemia episode was recorded, unless the positive blood culture was obtained ≥ 30 days (with blood culture clearance and resolution of clinical features of infection of the first episode) or

involved a different *Candida spp.* isolated from blood culture obtained ≥ 7 days after the first episode. Episodes involving > 1 *Candida spp.* isolated within 7 days of the first episode, defined as "mixed candidemia", were regarded as a single episode.

Microbiology and antifungal susceptibility testing

Candida spp. were isolated from blood using BD BAC-TEC™ FX (Becton, Dickinson and Company, Sparks, MD). The species were identified using MALDI Biotyper (BrukerDaltonik GmbH, Germany), morphology studies on cornmeal Tween 80 agar, and API 20C AUX (Biomerieux, Marcy l'Etoile, France). Isolates were stored in Microbank™ storage vials (Pro-Lab Diagnostics, Round Rock, TX, USA) at –70 °C until testing.

Antifungal susceptibility testing was performed using Sensititre YeastOne® YO10 panel (Trek Diagnostics System, West Sussex, England) according to manufacturer's recommendations. Minimum inhibitory concentrations (MICs) for amphotericin B, anidulafungin, caspofungin, micafungin, fluconazole, voriconazole, itraconazole, posaconazole and flucytosine were recorded. *Candida krusei* (*Issatchenkia orientalis*) ATCC 6258 and *C. parapsilosis* ATCC 22019 (American Type Culture Collection, Manassas, Virginia) were used as quality controls.

MICs were interpreted according to the current species-specific clinical breakpoints provided by the Clinical and Laboratory Standards Institute (CLSI) M27-S4 document [12]. Where clinical breakpoints were not available, the epidemiological cut-off values (ECV) were used to classify the isolates into wild-type or non-wild-type populations [13–15].

Detection of *fks* mutations

Isolates classified as intermediate or resistant to echinocandins were tested for the presence of mutations in the *fks* genes. Hot spots 1 and 2 regions of *fks1* and *fks2* (for *C. glabrata* only) genes were amplified using polymerase chain reaction (PCR), as described previously [16].

Clinical data collection

Clinical characteristics of patients with candidemia were obtained from inpatient charts and electronic medical records using a standardised case report form. Data extracted included demographics, hospitalisation history (previous hospital stay, previous intensive care unit (ICU) stay, length of hospital stay prior to candidemia), underlying medical conditions and prior exposure to invasive interventions (central lines, urinary catheters, drainage devices, invasive ventilation, dialysis, invasive surgery, total parenteral nutrition) and medical therapy (chemotherapy, immunosuppressive therapy, antibiotics, antifungal agents) within 30 days before the first positive blood culture. Charlson comorbidity index at the time of admission and Simplified Acute Physiology Score (SAPS) on the day of the first positive blood culture were also recorded. Information on the management of candidemia (choice and duration of antifungal agents) and outcome (in-hospital all-cause mortality within 30 days) were collected.

Data and statistical analyses

To calculate and analyse the incidence of candidemia, the number of candidemia episodes were obtained from the clinical microbiology laboratory computerised database, while inpatient-days were obtained from the hospital administrative database. Incidence data was available from 2008, hence trend analyses were performed for the period from 2008 to 2015. Incidence rates were calculated as the number of candidemia episodes per 1000 inpatient-days. Linear regression was used to determine trends over time in the incidences of candidemia.

Categorical variables were presented as numbers and percentages; and were compared using the X^2 or Fisher's exact test, as appropriate. Continuous variables were presented as mean ± SD or median and range; and were compared using the Student's t test, Mann–Whitney test, or Kruskal-wallis test, depending on the validity of the normality assumption.

A multivariable logistic regression model was used to identify predictors associated with 30-day mortality. Clinically plausible variables identified in the bivariate analysis were included in the multivariable logistic regression model if $p < 0.1$. Significant factors which may covary were grouped and only one factor from each group was selected for entry into the model. The final model was chosen on the basis of biologic plausibility.

Odds ratios (OR) and 95% confidence intervals (CI) were calculated to evaluate the strength of any association. For all calculations, a 2-tailed p value of less than 0.05 was considered to reveal a statistical significant difference. Statistical analyses were performed using IBM SPSS Statistics for Windows, Version 23.0 (IBM Corp., Armonk, NY).

Results

Incidence and species distribution

From 2012 to 2015, 261 candidemia episodes involving 254 patients and 272 isolates were analysed. Seven patients had two separate episodes each with distinct *Candida* species, while a patient had a repeated episode involving the same *Candida* species. The incidence was 0.14 episodes per 1000 inpatient-days during the study period. *C. glabrata* (82/261, 31.4%), *C. tropicalis* (78/261, 29.9%), *C. albicans* (62/261, 23.8%), and *C. parapsilosis* (36/261, 13.8%) accounted for majority of the episodes. Other species including *C. dubliniensis* ($n = 7$), *C. krusei* ($n = 3$), *C. guilliermondii (Meyerozyma guilliermondii)* ($n = 1$), *C. kefyr (Kluyveromyces marxianus)* ($n = 1$), *C. haemulonis* ($n = 1$) and *C. pseudohaemulonii* ($n = 1$) accounted for the remaining episodes. Of these 261 episodes, 11 (4.2%) were mixed candidemia episodes.

The incidence density and species distribution are displayed in Fig. 1. The overall incidence density was 0.15 (range 0.12–0.18) episodes/1000 inpatient-days and 0.89 (range 0.74–1.05) episodes/1000 admissions from 2008 to 2015. Analysing the incidence densities from 2008 to 2015, we found no significant change in the incidence density of candidemia [Coefficient 0.00009, confidence interval (CI) - 0.007–0.007, $p = 0.98$].

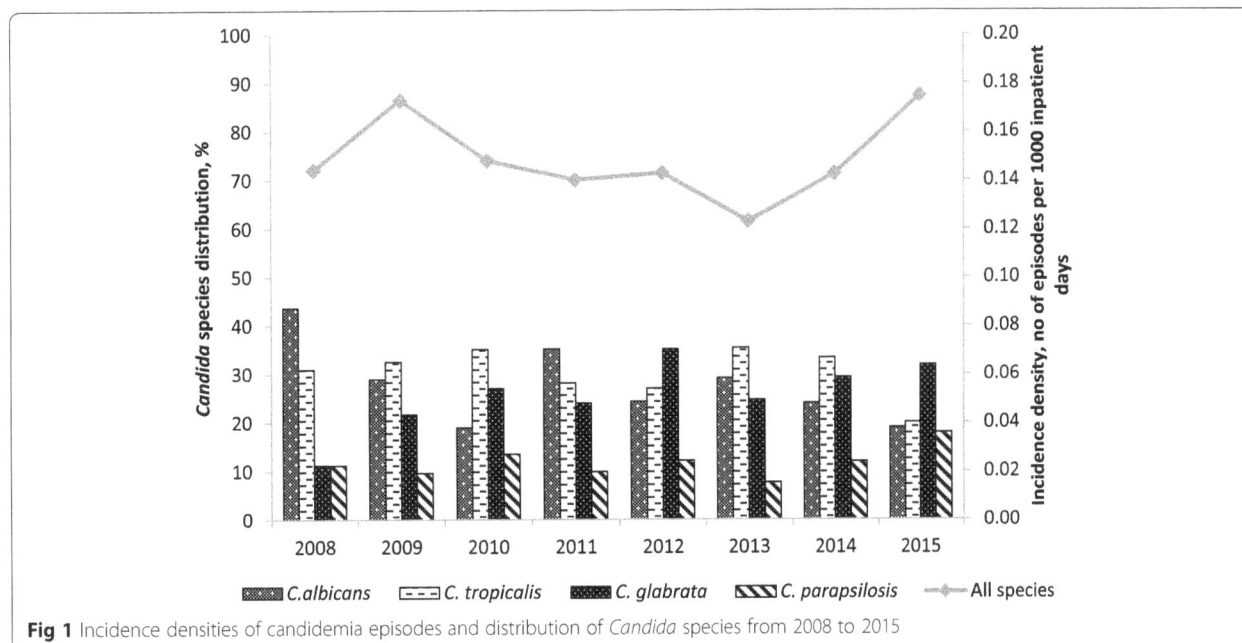

Fig 1 Incidence densities of candidemia episodes and distribution of *Candida* species from 2008 to 2015

However, we did note that the overall incidence density increased from 0.14 in 2014 to 0.18 episodes/1000 inpatient-days in 2015, suggesting the need for continual monitoring. There was a significant increasing trend in the incidence density of *C. glabrata* (Coefficient 0.004, CI 0–0.007, *p* = 0.04), while the incidence densities of the other *Candida spp.* remained stable. The proportions of *C. glabrata* increased from 11.3% in 2008 to 31.6% in 2015 and that of *C. albicans* decreased from 44% in 2008 to 19% in 2015.

Antifungal susceptibilities

Antifungal susceptibilities were available for 271 isolates, except for one *C. parapsilosis* (Table 1). Among isolates with available clinical breakpoints, overall susceptibility rates were 59.5% (153/257) for fluconazole, 86.9% (152/175) for voriconazole, 99.2% (255/257) for anidulafungin, 98.1% (252/257) for caspofungin and 98.9% (254/257) for micafungin. Using the clinical breakpoints, *C. albicans* and *C. parapsilosis* retained high susceptibility (>94%) to fluconazole and voriconazole. However, more than 20% of the *C. tropicalis* isolates were non-susceptible to fluconazole and voriconazole. The proportions of isolates classified as wild-type (MIC value less than or equals to ECV) for fluconazole, voriconazole, itraconazole and posaconazole were similar among *C. albicans*, *C. glabrata* and *C. parapsilosis* (ranged from 94–100%). Decreased susceptibilities (non wild-type; MIC value greater than ECV) to fluconazole and voriconazole were prominent in *C. tropicalis* isolates. Echinocandin resistance was rare, occurring only in three isolates (*C. albicans* = 1; *C. tropicalis* =1 and *C. glabrata* = 1) when assessed using both clinical breakpoints and ECVs. Most isolates had amphotericin B and flucytosine MICs below ECVs (96–100%), although a number of *C. parapsilosis* were classified as non-wild-type (20%). The amphotericin B MICs of these non-wild-type isolates were 2 µg/mL, which were just one dilution above the ECV (1 µg/mL) utilised in this study. Furthermore, the ECV used in this study was derived using the YeastOne® method and is one dilution lower than the ECVs for the other species (2 µg/mL) and the ECV derived from broth dilution methods.

fks mutations were detected in the echinocandin-resistant *C. albicans* (caspofungin MIC 4 µg/mL; anidulafungin MIC 0.25 µg/mL; micafungin MIC 2 µg/mL) and *C. tropicalis* (caspofungin MIC 2 µg/mL; anidulafungin MIC 0.5 µg/mL; micafungin 1 µg/mL) isolates. Both isolates harboured a point mutation (S645P in *C. albicans* and S80P in *C. tropicalis*) in the hotspot 1 region of the *fks1* gene. The two isolates remained susceptible to all other antifungals. Interestingly, *fks* mutations were not identified in the *C. glabrata* isolate which

was resistant (caspofungin MIC ≥ 8 µg/mL; anidulafungin MIC 4 µg/mL; micafungin MIC 4 µg/mL).

Clinical characteristics

The clinical characteristics of the candidemia episodes are summarised in Table 2. The median age of patients with candidemia was 65 years and incidence did not differ by gender (52.9% male *vs.* 47.1% female, *p* = 0.59). The episodes occurred primarily in the medical wards (42.1%), followed by intensive care units (ICUs) (38.3%), surgical wards (19.5%). Patients admitted to haematology-oncology (19.9%), internal medicine (19.5%) and general surgery units (12.3%) encountered the most episodes.

Most of the patients presented with multiple comorbidities (median Charlson score = 5, range 0–15), with many having malignancies (40.6%). Diabetes was also common among these patients (39.5%). Prior antibiotic exposure (90.4%), central venous catheter placement (73.6%), and surgery (65.1%) were common risk factors. A large number of patients were colonised or infected with *Candida* at other non-blood sites (45.2%) and had concurrent bacterial infections (48.7%). In addition, it appears that candidemia episodes caused by *C. tropicalis* were more commonly encountered in patients with haematological malignancies (*p* = 0.01), neutropenia (*p* < 0.001) and higher SAPS II scores (*p* = 0.02). Exposure to echinocandins was also associated with candidemia episodes caused by *C. parapsilosis* (*p* = 0.001).

Antifungal therapy and outcomes

Antifungal therapy was initiated in 225 (86.2%) episodes (Table 2). All but six of the 36 patients who did not receive treatment died before blood cultures flagged positive. Treatment was not initiated in four patients as they were conservatively managed. Interestingly, physicians elected not to initiate treatment in the remaining two patients.

Echinocandins were the initial treatment of choice (73.3%), followed by azoles (23.1%). Caspofungin (93.4%) was more commonly used, since it was the only echinocandin in the formulary until anidulafungin's inclusion in August 2015. Among the patients receiving treatment, 32 (14.2%) were already receiving antifungals as prophylaxis or empiric treatment on the day which cultures were taken. Fluconazole was the only azole used as initial treatment of candidemia in our institution. The median (range) time to initial treatment was 1 (0–9) days. Treatment was initiated in 73 (32.4%) patients on day of culture and in 172 (76.4%) patients within two days. The median (range) duration of therapy was 15 (1–140) days.

Patients with candidemia were moderately to severely-ill – 57.9% were having severe sepsis and the median (range) SAPS II score was 49 (14–103) at the time of culture. Many of these episodes (38.3%) occurred in

Table 1 Antifungal susceptibilities of major species of *Candida* isolates[a]

Antifungal	MIC$_{50}$ (µg/mL)	MIC$_{90}$ (µg/mL)	MIC Range (µg/mL)	%S[b]	%SDD/I[b]	%R[b]	%WT[c]
C albicans (n = 62)							
Fluconazole	0.5	2	≤0.12–>256	95.2	1.6	3.2	93.5
Itraconazole	0.06	0.12	≤0.015–>16	–	–	–	96.7
Posaconazole	0.015	0.06	≤0.08–>8	–	–	–	96.7
Voriconazole	≤0.008	0.03	≤0.008–>8	93.6	3.2	3.2	93.5
Anidulafungin	≤0.015	0.03	≤0.015–0.25	100	0	0	98.4
Caspofungin	0.03	0.06	0.015–4	98.4	0	1.6	98.4
Micafungin	≤0.008	0.015	≤0.008–2	98.4	0	1.6	98.4
Flucytosine	≤0.06	0.25	≤0.06–>64	–	–	–	96.7
Amphotericin B	0.5	1	≤0.12–1	–	–	–	100
C. glabrata (n = 82)							
Fluconazole	16	32	1–>256	–	92.8	7.2	97.6
Itraconazole	1	1	0.12–>16	–	–	–	93.9
Posaconazole	2	2	0.12–>8	–	–	–	95.1
Voriconazole	0.5	2	0.03–>8	–	–	–	97.6
Anidulafungin	0.03	0.06	≤0.015–4	98.8	0	1.2	98.7
Caspofungin	0.12	0.12	0.03–>8	96.4	2.4	1.2	96.3
Micafungin	0.015	0.015	≤0.008–4	98.8	0	1.2	98.7
Flucytosine	≤0.06	0.12	≤0.06–0.25	–	–	–	100
Amphotericin B	1	1	0.25–2	–	–	–	100
C. tropicalis (n = 78)							
Fluconazole	2	64	0.5–>256	78.2	5.1	16.7	84.6
Itraconazole	0.25	0.5	0.03–>16	–	–	–	96.1
Posaconazole	0.12	0.5	0.03–4	–	–	–	98.7
Voriconazole	0.12	4	≤0.008–>8	75.6	11.5	12.8	80.8
Anidulafungin	0.03	0.12	≤0.015–0.5	98.7	1.3	0	98.7
Caspofungin	0.03	0.06	0.015–2	98.7	0	1.3	98.7
Micafungin	0.03	0.03	≤0.008–1	98.7	0	1.3	98.7
Flucytosine	≤0.06	0.12	≤0.06–32	–	–	–	96.2
Amphotericin B	1	1	0.25–2	–	–	–	100
C. parapsilosis (n = 35)							
Fluconazole	0.5	2	0.25–4	97.1	2.9	0	100
Itraconazole	0.06	0.06	≤0.015–0.12	–	–	–	100
Posaconazole	0.03	0.06	0.015–0.12	–	–	–	100
Voriconazole	0.015	0.03	≤0.008–0.6	100	0	0	97.1
Anidulafungin	0.5	2	0.12–2	100	0	0	100
Caspofungin	0.25	0.5	0.06–1	100	0	0	100
Micafungin	0.5	2	0.12–2	100	0	0	100
Flucytosine	≤0.06	0.5	≤0.06–1	–	–	–	100
Amphotericin B	1	2	0.25–2	–	–	–	80.0

S susceptible, *SDD* susceptible dose-dependent, *I* intermediate, *R* resistant, *WT* wild-type

[a]MICs are only reflected for the predominant species

[b]Susceptibilities were assessed based on CLSI species-specific clinical interpretative breakpoints [12]. Clinical breakpoints are not available for itraconazole, posaconazole, flucytosine and amphotericin B for all species and voriconazole for *C. glabrata*

[c]ECVs were derived from [13, 14] and [15]

Table 2 Clinical characteristics of candidemia episodes

	All	C. glabrata	C. tropicalis	C. albicans	C. parapsilosis	p
	n = 261	n = 75 (28.6%)	n = 71 (27.1%)	n = 59 (22.6%)	n = 33 (12.6%)	
Demographics						
Male sex	138 (52.9)	37 (49.3)	39 (54.9)	32 (54.2)	22 (66.7)	0.42
Median age (range)	65 (22–101)	67 (24–95)	63 (28–90)	68 (27–101)	61 (28–86)	0.06
Ward type						0.83
Medical ward	110 (42.1)	30 (40.0)	35 (49.3)	23 (39.0)	14 (42.4)	
Surgical ward	51 (19.5)	16 (21.3)	10 (14.1)	14 (23.7)	7 (21.2)	
ICU	100 (38.3)	29 (38.7)	26 (36.6)	22 (37.3)	12 (36.4)	
Elective admission	27 (10.3)	12 (16.0)	5 (7.0)	5 (8.5)	4 (12.1)	0.32
Comorbidities						
Malignancies	106 (40.6)	34 (45.3)	29 (40.8)	23 (39.0)	12 (36.4)	0.81
Haematological	27 (10.3)	3 (4.0)	13 (18.3)	6 (10.2)	2 (6.1)	*0.03*
Oncological	84 (32.2)	32 (42.7)	17 (23.9)	18 (30.5)	11 (33.3)	0.11
With metastases	36 (13.8)	16 (21.3)	11 (15.5)	6 (10.2)	3 (9.1)	0.23
Diabetes	103 (39.5)	31 (41.3)	25 (35.2)	23 (39.0)	12 (36.4)	0.89
Chronic renal failure	67 (25.7)	17 (22.7)	22 (31.0)	14 (23.7)	8 (24.2)	0.67
Hepatobiliary disorders	58 (22.2)	17 (22.7)	20 (28.2)	8 (13.6)	8 (24.2)	0.25
Myocardial infarction	43 (16.5)	10 (13.3)	13 (18.3)	15 (25.4)	1 (3.0)	*0.04*
Cerebrovascular disease	29 (11.1)	12 (16.0)	8 (11.3)	4 (6.8)	4 (12.1)	0.44
Median (range) Charlson score	5 (0–15)	6 (0–15)	5 (0–14)	4 (0–12)	4 (0–9)	0.08
Risk factors						
Central venous catheter	192 (73.6)	47 (62.7)	55 (77.5)	46 (78.0)	26 (78.8)	0.11
Drain	60 (23.0)	22 (29.3)	14 (19.7)	16 (27.1)	6 (18.2)	0.43
Mechanical ventilation	111 (42.5)	26 (34.7)	31 (43.7)	25 (42.4)	16 (48.5)	0.52
Total parenteral nutrition	52 (19.9)	12 (16.0)	13 (18.3)	12 (20.3)	10 (30.3)	0.37
Surgery	170 (65.1)	51 (68.0)	44 (66.0)	39 (66.1)	20 (60.6)	0.83
Gastrointestinal surgery	41 (15.7)	18 (24.0)	5 (7.0)	9 (24.3)	5 (15.2)	0.05
Renal replacement therapy	85 (32.6)	16 (21.3)	28 (39.4)	21 (35.6)	12 (36.4)	0.10
Antimicrobial therapy	236 (90.4)	67 (89.3)	68 (95.8)	53 (89.8)	27 (81.8)	0.15
Antifungal therapy	51 (19.5)	13 (17.3)	15 (21.1)	8 (13.6)	11 (33.3)	0.13
Azole	24 (9.2)	5 (6.7)	10 (14.1)	6 (10.2)	2 (6.1)	0.41
Echinocandin	30 (11.5)	8 (10.7)	6 (8.5)	2 (3.4)	10 (30.3)	*0.001*
Immunosuppressive therapy	76 (29.1)	17 (22.7)	28 (39.4)	16 (27.1)	10 (30.3)	0.16
Neutropenia	21 (8.0)	3 (4.0)	13 (18.3)	2 (3.4)	2 (6.1)	*0.004*
Therapy						
Primary therapy						0.15
Echinocandin	165 (73.3)	45 (76.3)	49 (81.7)	32 (60.4)	22 (71.0)	
Azole	52 (23.1)	12 (20.3)	11 (18.3)	17 (32.0)	8 (25.8)	
Others	8 (3.1)	2 (3.3)	1 (1.7)	4 (6.8)	1 (3.2)	
None	36 (13.8)	16 (21.3)	10 (14.1)	6 (10.2)	2 (6.1)	
Median (range) time to primary therapy, days	1 (0–9)	2 (0–7)	1 (0–3)	2 (0–5)	1 (0–9)	*0.01*
Median (range) duration of therapy, days	15 (1–140)	16 (2–61)	11 (1–96)	16 (1–140)	15 (2–47)	*0.01*

Table 2 Clinical characteristics of candidemia episodes *(Continued)*

Infection Characteristics & Outcomes						
Median (range) time to positive culture, days	12 (0–282)	11 (0–282)	14 (0–123)	14 (0–79)	37 (0–104)	0.37
Median (range) time to reporting positive culture, days	2 (0–10)	3 (0–9)	1 (0–10)	2 (1–5)	2(1–3)	*<0.001*
Median (range) time to species identification, days	5 (2–22)	6 (2–12)	4 (2–12)	5 (2–9)	5 (3–7)	*<0.001*
Median (range) SAPS II score	49 (14–103)	48 (18–95)	55 (18–93)	48 (23–103)	44 (14–72)	*0.01*
Median (range) Pitts' bacteraemia score	3 (0–14)	2 (0–11)	3 (0–12)	3 (0–11)	2 (0–8)	0.86
Severe sepsis at time of culture	151 (57.9)	49 (65.3)	43 (60.6)	33 (55.9)	13 (58.0)	0.08
ICU stay	131 (50.2)	36 (48.0)	35 (49.3)	30 (50.8)	16 (48.5)	0.99
Concurrent infection	127 (48.7)	33 (44.0)	36 (57.0)	30 (50.8)	16 (48.5)	0.83
Candida colonization/infection at other sites	118 (45.2)	41 (54.7)	39 (54.9)	34 (57.6)	18 (54.5)	0.99
30-day in-hospital all-cause mortality	130 (49.8)	38 (50.7)	42 (59.2)	28 (47.5)	9 (27.3)	*0.03*

All variables are denoted as number of patients with the characteristic or belonging to the category [n (%)], unless otherwise stated
Sub-group analyses are shown only for episodes involving major *Candida spp.* and not for mixed candidemia and less common species
Comorbidities < 10% in occurrence are not reflected
Significant variables are reflected in bold and italics

critically-ill patients warded in the ICUs. We also observed that some patients (11.9%), who were initially in the general wards at the time of culture, required admission into the ICU after *Candida* isolation, suggesting that candidemia episodes can result in severe illness. Mortality occurred in 150 (57.4%) episodes during the admission. The 7-day, 14-day and 30-day in-hospital mortality rates were 28.3%, 39.8%, and 49.8%. The mortality rate was lowest in patients infected with *C. parapsilosis* (23.5%) ($p = 0.03$). Among the 225 patients who received treatment, the 30-day in-hospital mortality rate was 41.4%, while all but two (94.4%) of the non-treated episodes resulted in death.

Predictors of mortality

The characteristics of survivors and non-survivors at 30 days are depicted in Table 3. Based on the multivariable logistic regression model, high SAPS II score (Odds ratio, OR 1.08; 95% confidence interval, CI 1.06–1.11) and renal replacement therapy (OR 4.31; CI 2.24–8.28) were the only factors associated with 30-day mortality. Presence of drains was a protective factor (OR 0.45; CI 0.21–0.94). Mortality occurred rapidly in many of the non-survivors, hence receipt/type of antifungal therapy was not included in this model, since antifungal therapy could not be initiated in this subset of patients. To examine the impact of initial antifungal therapy on 30-day mortality, a separate analysis was performed for candidemia episodes where treatment was administered. Results were similar when non-treated episodes were excluded. High SAPS II score, renal replacement therapy

and drains placement were significant factors in the multivariable regression model (Table 4). The choice and timing of initial antifungal therapy was not associated with mortality.

Discussion

We report here a comprehensive epidemiological study of candidemia conducted at a large tertiary regional referral centre, which included the clinical characteristics, antifungal treatment, species distribution, antifungal susceptibilities and outcomes of candidemia. Our study showed that the incidence density of candidemia in our institution has remained fairly stable since 2008. This concurs with the general trend of stability in incidence reported in other developed countries, such as the United States and Europe [2, 17]. A recent study comparing candidemias among sites in Asia indicated that rates in Singapore (0.15 episodes per 1000 patient-days) were comparable with most other Asian countries, with the exception of Taiwan (0.37 per 1000 patient-days) and India (1.24 per 1000 patient-days) [10]. On a more global scale, our rates were lower than those in Italy (0.33 per 1000 patient-days) [18], and Brazil (0.37 per 1000 patient-days) [19]. It appears that the species distribution in our institution is changing. Previous local studies reported a predominance of *C. tropicalis*, a finding commonly observed in tropical regions [10, 20]. We observed an increasing proportion of *C. glabrata* from 11% in 2008 to 31% in 2015, overtaking *C. tropicalis* as the predominant species.

Table 3 Characteristics of survivors vs. non-survivors

	Survivors n = 134	Non-survivors n = 127	p
Demographics			
Male sex	73 (54.5)	65 (51.2)	0.59
Median age (range)	64 (22–95)	65 (24–101)	0.81
Ward type			<0.001[a]
Medical ward	66 (49.3)	44 (34.6)	
Surgical ward	37 (27.6)	14 (11.0)	
ICU	31 (23.1)	69 (54.3)	
Elective admission	14 (10.4)	13 (10.2)	0.96
Comorbidities			
Malignancies	58 (43.3)	48 (51.6)	0.37
Diabetes	53 (39.6)	50 (39.4)	0.97
Chronic renal failure	22 (16.4)	45 (35.4)	<0.001
Hepatobiliary disorders	25 (18.7)	33 (26.0)	0.16
Myocardial infarction	19 (14.2)	24 (18.9)	0.30
Cerebrovascular disease	11 (8.2)	18 (14.2)	0.13
Median (range) Charlson score	4 (0–15)	5 (0–14)	0.09[a]
Median (range) SAPS II score	43 (14–82)	58 (27–103)	<0.001[a]
Risk factors			
Central venous catheter	89 (66.4)	103 (81.1)	0.007[a]
Drain	37 (27.6)	23 (18.1)	0.07[a]
Mechanical ventilation	47 (35.1)	64 (50.4)	0.01[a]
Total parenteral nutrition	28 (20.9)	24 (18.9)	0.69
Surgery	81 (60.4)	89 (70.1)	0.10
Gastrointestinal surgery	20 (14.9)	21 (16.5)	0.72
Renal replacement therapy	23 (17.2)	62 (48.8)	<0.001[a]
Antimicrobial therapy	116 (86.6)	120 (94.5)	0.30
Antifungal therapy	27 (20.1)	24 (18.9)	0.79
Immunosuppressive therapy	33 (24.6)	43 (33.9)	0.10
Neutropenia	10 (7.5)	11 (8.7)	0.72
Therapy			
Initial therapy			<0.001[b]
Echinocandin	89 (66.4)	76 (59.8)	
Azole	40 (29.9)	12 (9.4)	
Others (Amphotericin or combination)	3 (2.2)	5 (3.9)	
None	2 (1.5)	34 (26.8)	
Received initial therapy within 24 h	58 (43.2)	64 (50.4)	<0.001[b]
Infection Characteristics			
Species			0.04[a]
C. albicans	32 (23.9)	27 (21.3)	
C. glabrata	39 (29.1)	36 (28.3)	
C. tropicalis	29 (21.6)	42 (33.1)	
C. parapsilosis	24 (17.9)	9 (7.1)	

Table 3 Characteristics of survivors vs. non-survivors *(Continued)*

Median (range) time to reporting positive culture, days	2 (0–10)	2 (0–10)	0.08[a]
Median (range) time to species identification, days	5 (2–16)	5 (2–22)	***0.001**[a]*
Median (range) Candida score	2 (0–5)	3 (0–5)	***0.01***
Median (range) Pitts' bacteraemia score	2 (0–11)	5 (0–14)	*<**0.001**[a]*
Severe sepsis at time of culture	64 (47.8)	87 (68.5)	***0.001**[a]*
Concurrent bacterial infection	59 (46.5)	68 (53.5)	0.12
Candida colonization/infection at other sites	61 (45.5)	57 (44.9)	0.92

All variables are denoted as number of patients with the characteristic or belong to the category n (%), unless otherwise stated
Significant variables are reflected in bold and italics
[a]Factors entered into multivariable logistic regression model
[b]Additional factors entered into multivariable logistic regression model including only treated episodes

With respect to antifungal susceptibilities, while *C. albicans* and *C. parapsilosis* remained mostly susceptible, fluconazole resistant rates of *C. tropicalis* was 17%. Notably, the fluconazole MIC_{90} of *C. tropicalis* increased from 2 μg/mL in 2007 to 64 μg/mL reported in our study [20]. This MIC uptrend suggests that *C. tropicalis*, one of the predominant species in our context, is increasingly becoming less susceptible. Further molecular investigations are underway to understand the mechanisms related to azole resistance in these isolates.

Another noteworthy finding of our study was the emergence of echinocandin resistance in the Southeast Asia region. In the post-echinocandin era, there have been increasing reports of echinocandin treatment failures in most clinically-relevant species, especially in *C. glabrata* [7, 21–24]. Fortunately, resistance rates remained rare in the local context. There were only three (1.1%) isolates which were echinocandin-resistant, of which two had *fks* mutations. To the best of our knowledge, this is the first incidence of *fks* mutations in *Candida* bloodstream isolates other than *C. glabrata* identified locally. While the *fks* mutations identified in our isolates have been previously described, it is interesting to note that resistance developed rapidly (within 4 days of exposure to caspofungin) in one of the patients. Development in resistance has been primarily related to prolonged use of echinocandins, which was observed in the other patient, who had received 30 days of caspofungin prior to *Candida* isolation [22].

Our study observed a high 30-day mortality rate of 49%. Like many previous studies, we found that mortality was associated with severity of illness at onset of

Table 4 Multivariable logistic regression model for mortality in treated cases (*n* = 225)

Variable	OR (95% CI)
SAPS II score	1.08 (1.05–1.11)
Presence of drains	0.44 (0.19–0.99)
Renal replacement therapy	5.54 (2.80–10.97)

candidemia, suggesting that the poor outcomes of patients with candidemia is likely related to the poor prognosis of these patients with multiple comorbidities [25]. Receipt of renal replacement therapy was also associated with 30-day mortality. This could be an indication of the underlying organ dysfunction contributing to severity of illness. Drains placement prior to *Candida* isolation was found to be protective, suggesting that perhaps source control could contribute to better survival in patients with secondary candidemia.

Initial antifungal choice did not appear to be associated with mortality in our study. Although the Infectious Diseases Society of America guidelines have recommended the use of an echinocandin as a first-line agent, randomised controlled trials conducted so far have yet to conclusively demonstrate superiority of one agent over another [26–28]. A recent study has also illustrated that clinical severity, rather than initial antifungal strategy, was significantly correlated with mortality [25]. One reason why we were unable to detect any association of initial antifungal choice with mortality could be because we did not account for the appropriateness of the therapy in terms of dosing. Furthermore, pharmacokinetic variability can result in fluctuating antifungal levels in individual patients [29]. Perhaps, the impact of initial antifungal choice on treatment outcomes can be better elucidated if antifungal dosing was individualised, such as through the use of therapeutic drug monitoring. This therapeutic approach is currently being explored in our institution.

Although a large number of our patients received antifungals in a timely fashion, there was still a delay in therapy for some patients, with some receiving antifungals more than a week after cultures were taken. The time to administration of antifungals could be limited by the lack of rapid diagnostic tests available in our institution. It takes an average of two days to report a positive *Candida* blood culture, and in some instances even up to a week.

Our study was not without limitations. This was a single-centre study and our results might not be extrapolated to other institutions as the epidemiology of candidemia can be highly institution-specific. The retrospective nature of the study also precluded the analysis of impact of time of catheter removal on mortality. Nevertheless, this study provides important epidemiological findings which are instrumental in designing strategies for better management of candidemia in our institution.

Conclusions

While incidence of candidemia appeared to be stable, incidence of *C. glabrata* is increasing. *C. glabrata* and *C. tropicalis* contributed to majority of the candidemia cases in our institution. Decreasing azole susceptibilities to *C. tropicalis* and the emergence of echinocandin resistance suggests that susceptibility patterns may no longer be sufficiently predicted by speciation in our institution. Routine antifungal susceptibility, particularly for *C. tropicalis*, might be essential to guide clinician to effectively manage patients with invasive *Candida* infections. Candidemia was associated with high mortality, and antifungal stewardship efforts in individualising antifungal dosing through therapeutic drug monitoring should be further explored to improve outcomes in this population.

Abbreviations
ATCC: American Type Culture Collection; CI: Confidence interval; CLSI: Clinical and Laboratory Standards Institute; ECV: Epidemiological cut-off values; ICU: Intensive care unit; MIC: Minimum inhibitory concentration; OR: Odds ratio; PCR: Polymerase chain reaction; SAPS: Simplified acute physiology score; SGH: Singapore General Hospital

Acknowledgements
The authors acknowledge the excellent assistance of lab members of the Pathology Lab, in particular Ms Tan Mei Gie, and Pharmacy Research Lab, Singapore, in the collection of the isolates.

Funding
This study was funded by grants from National Medical Research Council (NMRC/TA/0025/2013 and NMRC/CG/016/2013); SGH Supplementary Research Grant (SRG #15/20); and Pfizer Inc. (WS2347894). The grant agencies had no involvement in the study design, in the collection, analysis and interpretation of the data, or in the decision to submit the article for publication.

Authors' contributions
JQT, SRC, SJL, SYC, HL, TPL and ALT participated in the microbiological and/or molecular experiments. JQT, SRC, HPN, KWL, YC and WL collected clinical data. SRC prepared the initial draft of the manuscript. JQT and ALK conceived the study, interpreted the results, revised the manuscript and wrote the manuscript. RPE participated in the design of the study and revised the manuscript. All authors read and approved the final manuscript.

Competing interests
The authors declare that they have no competing interests.

Consent for publication
Not applicable.

Author details
[1]Department of Pharmacy, Singapore General Hospital, Blk 8 Level 2, Outram Road, Singapore 169608, Singapore. [2]Department of Microbiology, Singapore General Hospital, Outram Road, Singapore 169608, Singapore. [3]Department of Pharmacy, National University of Singapore, 18 Science Drive 4, Singapore 117543, Singapore. [4]SingHealth Duke-NUS Medicine Academic Clinical Programme, 20 College Rd, Singapore 169856, Singapore. [5]Emerging Infectious Diseases, Duke-NUS Medical School, 8 College Rd, Singapore 169857, Singapore. [6]Present address: Tan Tock Seng Hospital, 11 Jalan Tan Tock Seng, Singapore 308433, Singapore.

References
1. Magill SS, Edwards JR, Bamberg W, Beldavs ZG, Dumyati G, Kainer MA, Lynfield R, Maloney M, McAllister-Hollod L, Nadle J, Ray SM, Thompson DL, Wilson LE, Fridkin SK. Emerging Infections Program Healthcare-Associated I, Antimicrobial Use Prevalence Survey T. Multistate point-prevalence survey of health care-associated infections. N Engl J Med. 2014;370(13):1198–208.
2. Bassetti M, Merelli M, Ansaldi F, de Florentiis D, Sartor A, Scarparo C, Callegari A, Righi E. Clinical and therapeutic aspects of candidemia: a five year single centre study. PLoS One. 2015;10(5):e0127534.
3. Pfaller M, Neofytos D, Diekema D, Azie N, Meier-Kriesche HU, Quan SP, Horn D. Epidemiology and outcomes of candidemia in 3648 patients: data from the Prospective Antifungal Therapy (PATH Alliance(R)) registry, 2004–2008. Diagn Microbiol Infect Dis. 2012;74(4):323–31.
4. Diekema D, Arbefeville S, Boyken L, Kroeger J, Pfaller M. The changing epidemiology of healthcare-associated candidemia over three decades. Diagn Microbiol Infect Dis. 2012;73(1):45–8.
5. Hassan I, Powell G, Sidhu M, Hart WM, Denning DW. Excess mortality, length of stay and cost attributable to candidaemia. J Infect. 2009;59(5):360–5.
6. Falagas ME, Apostolou KE, Pappas VD. Attributable mortality of candidemia: a systematic review of matched cohort and case–control studies. Eur J Clin Microbiol Infect Dis. 2006;25(7):419–25.
7. Alexander BD, Johnson MD, Pfeiffer CD, Jimenez-Ortigosa C, Catania J, Booker R, Castanheira M, Messer SA, Perlin DS, Pfaller MA. Increasing echinocandin resistance in Candida glabrata: clinical failure correlates with presence of FKS mutations and elevated minimum inhibitory concentrations. Clin Infect Dis. 2013;56(12):1724–32.
8. Montagna MT, Lovero G, Borghi E, Amato G, Andreoni S, Campion L, Lo Cascio G, Lombardi G, Luzzaro F, Manso E, Mussap M, Pecile P, Perin S, Tangorra E, Tronci M, Iatta R, Morace G. Candidemia in intensive care unit: a nationwide prospective observational survey (GISIA-3 study) and review of the European literature from 2000 through 2013. Eur Rev Med Pharmacol Sci. 2014;18(5):661–74.
9. Guinea J. Global trends in the distribution of Candida species causing candidemia. Clin Microbiol Infect. 2014;20 Suppl 6:5–10.
10. Tan BH, Chakrabarti A, Li RY, Patel AK, Watcharananan SP, Liu Z, Chindamporn A, Tan AL, Sun PL, Wu UI, Chen YC. Asia Fungal Working G. Incidence and species distribution of candidaemia in Asia: a laboratory-based surveillance study. Clin Microbiol Infect. 2015;21(10):946–53.
11. Tan TY, Hsu LY, Alejandria MM, Chaiwarith R, Chinniah T, Chayakulkeeree M, Choudhury S, Chen YH, Shin JH, Kiratisin P, Mendoza M, Prabhu K, Supparatpinyo K, Tan AL, Phan XT, Tran TT, Nguyen GB, Doan MP, Huynh VA, Nguyen SM, Tran TB, Van Pham H. Antifungal susceptibility of invasive Candida bloodstream isolates from the Asia-Pacific region. Med Mycol. 2016;54(5):471–7.
12. CLSI. Reference Method for Broth Dilution Antifungal Susceptibility Testing of Yeasts; Fourth Informational Supplement. CLSI document M27-S4. Wayne: Clinical and Laboratory Standards Institute; 2012.
13. Canton E, Peman J, Hervas D, Iniguez C, Navarro D, Echeverria J, Martinez-Alarcon J, Fontanals D, Gomila-Sard B, Buendia B, Torroba L, Ayats J, Bratos A, Sanchez-Reus F, Fernandez-Natal I. Comparison of three statistical methods for establishing tentative wild-type population and epidemiological cutoff values for echinocandins, amphotericin B, flucytosine, and six Candida species as determined by the colorimetric Sensititre YeastOne method. J Clin Microbiol. 2012;50(12):3921–6.
14. Canton E, Peman J, Iniguez C, Hervas D, Lopez-Hontangas JL, Pina-Vaz C, Camarena JJ, Campos-Herrero I, Garcia-Garcia I, Garcia-Tapia AM, Guna R, Merino P, Perez del Molino L, Rubio C, Suarez A, Group FS. Epidemiological

cutoff values for fluconazole, itraconazole, posaconazole, and voriconazole for six Candida species as determined by the colorimetric Sensititre YeastOne method. J Clin Microbiol. 2013;51(8):2691–5.

15. Espinel-Ingroff A, Alvarez-Fernandez M, Canton E, Carver PL, Chen SC, Eschenauer G, Getsinger DL, Gonzalez GM, Govender NP, Grancini A, Hanson KE, Kidd SE, Klinker K, Kubin CJ, Kus JV, Lockhart SR, Meletiadis J, Morris AJ, Pelaez T, Quindos G, Rodriguez-Iglesias M, Sanchez-Reus F, Shoham S, Wengenack NL, Borrell Sole N, Echeverria J, Esperalba J, Gomez GPE, Garcia Garcia I, Linares MJ, Marco F, Merino P, Peman J, Perez Del Molino L, Rosello Mayans E, Rubio Calvo C, Ruiz Perez de Pipaon M, Yague G, Garcia-Effron G, Guinea J, Perlin DS, Sanguinetti M, Shields R, Turnidge J. Multicenter study of epidemiological cutoff values and detection of resistance in Candida spp. to anidulafungin, caspofungin, and micafungin using the Sensititre YeastOne colorimetric method. Antimicrob Agents Chemother. 2015;59(11):6725–32.

16. Desnos-Ollivier M, Bretagne S, Raoux D, Hoinard D, Dromer F, Dannaoui E. Mutations in the fks1 gene in Candida albicans, C. tropicalis, and C. krusei correlate with elevated caspofungin MICs uncovered in AM3 medium using the method of the European Committee on Antibiotic Susceptibility Testing. Antimicrob Agents Chemother. 2008;52(9):3092–8.

17. Cleveland AA, Harrison LH, Farley MM, Hollick R, Stein B, Chiller TM, Lockhart SR, Park BJ. Declining incidence of candidemia and the shifting epidemiology of Candida resistance in two US metropolitan areas, 2008–2013: results from population-based surveillance. PLoS One. 2015;10(3):e0120452.

18. Posteraro B, Spanu T, Fiori B, De Maio F, De Carolis E, Giaquinto A, Prete V, De Angelis G, Torelli R, D'Inzeo T, Vella A, De Luca A, Tumbarello M, Ricciardi W, Sanguinetti M. Antifungal Susceptibility Profiles of Bloodstream Yeast Isolates by Sensititre YeastOne over Nine Years at a Large Italian Teaching Hospital. Antimicrob Agents Chemother. 2015;59(7):3944–55.

19. Colombo AL, Nucci M, Park BJ, Nouer SA, Arthington-Skaggs B, da Matta DA, Warnock D, Morgan J. Brazilian Network Candidemia S. Epidemiology of candidemia in Brazil: a nationwide sentinel surveillance of candidemia in eleven medical centers. J Clin Microbiol. 2006;44(8):2816–23.

20. Tan TY, Tan AL, Tee NW, Ng LS, Chee CW. The increased role of non-albicans species in candidaemia: results from a 3-year surveillance study. Mycoses. 2010;53(6):515–21.

21. Ruggero MA, Topal JE. Development of echinocandin-resistant Candida albicans candidemia following brief prophylactic exposure to micafungin therapy. Transpl Infect Dis. 2014;16(3):469–72.

22. Jensen RH, Justesen US, Rewes A, Perlin DS, Arendrup MC. Echinocandin failure case due to a previously unreported FKS1 mutation in Candida krusei. Antimicrob Agents Chemother. 2014;58(6):3550–2.

23. Pfeiffer CD, Garcia-Effron G, Zaas AK, Perfect JR, Perlin DS, Alexander BD. Breakthrough invasive candidiasis in patients on micafungin. J Clin Microbiol. 2010;48(7):2373–80.

24. Garcia-Effron G, Kontoyiannis DP, Lewis RE, Perlin DS. Caspofungin-resistant Candida tropicalis strains causing breakthrough fungemia in patients at high risk for hematologic malignancies. Antimicrob Agents Chemother. 2008;52(11):4181–3.

25. Murri R, Scoppettuolo G, Ventura G, Fabbiani M, Giovannenze F, Taccari F, Milozzi E, Posteraro B, Sanguinetti M, Cauda R, Fantoni M. Initial antifungal strategy does not correlate with mortality in patients with candidemia. Eur J Clin Microbiol Infect Dis. 2016;35(2):187–93.

26. Pappas PG, Kauffman CA, Andes DR, Clancy CJ, Marr KA, Ostrosky-Zeichner L, Reboli AC, Schuster MG, Vazquez JA, Walsh TJ, Zaoutis TE, Sobel JD. Clinical Practice Guideline for the Management of Candidiasis: 2016 Update by the Infectious Diseases Society of America. Clin Infect Dis. 2016;62(4):e1–50.

27. Reboli AC, Rotstein C, Pappas PG, Chapman SW, Kett DH, Kumar D, Betts R, Wible M, Goldstein BP, Schranz J, Krause DS, Walsh TJ, Anidulafungin SG. Anidulafungin versus fluconazole for invasive candidiasis. N Engl J Med. 2007;356(24):2472–82.

28. Krause DS, Simjee AE, van Rensburg C, Viljoen J, Walsh TJ, Goldstein BP, Wible M, Henkel T. A randomized, double-blind trial of anidulafungin versus fluconazole for the treatment of esophageal candidiasis. Clin Infect Dis. 2004;39(6):770–5.

29. Lewis RE. Current concepts in antifungal pharmacology. Mayo Clin Proc. 2011;86(8):805–17.

15

Virucidal efficacy of peracetic acid for instrument disinfection

Britta Becker[1], Florian H. H. Brill[1], Daniel Todt[2] ⓘ, Eike Steinmann[2], Johannes Lenz[3], Dajana Paulmann[1], Birte Bischoff[1] and Jochen Steinmann[1*]

Abstract

Background: Various peracetic-acid (PAA)-based products for processing flexible endoscopes on the market are often based on a two-component system including a cleaning step before the addition of PAA as disinfectant. The peracetic acid concentrations in these formulations from different manufacturers are ranging from 400 to 1500 ppm (part per million). These products are used at temperatures between 20 °C and 37 °C. Since information on the virus-inactivating properties of peracetic acid at different concentrations and temperature is missing, it was the aim of the study to evaluate peracetic acid solutions against test viruses using the quantitative suspension test, EN 14476. In addition, further studies were performed with the recently established European pre norm (prEN 17111:2017) describing a carrier assay for simulating practical conditions using frosted glass.

Methods: In the first step of examination, different PAA solutions between 400 and 1500 ppm were tested at 20 °C, 25 °C, and 35 °C with three test viruses (adenovirus, murine norovirus and poliovirus) necessary for creating a virucidal action according to the European Norm, EN 14476. A second step for simulating practical conditions based on prEN 17111:2017 followed by spreading a test virus together with soil load onto a glass carrier which was immerged into a peracetic acid solution. A fixed exposure time of five minutes was used in all experiments.

Results: In the quantitative suspension test 1500 ppm PAA solution was needed at 35 °C for five minutes for the inactivation of poliovirus, whereas only 400 ppm at 20 °C for adeno- and murine norovirus were necessary. In the carrier assay 400 ppm peracetic acid at 20 °C were sufficient for adenovirus inactivation, whereas 600 ppm PAA were needed at 25 °C and 35 °C and 1000 ppm at 20 °C for murine norovirus. A PAA solution with 1000 ppm at 35 °C was required for complete inactivation of poliovirus. However, a dramatically decrease of titer after the drying and immerging could be observed. In consequence, a four log reduction of poliovirus titer could not be achieved in the carrier test.

Conclusion: In summary, 1500 ppm PAA at 35 °C was necessary for a virucidal action in the quantitative suspension test. After passing the requirements of the suspension test, additional examinations with adeno- and murine norovirus on glass carriers based on prEN 17111:2017 will not additionally contribute to the final claim of an instrument disinfectant for virucidal efficacy. This is due to the great stability of poliovirus in the preceded quantitative suspension test and the fact that poliovirus could not serve as test virus in the following carrier assay.

Keywords: Peracetic acid, Virucidal efficacy, Instrument disinfection

* Correspondence: jochen.steinmann@brillhygiene.com
[1]Dr. Brill + Partner GmbH Institute for Hygiene and Microbiology, Norderoog 2, DE-28259 Bremen, Germany

Background

Peracetic acid (PAA) is often incorporated as active ingredient of instrument disinfectants for reprocessing flexible endoscopes in manual and automatic procedures. Such instrument disinfectants are often used between room temperature and 40 °C with short exposure times. By introducing PAA as active ingredient, a broad range of virucidal efficacy for instrument disinfectants can be achieved, as requested by the Commission for Hospital Hygiene and Infection Prevention (Kommission für Krankenhaushygiene und Infektionsprävention, KRINKO) [1]. There is only a minor temperature stress for the instruments when using short exposure times with PAA and only aldehydes are able to demonstrate a comparative range of efficacy against viruses. But for aldehydes, higher temperatures are necessary in general for reaching a sufficient virucidal action resulting in a claim of these chemicals against enveloped and non-enveloped viruses.

The virus-inactivating properties of PAA had been demonstrated earlier in detail by the group of Prößig [2, 3]. Later it was questioned whether peracetic-acid-based formulations are suited for the cleaning step when reprocessing flexible endoscopes due to the fixation potential of PAA [4]. Current formulations on the market are always based on a two-step procedure including a cleaning step before the addition of PAA.

The concentrations of PAA in the products for reprocessing endoscopes differ and there are only few data on the behaviour of PAA in test methods developed as European Norms (EN). Therefore, we evaluated the virucidal activity of PAA solutions in clean conditions according to a quantitative suspension test (phase 2/step 1) which is described as EN 14476 with a short exposure time [5]. This was followed by a phase 2/step 2 carrier test, simulating practical conditions recently established as prEN 17111:2017 for instrument disinfectants in Europe [6].

Methods

For the examination of the virucidal efficacy of different concentrations of PAA a quantitative suspension test according to the European Guideline EN 14476 with poliovirus (PV), adenovirus (AdV) and murine norovirus (MNV) as surrogate of human norovirus was used [5]. Subsequently, a quantitative carrier assay using frosted glass based on prEN 17111:2017 [6] was run with identical conditions regarding exposure time and test temperature with AdV and MNV and PV [6]. For all tests, clean conditions (0.3 g/L bovine serum albumin) and a fixed exposure time of five minutes were used.

PAA was supplied by AppliChem GmbH (order number 143495, 15% solution) (Ottoweg 4, DE-64291 Darmstadt). Dilutions of PAA were prepared with hard water according to the European norms immediately before the inactivation tests started.

PV type 1 strain LSc-2ab (Chiron-Behring) was obtained from PD Dr. O. Thraenhart, Eurovir, DE-14943 Luckenwalde. AdV type 5 strain Adenoid 75 (ATCC VR-5) from PD Dr. A. Heim, Institute of Medical Virology, Hannover Medical School, DE-30625 Hannover. MNV S99 was obtained from PD Dr. E. Schreier at the Robert Koch-Institute (RKI) in DE-13302 Berlin (now available at the Friedrich-Loeffler-Institute Bundesforschungsinstitut für Tiergesundheit, Ile of Riems).

The test virus suspensions were prepared by infecting monolayers of the respective cell lines. The virus titers of these suspensions ranged from 10^8 to 10^9 $TCID_{50}$/mL (tissue culture infectious dose 50). PV type 1 was propagated in BGM cells (buffalo green monkey kidney cell line; supplied by Prof. Dr. Lindl, Institute for Applied Cell Culture, DE-81669 München) in Dulbecco's Modified Eagle's Medium (DMEM) with 1 g/L glucose. AdV type 5 replication was performed in A549 cells (human lung epithelial carcinoma cells). The A549 cells originated from the Institute of Medical Virology, Hannover Medical School, DE-30625 Hannover and were cultivated in Eagle's Minimum Essential Medium with Earle's BSS (EMEM). MNV strain S99 was propagated in RAW 264.7 cells (a macrophage-like, Abelson leukemia virus transformed cell line derived from BALB/c mice, ATCC TIB-71) in DMEM with 1 g/L glucose.

Tests according to EN 14476 were run with PV, AdV and MNV as test viruses of the EN 14476 in clean conditions with a fixed exposure time of five minutes [5]. 20 °C, 25 °C and 35 °C were used as test temperatures. Hard water was added as a control instead of PAA and cytotoxicity was additionally determined by addition of hard water instead of virus suspension. Infectivity was stopped by immediate serial dilution with ice-cold medium according to the standards of the European Committee for Normalisation [5, 6]. Of each dilution, 100 μL were placed in eight wells of a sterile polystyrene flat bottomed 96-well microtiter plate containing 100 μL cell suspension. Cultures were observed for cytopathic effects (CPE) after 4–10 days of inoculation depending on the cell culture system used.

The virus titers were determined using the Spearman and Kaerber method [7, 8] and expressed as $\log_{10}TCID_{50}$/mL with 95% confidence interval (CI). Titer reduction caused by the biocide is presented as the difference between the virus titer after defined contact time with the water control and the disinfectant and defined as reduction factor (RF). A reduction of infectivity of ≥4 $\log_{10}$ steps (inactivation ≥99.99%, RF = 4) is regarded as evidence of virucidal activity.

The quantitative carrier test based on prEN 17111:2017 was performed in clean conditions with AdV and MNV and additionally with PV [6]. The surface sandblasted frosted glass carriers (15 mm × 60 mm × 1 mm, manufacturer: Zell Quarzglas und Technische Keramik Technologie GmbH, DE-21502 Geesthacht) were prepared as described in the prEN 17111:2017. One volume of interfering substance was mixed with nine volumes of test virus suspension (virus inoculum); 50 μL of this virus inoculum were pipetted on the inoculation square of the carrier followed by drying [6].

Ten mL of the different PAA solutions in a cylindrical screw tube were placed in a water bath at the chosen test temperature. After the drying process had been finished, the inoculated carrier was immersed in the prepared PAA solution (or hard water as control). Immediately at the end of the exposure time the carrier was transferred into a second screw tube with medium and glass beads and mixed for 60 s. After five minutes a second mixture was started for 60 s. Virus titer was determined by end point dilution titration in microtiter plates. Of each dilution 100 μL were placed in eight wells of a sterile polystyrene flat bottomed 96-well microtiter plate containing 100 μL cell suspension. Cultures were observed for cytopathic effects (CPE) after 4–10 days of inoculation depending on the cell culture system.

As in the suspension assay the method of Spearman and Kaerber [7, 8] was used for calculating virus titers. These were expressed as $\log_{10}TCID_{50}$/mL with 95% CI. Titer reduction caused by the biocide is also presented as the difference between the virus titer after defined contact time with the water control and the disinfectant. As in the suspension test a reduction of infectivity of ≥4 $\log_{10}$ steps (inactivation ≥99.99%, RF = 4) is regarded as virucidal activity.

Linear regression analyses and statistical testing of differences between slopes and Y-intercepts were performed using GraphPad Prism v7.03. For individual linear regression per temperature, infectivity values between 400 and 1500 ppm PAA were taken into account (****$P < 0.0001$, **$P < 0.01$). Slopes and Y-intercepts are depicted in separate plots with 95% CI indicated by vertical lines.

Results

The PAA solutions between 400 ppm to 1500 ppm were examined in the suspension test according to the European Standard EN 14476 [5]. A four $\log_{10}$ reduction of the titer of PV was only achieved with 1500 ppm PAA at 35 °C when the initial titer of 8.38 $\log_{10}TCID_{50}$/mL dropped to ≤3.63 $\log_{10}TCID_{50}$/mL (RF = ≥ 4.75 ± 0.64) as depicted in Fig. 1. Lower concentrations (between 400 ppm and 1200 ppm) and lower temperatures (20 °C and 25 °C) were not successful in inactivating this respective test virus. These results were also visualized by a linear

regression analysis and statistical testing of differences between slopes and Y-intercepts (Fig. 1). For inactivation of AdV, in nearly all cases no residual virus could be detected. The initial virus titre of 7.63 $\log_{10}TCID_{50}$/mL at all temperatures tested decreased to ≤2.50 $\log_{10}TCID_{50}$/mL (lower detection limit) resulting in a maximum RF of ≥5.13 ± 0.25. Likewise for MNV, 400 ppm PAA was able to inactivate the test virus at 20 °C. After five minutes exposure the titer was ≤3.50 $\log_{10}TCID_{50}$/ml (initial virus titre 8.00 $\log_{10}TCID_{50}$/mL, RF = ≥ 4.50 ± 0.52). In contrast to AdV, for all concentrations tested residual MNV could be detected except with 1500 ppm (Fig. 1).

In the test simulating practical conditions based on the prEN 17111:2017, the initial titer of PV dropped from 7.63 to 3.63 $\log_{10}TCID_{50}$/mL at 20 °C, to 3.88 $\log_{10}TCID_{50}$/mL at 25 °C and to 3.19 $\log_{10}TCID_{50}$/mL at 35 °C in the virus controls, respectively, during the drying process and the additional incubation of the carrier in hard water (Fig. 2). Therefore, it was impossible with such a virus inoculum to demonstrate a four $\log_{10}$ reduction due to the virus loss. Nevertheless, no residual PV could be detected with 1000 ppm PAA at 35 °C. The initial virus titer of 3.19 ± 0.17 $\log_{10}TCID_{50}$/mL dropped to ≤0.50 $\log_{10}TCID_{50}$/mL (max. RF = ≥ 2.69 ± 0.17). For AdV 400 ppm PAA at 20 °C was sufficient for a four log reduction (Fig. 2). MNV was more stable than AdV in the carrier test requiring 1000 ppm PAA at 20 °C (RF = ≥ 4.19 ± 0.52) and 600 ppm PAA at 25 °C (RF = 4.13 ± 0.35) and 37 °C (RF = ≥ 4.87 ± 0.50) (Fig. 2).

Discussion

There are some peracetic-acid-based products on the European market as recently listed by Kampf et al. [4] with different PAA concentrations and different exposure temperatures. They are used for instrument disinfection with a virucidal action presumably based on quantitative suspension tests. Currently, a European standardized test simulating practical conditions for reaching a virus inactivation is only being drafted with AdV and MNV as presumed test viruses [6]. PV is not included in this European normalisation assay due to problems of virus loss during drying.

In Europe, an instrument disinfectant has to pass first the quantitative suspension test followed by the carrier test. Therefore we used both test methods for evaluating the virus-inactivating properties of PAA.

Kline and Hull already demonstrated in 1960 for the first time, the strong virus-inactivating properties of PAA [9]. They showed that a 400 ppm PAA solution was able to produce a 7.5 $\log_{10}$ step reduction of PV after five minutes exposure time without any soil loading in a suspension test. Interestingly, they pointed out that formaldehyde showed an identical activity as a 5% solution after 20 min [9].

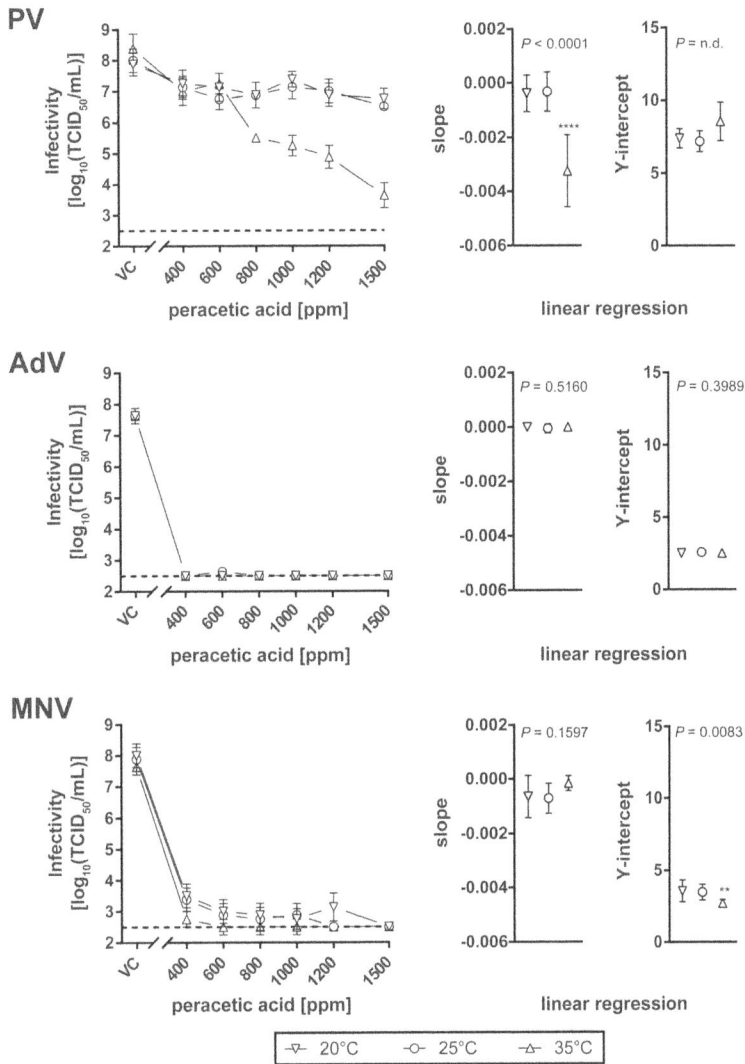

Fig. 1 Inactivation of poliovirus (PV), adenovirus (AdV) and murine norovirus (MNV) by different peracetic acid concentrations at 20 °C (inverted triangles), 25 °C (inverted triangles) and 35 °C (triangles) in the quantitative suspension test depicted on the left as $\log_{10}\mathrm{TCID}_{50}$/mL. Exposure time was five minutes. The dotted line represents the detection limit of the assay. Slopes (± 95% CI) and Y-intercepts (± 95% CI) of respective linear regression analyses are shown in the right panels. ****$P < 0.0001$, **$P < 0.01$, n.d.n.d.*not determined* not determined

Additional data were published on solutions of PAA often in alcohol by Sprößig and Mücke [2, 3]. Furthermore, they introduced PAA as a disinfectant in human medicine [3]. The mechanism of PAA on viruses is characterised by disruption of the capsid and a RNA fragmentation as shown with PV type 1 [10].

Our data show that among the test viruses of the European norm EN 14476, the PV was much more stable than adenovirus and MNV that miss the strong hydrophilic character of PV. In contrast to the older data of Kline and Hull [9], higher concentrations were required but the experimental design between their study and our experiments is difficult to compare mainly related to the ratio of biocide to virus suspension and the soil loading.

Sauerbrei et al. found in comparative studies with PV type 1 and echovirus type 1 that 0.05% PAA was not active in clean and dirty conditions against PV, whereas 0.5% was virucidal within 10–30 min exposure time, thus showing similar data in comparison to our study [11]. For AdV type 5, Sauerbrei et al. found that 0.1% and 0.2% PAA were necessary to inactivate the AdV after 15 and 5 min, respectively [12]. But these tests were run with a higher soil load (10% foetal calf serum) according to the DVV Guideline in contrast to clean conditions.

In our suspension tests, AdV and MNV showed a similar behaviour. There might be a difference in stability between both viruses at concentrations lower that 400 ppm, However, we did not use lower concentrations

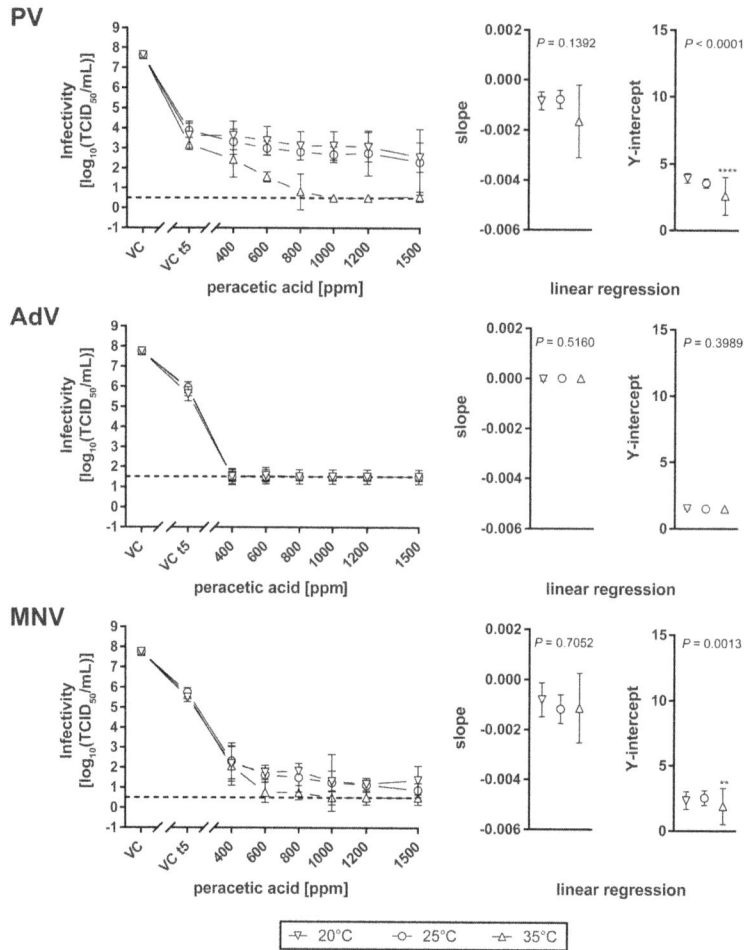

Fig. 2 Inactivation of poliovirus (PV), adenovirus (AdV) and murine norovirus (MNV) by different peracetic acid concentrations at 20 °C (inverted triangles), 25 °C (inverted triangles) and 35 °C (triangles) in the carrier test depicted on the left as $\log_{10}TCID_{50}/mL$. Exposure time was five minutes. The dotted line represents the detection limit of the assay. Slopes (± 95% CI) and Y-intercepts (± 95% CI) of respective linear regression analyses are shown in the right panels. ****$P < 0.0001$, **$P < 0.01$

because the concentration of PAA in the instrument disinfectant on the market in general is higher.

The greater stability of PV in contrast to AdV and MNV was also found performing test simulated practical conditions. Due to a high loss of virus titer for PV during drying and immerging, a four $\log_{10}$ reduction could not be observed with this virus. It can only be mentioned that 35 °C and at least 1000 ppm PAA were necessary to detect no residual PV. Here, in the test simulating practical conditions MNV was more stable than AdV. At 20 °C the required concentration of PAA for MNV was 1000 ppm in comparison to 400 ppm for AdV.

An identical procedure as shown here with frosted glass carriers was performed with PAA testing vaccinia virus strain Elstree and polyomavirus SV40 strain 777 by Strohhäcker und Eggers [13]. They found that even 0.05% PAA was sufficient for virus inactivation of both viruses within five minutes in clean and dirty conditions.

Following the procedure of virucidal testing in Europe, first the requirements of the suspension test have to be fulfilled. Then the phase 2/step 2 test must follow. According to our data with PAA and PV, it is much more difficult to reach an inactivation with PV, AdV and MNV in the quantitative suspension test due to the great stability of PV than to be successful with AdV and MNV in the carrier test based on prEN 17111:2017 simulating practical conditions. Therefore, it should be put into consideration in the future in Europe to include the stable murine parvovirus as a test virus in the phase 2/step 2 procedure even when using temperature < 40 °C. At the moment murine parvovirus is only used as sole test virus for instrument disinfectants at temperature ≥ 40 °C.

Conclusion

In summary, 1500 ppm peracetic acid at 35 °C was necessary for a virucidal action in the quantitative suspension test. After passing the requirements of the suspension test, additional examinations with adeno- and murine norovirus on glass carriers based on prEN 17111:2017 will not additionally contribute to the final claim of an instrument disinfectant to have sufficient virucidal efficacy. This is due to the great stability of poliovirus in the preceded quantitative suspension test and the fact that poliovirus could not serve as test virus in the carrier assay.

Abbreviation

AdV: Adenovirus; CI: Confidence interval; CPE: Cytopathic effect; DMEM: Dulbecco's modified Eagle medium; EN: European Norm; KRINKO: Kommission für Krankenhaushygiene und Infektionsprävention; MNV: Murine norovirus; n.d.: Not determined; PAA: Peracetic acid; ppm: Part per million; prEN: European pre norm; PV: Poliovirus; RF: Reduction factor; RKI: Robert Koch-Institute; TCID50: Tissue culture infectious dose 50

Acknowledgements
Not applicable.

Funding
This study was supported by Chemische Fabrik Dr. Weigert GmbH & Co.KG, Germany. E. S. was supported by the Helmholtz Centre for Infection Research, Hannover Germany.

Authors' contributions
JS and JL together with FB and ES formulated the study questions and designed the study. BB, DP and BB were responsible performing all experimental data. DT was responsible for data evaluation. All authors read and approved the final manuscript.

Consent for publication
Not applicable.

Competing interests
JL is employee of Chemische Fabrik Dr. Weigert GmbH & Co.KG. The other authors declare that they have no competing interests.

Author details
[1]Dr. Brill + Partner GmbH Institute for Hygiene and Microbiology, Norderoog 2, DE-28259 Bremen, Germany. [2]Institute for Experimental Virology, TWINCORE Centre for Experimental and Clinical Infection Research; a joint venture between the Medical School Hannover (MHH) and the Helmholtz Centre for Infection Research (HZI), Hannover, Germany. [3]Chemische Fabrik Dr. Weigert GmbH & Co.KG, Hamburg, Germany.

References

1. Commission for Hospital Hygiene and Infection Prevention (KRINKO); Federal Institute for Drugs and Medical Devices (BfArM). Hygiene requirements for the processing of medical devices. Recommendation of the Commission for Hospital Hygiene and Infection Prevention (KRINKO) at the Robert Koch Institute (RKI) and the Federal Institute for Drugs and Medical Devices (BfArM). Bundesgesundheitsbl. 2012;55:1244–310.

2. Sprößig M, Mücke H. Über die stark viruzide Eigenschaft eines praktisch anwendbaren Alkohol-Peressigsäure-Gemisches. Wiss Ztschr der Karl-Marx-Universität Leipzig, Math-Naturwiss R. 1964;13:1167–9.

3. Sprößig M, Mücke H. Über die antimikrobielle Wirkung der Peressigsäure. 5. Mitteilung. Untersuchungen zur viruziden Wirkung. Die Pharmazie. 1968;23:665–7.

4. Kampf G, Fliss PM, Martiny H. Is peracetic acid suitable for the cleaning step of reprocessing flexible enodcopes. World J Gastrointest Endosc. 2014;6(9):390–406.

5. DIN EN 14476:2013. Chemical disinfectants and antiseptics. Virucidal quantitative suspension test for chemical disinfectants and antiseptics used in human medicine. Test method and requirements (phase 2, step 1). Brussels: CEN-Comité Européen de Normalisation; 2013.

6. CEN 216 prEN 17111:2017. Chemical disinfectants and antiseptics. Quantitative carrier test for the evaluation of virucidal activity used in the medical area – test method and requirements (phase 2, test 2). Brussels: CEN-Comité Européen de Normalisation; 2017.

7. Spearman C. The method of right and wrong cases (constant stimuli) without Gauss's formulae. Brit J. Psychology. 1908;2:227–42.

8. Kärber G. Beitrag zur kollektiven Behandlung pharmakologischer Reihenversuche. Arch Exp Path Pharmakol. 1931;162:480–3.

9. Klein L, Hull RH. The virucidal properties of peractic acid. Am J Clin Path 2060;33:30-33.

10. Sporkenbach-Höffler J, Wiegers KJ, Dernick R. Untersuchungen zum Mechanismus der Virusinaktivierung durch Persäuren. Zbl Bakt Hyg, I Abt Orig B. 1983;177:469–81.

11. Sauerbrei A, Eschrich W, Brandstädt, Wutzler P. Sensitivity of poliovirus type 1 and echovirus type 1 to different groups of chemical biocides. J Hosp Infect. 2009;72:277–9.

12. Sauerbrei A, Sehr K, Brandstädt A, et al. Sensitivity of human adenovirus to different groups of chemical biocides. J Hosp Infect. 2004;57:59–66.

13. Strohhäcker J, Eggers M. Praxisnaher Test zur Prüfung der viruziden Wirksamkeit von chemischen Instrumentendesinfektionsmitteln zur Aufbereitung von transvaginalen Ultraschallsonden. Hyg Med. 2012;37(7/8):320–9.

16

Risk factors for *Clostridium difficile* infection in surgical patients hospitalized in a tertiary hospital in Belgrade, Serbia

Vesna Šuljagić[1,2*], Ivan Miljković[3], Srđan Starčević[2,4], Nenad Stepić[2,5], Zoran Kostić[2,6], Dragutin Jovanović[7], Jelena Brusić-Renaud[8], Biljana Mijović[9] and Sandra Šipetić-Grujičić[10]

Abstract

Background: The objective of this study was to investigate independent risk factors (RFs) connected with healthcare-associated (HA) *Clostridium difficile* infection (CDI) in surgical patients, its frequency per surgical wards and in-hospital-mortality at a single hospital.

Methods: Risk factors for the infection were prospectively assessed among surgical patients with laboratory confirmed HA CDI and compared with a control group without HA CDI.

Results: The overall incidence rate of HA CDI was 2.6 per 10000 patient-days. Significant independent RFs for HA CDI were the use of carbapenems ($P = 0.007$, OR: 10.62, 95% CI: 1.93–58.4), the admission to intensive care unit ($P = 0.004$, OR:3.00, 95% CI:1.41–6.40), and the administration of 3rd generation cephalosporins ($P = 0.014$, OR:2.27, 95% CI:1.18–4.39). Patients with HA CDI had significantly higher in–hospital mortality compared to controls (P: 0.007; OR: 8.95; 95% CI: 1.84–43.43).

Conclusions: CDI is an important HA infection in population of surgical patients and this study emphasizes the importance of the wise use of antibiotics, and other infection control strategies in order to prevent HA CDI, and to decrease the incidence and in-hospital mortality rate.

Keywords: *Clostridium difficile*, Incidence, Risk factors, In-hospital mortality, Surgical patients

Background

During the current century the epidemiology of *Clostridium difficile* (*C.difficile*) infections (CDI) has changed rapidly, with increases noted in the incidence of diseases internationally, and in the reports of CDI outbreaks within healthcare institutions in the USA, Canada and Europe. The increase of CDI incidence was partly associated with the epidemic emergence of a new C. difficile ribotype 027, which was also described to cause more severe infections [1]. CDI became one of the most common healthcare-associated (HA) infections in modern medicine. CDI results in a wide spectrum of clinical conditions, including an asymptomatic carrier state; mild, self-limited diarrhea; pseudomembranous colitis; and fulminant colitis. It is associated with the increased morbidity, in-hospital mortality, prolonged hospitalization, and increased costs. The main risk factors for CDI include the administration of antibiotics, patients older than 65 years, multiple co-morbid conditions, previous hospitalization, medical procedures, and long stay in hospitals [2–4]. The reported incidence of HA CDI varies according to the country, the size of institution and ward location, the type of population studied [5–11]. Patients undergoing surgical procedures are at risk of the postoperative HA CDI development. Most studies of risk factors (RFs) for CDI in surgical patients have been conducted in the USA or Western European countries, which

---
* Correspondence: suljagicv@gmail.com
[1]Department of Nosocomial Infections Control, Military Medical Academy, 11 000 Belgrade, Serbia
[2]Faculty of Medicine of Military Medical Academy University of Defence, 11000 Belgrade, Serbia

are characterized by the well-developed healthcare systems [8–10, 12]. In contrast, the burden of CDI in Serbia, a country in socioeconomic transition and with a resource-limited healthcare system, is less well studied [3, 11]. The burden of CDI in surgical patients in Serbia is unclear.

The aim of this study was to investigate independent RFs associated with HA CDI in surgical patients, its frequency per surgical wards and in-hospital-mortality in a tertiary healthcare centre in Serbia.

Methods

Patients and databases

The Military Medical Academy (MMA), Belgrade, Serbia, a teaching hospital of the University of Defense, is a 1200-bed tertiary healthcare centre divided into 27 departments. The department of Infection Control performs continuous surveillance of the MMA patients. The surveillance of HA infections, including CDI, covered patients in surgical clinics of the MMA: Urology, General Surgery, Orthopedics/Traumatology, Neurosurgery, Maxillofacial Surgery, Plastic Surgery/Burns, Vascular Surgery, Thoracic Surgery, Cardio Surgery, Otorhinolaryngology, and Ophthalmology.

Through regular hospital surveillance of surgical patients we prospectively identified all patients who had new HA, laboratory confirmed postoperative CDI during the study period, from 1st January 2011 to 31st December 2012. Reviewing the clinical chart information on patient characteristics, RFs related to healthcare were collected. We gathered data on the following variables: intrinsic factors (existing at admission) sex, age, *Diabetes mellitus*, malignancy, and factors related to healthcare including previous hospitalization in other hospitals, intensive care unit (ICU) admission, duration of treatment in ICU, mechanical ventilation, nasogastric tubes, previous use of corticosteroids, histamine-2-receptor antagonists (H2RAs), proton-pump inhibitors (PPIs) and antibiotics (number, type, and duration of used antibiotics). Also, data about in-hospital mortality were recorded.

In the case–control study, every surgical patient with HA CDI was compared with two control patients without CDI. HA CDI was defined as diarrhea (≥3 daily) which was acquired more than three days after admission to the surgical department and detection of *C. difficile* toxins A and B in a stool sample, which was derived more than three days after admission. Control patients were matched to the cases according to the inpatient ward, gender, age (±5 years), and date of surgical operation.

Microbiological testing

Microbiological testing was performed at the Institute of Medical Microbiology at the MMA. Enzyme immunoassay

kits for *C. difficile* toxins A and B were used (*BIOMER-IEUX-VIDAS Clostridium difficile toxins A&B CDAB*). Only patients who had never been diagnosed with CDI at the MMA were included in the control group, and only those who had not been diagnosed with CDI before enrolling in the study, were included in the case group, respectively. The Research Ethics Board of the MMA approved the research protocol. All study participants provided the informed written consent.

Statistical analysis

Incidence rate (IR) was defined as the number of HA CDIs per 10000 patient-days and per 1000 patients treated. The rate of testing (TR) was defined as the number of *C. difficile* toxin tests performed per 10000 patient-days. The in-hospital mortality rate was defined as the number of deaths per 100 patients. Data analyses were performed with SPSS, version 21.0 (SPSS, Inc, Chicago, IL). Results were expressed as the mean ± SD or as the proportion of the total number of patients. The χ^2 test or Fischer exact test were used for categorical variables and relative risk, and their corresponding 95% confidence intervals (CI) were calculated. For parametric continuous variables, mean values were compared using the Student t test. For nonparametric continuous variables the Mann–Whitney U test was used. RF independently associated with CDI were identified by stepwise logistic regression analysis of variables selected by univariate analysis, with a limit for enetering and removing variables from the model at 0.05.

Results

During 2011–2012 in the MMA 29033 surgical patients were treated during 255431 patient-days. A total of 67 surgical patients with CDI were registered (IR: 2.6 per 10000 patient-days or 2.3 per 1000 patients, TR: 8.5 per 10000 patient-days) (Table 1).

Demographic and clinical characteristics of patients in the case and control groups according to ULRA are shown in Table 2. MLRA identified three independent RFs associated with CDI in surgical patients: the previous administration of carbapenems ($P = 0.007$, OR:10.62, 95% CI:1.93–58.4), the 3rd generation of cephalosporins ($P = 0.014$, OR:2.27, 95% CI:1.18–4.39) and admission to the ICU ($P = 0.004$, OR:3.00, 95% CI:1.41–6.40). According to the ULRA, PPIs usage was a significant RF for HA CDI ($P = 0.05$), but it was not a significant independent RF according to MLRA ($P = 0.051$, OR:2.7, 95% CI:1.00–7.19).

In hospital-mortality was significantly higher by 9-fold in HA CDI compared to control (12% *vs* 1.5%, P: 0.007; OR: 8.95; 95% CI: 1.84–43.43). Of 8 deaths in the case group, 6 or 75% were in the older than 65.

Table 1 Incidence rates of *Clostridium difficile* infections in 11 surgical wards of Military Medical Academy during 2011–2012

Ward	Hospital Inpatient Days/ Number of patients treated	New cases per 10000 patient-days	New cases per 1000 patients	Testing frequency per 10000 patient-days
Urology	39022/5968	1.5	1.0	6.7
General Surgery	42063/4358	1.7	1.6	6.4
Traumatology/Orthopaedics	44139/3716	6.1	7.2	12.5
Neurosurgery	22546/2639	0	0	4.4
Maxillofacial Surgery	16829/2242	0.6	0.4	2.4
Plastic Surgery and Burns	24019/2414	4.6	4.6	11.2
Vascular Surgery	20175/1631	1.5	1.8	16.9
Thoracic Surgery	12408/1191	0.8	0.8	7.3
Cardiosurgery	13842/827	6.5	10.9	14.5
Otorhinolaryngology	20388/4047	1.0	0.5	2.0
Overall	255431/29033	2.6	2.3	8.5

Discussion

Most of epidemiological data about CDI in surgical patients have been limited to North America and West Europe [8–10, 12]. This study provides data about IR, RF and in-hospital-mortality of HA CDI in surgical patients admitted to the tertiary healthcare centre in the South East Europe.

The overall IR of HA CDI was 2.6 per 10000 patient-days, varied by different wards from 0 in Neurosurgery to more than 6 per 10000 patient-days in Orthopedics/Traumatology and Cardio Surgery. The overall TR was 8.5 per 10000 patient-days varied by different wards from 2.0 in Otorhinolaryngology to 16.9 per 10000 patient-days in Vascular Surgery. Our results of IR were similar to data reported by a coordinating laboratory for Portugal (2.9 for 2011–2012 and 3.0 for 2012–2013), but lower than mean IR of 7.0 of HA CDI (country range 0.7–28.7) in a European, multicentre, prospective, biannual point-prevalence study of CDI in hospitalized patients with diarrhea (EUCLID) (4). In our hospital we have the practice of routine testing of all submitted diarrheal inpatient samples, but our TR in surgical patients in the two-year period was far lower than mean TR in European hospitals (65.8 tests, country range 4.6–223.3) (4).

An association between female gender and CDI has been reported by previous population-based studies from the USA [5]. Similarly to the report of Rodrigues et al. [9], our results showed no significant association between gender and CDI. Advance age is an independent RF for CDI in many studies [5, 9, 10]. RFs specific to older adults are frequent interactions with healthcare systems and age-related changes in physiology, including immune senescence and changes of the gut microbiome [13]. In our study majority of CDI occurred in patients older than 40 years and half in patients older than 65 years. We did not analyze age and sex in the model of MLRA because cases and controls were matched according to those variables.

Among the main findings of this study are the identification of significant independent RFs for CDI in surgical patients, including carbapenems, admission to ICU and the 3rd generation of cephalosporins. The disruption of the normal flora caused by antibiotics allows *C. difficile* to colonize and overgrow within the gastrointestinal tract. Nearly all antibiotics have been implicated in CDI, but certain classes seem to cause higher risk for CDI. Stojanović confirmed in his study that all the groups of antibiotics, except for tetracycline, and trimetoprim-sulfamethoxazole, were statistically significant RFs for CDI [3]. The administration of quinolones emerged as the most important RF for CID in Quebec during an epidemic caused by a hipervirulent strain of *C. difficile* [14]. A recent study from England showed that restricting quinolones prescribing was associated with a decline in incidence of CDI [15]. The majority of patients in our study received at least one class of antibiotic. The third-generation cephalosporins were the most commonly used antibiotics in both groups and an independent RF for CDI. The study of Korean authors showed that the use of cephalosporins increased the risk for CDI [4]. Also, the use of carbapenems, in addition to having the higher frequency in the case group, was an independent RF for CDI in our study. The study of Metzger et al. showed that carbapenems usage was associated with CDI in ULRA, but didn't retain significance as an independent RF in MLRA [16].

The admission to ICU was significantly associated with CDI in our patients as reported before [4, 9]. Critically ill patients in ICU share many of the RFs for developing CDI such as: severe underlying diseases, antibiotic exposure, gastric acid suppression with H2RAs or PPIs, the use of mechanical ventilation, and nasogastric tubes [17].

However, in a meta-analysis, Kwok et al. demonstrated the possible association between the PPI use and the incident and recurrent CDI. This risk was further

Table 2 Distribution of cases and controls according to their demographic and clinical characteristics: results of univariate analysis

Variable	Case N° (%) n = 67	Controls N° (%) n = 134	p value
Male	32 (47.8)	64 (47.8)	1.00
Age			
≤ 40	2 (2.9)	5 (3.7)	0.786
41–64	32 (47.8)	58 (43.3)	0.547
≥ 65 years	33 (49.2)	71 (52.9)	0.618
Diabetes mellitus	10 (14.9)	15 (11.2)	0.451
Malignacy	14 (20.9)	22 (16.4)	0.436
Previous hospitalization	13 (19.4)	19 (14.1)	0.342
ICU admission	22 (32.8)	19 (14.1)	0.003
≥ 5 days in ICU	67 (100.0)	121 (90.3)	0.051
Nasogastric tube	5 (7.4)	1 (0.7)	0.032
Mechanical ventilation	4 (5.9)	0 (0.0)	0.032
Proton-pump inhibitors	13 (19.4)	8 (5.9)	0.005
H2 receptor antagonist	40 (59.7)	62 (46.2)	0.074
Corticosteroides	4 (5.9)	1 (0.7)	0.059
One antibiotic	32 (47.8)	85 (63.4)	0.035
Days of usage an antibiotic	5.13 ± 2.14	4.40 ± 2.27	0.120
Two antibiotics	20 (29.9)	27 (20.1)	0.128
Days of usage two antibiotics	5.85 ± 3.79	4.63 ± 2.13	0.167
Three antibiotics	9 (13.4)	5 (3.7)	0.017
Days of usage three antibiotics	7.89 ± 5.89	5.60 ± 2.07	0.423
Four antibiotics	4 (6.0)	2 (1.5)	0.103
Days of usage four antibiotics	8.75 ± 4.35	7.00 ± 2.83	0.642
Cephalosporins 1st gen.	15 (22.4)	33 (24.6)	0.726
Days of usage cephalosporins 1st gen.	1.15 ± 2.47	1.04 ± 2.16	0.742
Cephalosporins 2nd gen.	14 (20.9)	25 (18.7)	0.705
Days of usage cephalosporins 2nd gen.	1.18 ± 2.50	0.96 ± 2.25	0.537
Cephalosporins 3rd gen.	42 (62.7)	62 (46.3)	0.029
Days of usage cephalosporins 3rd gen.	4.39 ± 4.59	2.51 ± 3.25	0.001
Aminiglycosides	7 (10.4)	18 (13.4)	0.546
Days of usage Aminoglycosides	0.91 ± 3.58	0.66 ± 2.10	0.528
Quinolones	6 (8.9)	4 (3.0)	0.080
Days of usage Quinolones	0.52 ± 1.76	0.16 ± 0.94	0.056
Sulfonamides	3 (4.5)	5 (3.7)	0.799
Days of usage Sulfonamides	0.25 ± 1.26	0.15 ± 0.86	0.491
Carbapenems	6 (9.0)	2 (1.5)	0.024
Days of usage Carbapenems	0.62 ± 2.10	0.10 ± 0.85	0.014

increased by concomitant use of antibiotics and PPI, whereas H2RAs may be less harmful [18]. In our study, according to ULRA, both groups of patients received H2RAs (59.7% of cases and 46.2% controls) more frequently than PPIs (19.4% and 5.9%), but only PPIs significantly increased the risk of CDI without being a significant independent RF. Also, mice model demonstrated that PPIs administration can increase the severity of CDI induced by an antibiotic cocktail [19]. Medications that suppress gastric acid have been associated with the alteration of gastrointestinal flora and the increased susceptibility to gastrointestinal infections [20].

The mortality rate in patients with CDI in this study was 12.1% and significantly higher than in the control group. Also, it is higher than it was reported in Veterans Health Administration (12.1% vs 5.3%) [8]. This difference is explained by the different levels of healthcare and treatment of patients in hospitals in Serbia and the USA.

Of 8 deaths in the case group, 6 or 75% were in the older than 65. CDI was not the primary cause of death but it was mentioned in the clinical chart information. A systematic review of unfavorable outcomes of CDI (68 studies), based on publications from 1978 until 2013, showed that mortality was associated with age, co-morbidities, hypo-albuminemia, leucocytosis, acute renal failure, and infection with ribotype 027 [21].

Last data from a European, multicentre, prospective, biannual point-prevalence study of CDI showed that overall prevalence of ribotype 027 has risen more than three-fold (from 5% to 18%) and high endemicity of ribotype 027 has shifted from the UK and Ireland in 2008, to Germany and Eastern Europe in 2012–13 [6, 7]. The study of Rupnik et al. analyzed PCR ribotype distribution of 249 *C. difficile* isolates received for typing from six hospital settings from South Europe (the MMA was not included) in time period from 2008 to 2015 and showed that PCR ribotype 027 and related ribotype 176 were detected in outbreaks in Croatia, Bosnia and Herzegovina and Serbia [22]. Some PCR ribotypes are more often associated with severe diseases and/or are easily transmitted and linked to outbreaks. In our study we did not know if all those cases were from the outbreak because of the inability of laboratory pathogen isolation and the impossibility of determining its ribotype.

Important limitation of this study is that CDI testing was based on toxin A/B enzyme immunoassay (EIA) as the only diagnostic procedure in laboratory (no EIA detecting glutamate dehydrogenase, no nucleic acid amplification tests, no isolation of *C. difficile* and detection of toxigenic isolates). This procedure has shown poor sensitivity of less than 50% in studies of Shin [23] and Swindells [24]. The meta-analysis of Crobach et al. showed that no single test can be used as a stand-alone test for diagnosed CDI as a result of inadequate positive predictive values at low CDI prevalence [25]. *C. difficile* toxins can degrade at room temperature and the quality of CDI diagnostic also depends on transport time of the samples in the respective settings of the MMA. Both, the low rate of test performance in general and limitations of diagnostic test system, which we used, make it very likely that the actual incidence of CDI in our study was markedly higher.

Another limitation is the possibility of confounding variables that were not examined in our study. Although confounding variables were chosen after an exhaustive search of the literature, the potential for oversight and exclusion does exist. We tried to find all of the data in order to gain an understanding of the RF; we did not include some parameters, namely the diagnosis upon admission, all co-morbidities, durations of the hospital stays, PPIs exposure in previous 30 days, the duration of PPIs and H2RA use, and outpatient antibiotic use, and analyzing these factors could have enhanced the relevance of our results. Furthermore, we did not evaluate the CDI cases and the controls in relation to the sex, age and wards in which they had undergone treatment, because CDI cases and controls were matched according to them.

Another limitation is that we performed case–control study and that we have small sample size.

The strengths of our study include its setting in a teaching hospital, and its 2-year duration. ULRA and MLRA strengthened the evidence.

Conclusions

The results of the present study are valuable in documenting the relations between RFs and CDI in patients undergoing surgery and contribute to improve quality of health care. CDI is an important HA infection in population of surgical patients and this study emphasizes the importance of the wise use of antibiotics, and other infection control strategies to prevent HA CDI, decrease incidence and in- hospital mortality rate.

Abbreviations

C.difficile: *Clostridium difficile*; CDI: *Clostridium difficile* infection; CI: Confidence intervals; H2RAs: Histamine-2-receptor antagonists; HA: Healthcare-associated; ICU: Intensive care unit; IR: Incidence rate; MLRA: Multivariate logistic regression analysis; MMA: Military Medical Academy; PPIS: Proton-pump inhibitors; RF: Risk factors; TR: Testing rate

Acknowledgments
Not applicable.

Funding
This study was supported by internal funding of the Military Medical Academy.

Authors' contributions
ŠV, ŠGS, KZ participated in design of study. MI, SS, SN, BRJ took part in acquisition of data. JD carried out the enzyme immunoassay for *C. difficile* toxins A and B. MB and ŠGS performed the statistical analysis. ŠV coordination and helped to draft the manuscript. All authors read and approved the final manuscript.

Competing interests
The authors declare that they have no competing interests.

Consent for publication
Not applicable.

Author details
[1]Department of Nosocomial Infections Control, Military Medical Academy, 11 000 Belgrade, Serbia. [2]Faculty of Medicine of Military Medical Academy University of Defence, 11000 Belgrade, Serbia. [3]Institute of Epidemiology, Military Medical Academy, 11 000 Belgrade, Serbia. [4]Clinic for Orthopedic Surgery and Traumatology, Military Medical Academy, 11 000 Belgrade, Serbia. [5]Clinic for Plastic Surgery and Burns, Military Medical Academy, 11 000 Belgrade, Serbia. [6]Clinic for General Surgery, Military Medical Academy, 11 000 Belgrade, Serbia. [7]Institute of Microbiology Military Medical Academy, 11 000 Belgrade, Serbia. [8]Sector for Pharmacy, Military Medical Academy, 11 000 Belgrade, Serbia. [9]Faculty of Medicine, University of East Sarajevo, 73300 Foča, Republic of Srpska, Bosnia and Herzegovina. [10]Institute of Epidemiology, Faculty of Medicine, University of Belgrade, 11000 Belgrade, Serbia.

References
1. Freeman J, Bauer MP, Baines SD, Corver J, Fawley WN, Goorhuis B, et al. The changing epidemiology of Clostridium difficile infections. Clin Microbiol Rev. 2010;23:529–49.
2. Magee G, Strauss ME, Thomas SM, Brown H, Baumer D, Broderick KC. Impact of Clostridium difficile-associated diarrhea on acute care length of stay, hospital costs, and readmission: A multicenter retrospective study of inpatients, 2009–2011. Am J Infect Control. 2015;43(11):1148–53.
3. Stojanović P. Analysis of risk factors and clinical manifestations associated with Clostridium difficile disease in Serbian hospitalized patients. Braz J Microbiol. 2016;47(4):902–10.
4. Cho SM, Lee JJ, Yoon HJ. Clinical risk factors for Clostridium difficile-associated diseases. Braz J Infect Dis. 2012;16:256–61.
5. Lessa FC, Mu Y, Bamberg WM, Beldavs ZG, Dumyati GK, Dunn JR, et al. Burden of Clostridium difficile infection in the United States. N Engl J Med. 2015;372:825–34.
6. Davies KA, Longshaw CM, Davis GL, Bouza E, Barbut F, Barna Z, et al. Underdiagnosis of Clostridium difficile across Europe: the European, multicentre, prospective, biannual, point-prevalence study of Clostridium difficile infection in hospitalised patients with diarrhoea (EUCLID). Lancet Infect Dis. 2014;14:1208–19.
7. Bauer MP, Notermans DW, van Benthem BH, Brazier JS, Wilcox MH, Rupnik M, ECDIS Study Group, et al. Clostridium difficile infectioninEurope: a hospital-based survey. Lancet. 2011;377:63–73.
8. Li X, Wilson M, Nylander W, Smith T, Lynn M, Gunnar W. Analysis of Morbidity and Mortality Outcomes in Postoperative Clostridium difficile Infection in the Veterans Health Administration. JAMA Surg. 2015;25:1–9.
9. Rodrigues MA, Brady RR, Rodrigues J, Graham C, Gibb AP. Clostridium difficile infection in general surgery patients; identification of high-risk populations. Int J Surg. 2010;8:368–72.
10. Abdelsattar ZM, Krapohl G, Alrahmani L, Banerjee M, Krell RW, Wong SL, et al. Postoperative Burden of Hospital-Acquired Clostridium difficile Infection. Infect Control Hosp Epidemiol. 2015;36:40–6.
11. Šuljagić V, Đorđević D, Lazić S, Mijović B. Epidemiological characteristics of nosocomial diarrhea caused by *Clostridium difficile* in a tertiary level hospital in Serbia. Srp Arh Celok Lek. 2013;141:482–9.
12. Skovrlj B, Guzman JZ, Silvestre J, Al Maaieh M, Quereshi SA. *Clostridium difficile* colitis in patients undergoing lumbar spine surgery. Spine. 2014;39:E1167–1173.

13. Jump RL. Clostridium difficile infection in older adults. Aging health. 2013;9(4):403–14.

14. Pépin J, Saheb N, Coulombe MA, Alary ME, Corriveau MP, Authier S, et al. Emergence of fluoroquinolones as the predominant risk factor for Clostridium difficile–associated diarrhea: a cohort study during an epidemic in Quebec. Clin Infect Dis. 2005;41(9):1254–60.

15. Dingle KE, Didelot X, Quan TP, Eyre DW, Stoesser N, Golubchik T, et al. Effects of control interventions on Clostridium difficile infection in England: an observational study. Lancet Infectious Diseases. 2017

16. Metzger R, Swenson BR, Bonatti H, Hedrick TL, Hranjec T, Popovsky KA, et al. Identification of risk factors for the development of Clostridium difficile-associated diarrhea following treatment of polymicrobial surgical infections. Ann Surg. 2010;251(4):722–7.

17. Riddle DJ, Dubberke ER. Clostridium difficile infection in the intensive care unit. Infect Dis Clin North Am. 2009;23(3):727–43.

18. Kwok CS, Arthur AK, Anibueze CI, Singh S, Cavallazzi R, Loke YK. Risk of Clostridium difficile infection with acid suppressing drugs and antibiotics: meta-analysis. Am J Gastroenterol. 2012;107:1011–9.

19. Hung YP, Ko WC, Chou PH, Chen YH, Lin HJ, Liu YH, et al. Proton pump inhibitor exposure aggravates *Clostridium difficile* associated colitis: evidences from a mouse model. J Infect Dis. 2015;212:654–63.

20. Williams C. Occurrence and significance of gastric colonization during acid-inhibitory therapy. Best Pract Res Clin Gastroenterol. 2001;15(3):511–21.

21. Chakra CN, Pepin J, Sirard S, Valiquette L. Risk factors for recurrence, complications and mortality in Clostridium difficile infection: a systematic review. PLoS One. 2014;9(6):e98400.

22. Rupnik M, Andrasevic AT, Dokic ET, Matas I, Jovanovic M, Pasic S, et al. Distribution of Clostridium difficile PCR ribotypes and high proportion of 027 and 176 in some hospitals in four South Eastern European countries. Anaerobe. 2016;42:142–4.

23. Shin S, Kim M, Kim M, Lim H, Kim H, Lee K, et al. Evaluation of the Xpert Clostridium difficile assay for the diagnosis of Clostridium difficile infection. Ann Lab Med. 2012;32:355e8.

24. Swindells J, Brenwald N, Reading N, Oppenheim B. Evaluation of diagnostic tests for Clostridium difficile infection. J Clin Microbiol. 2010;48:606e8.

25. Crobach MJ, Planche T, Eckert C, Barbut F, Terveer EM, Dekkers OM, Wilcox MH, Kuijper EJ. European Society of Clinical Microbiology and Infectious Diseases: update of the diagnostic guidance document for Clostridium difficile infection. Clin Microbiol Infect. 2016;22:S63–81.

17

The Tigecycline Evaluation and Surveillance Trial; assessment of the activity of tigecycline and other selected antibiotics against Gram-positive and Gram-negative pathogens from France collected between 2004 and 2016

Jean-Winoc Decousser[1*], Paul-Louis Woerther[1], Claude-James Soussy[1], Marguerite Fines-Guyon[2] and Michael J. Dowzicky[3]

Abstract

Background: A high level of antibiotic consumption in France means antimicrobial resistance requires rigorous monitoring. The Tigecycline Evaluation and Surveillance Trial (T.E.S.T.) is a global surveillance study that monitors the *in vitro* activities of tigecycline and a panel of marketed antimicrobials against clinically important Gram-positive and Gram-negative isolates.

Methods: Annually clinically relevant strains were prospectively included in the survey through a national network of hospital-based laboratories. MICs were determined locally by broth microdilution using CLSI guidelines. Antimicrobial susceptibility was assessed using European Committee on Antimicrobial Susceptibility Testing breakpoints.

Results: Thirty-three centres in France collected 26,486 isolates between 2004 and 2016. *Enterococcus* species were highly susceptible (≥94.4%) to linezolid, tigecycline and vancomycin. *Staphylococcus aureus*, including methicillin-resistant *S. aureus* (MRSA), were susceptible (≥99.9%) to tigecycline, vancomycin and linezolid. Between 2004 and 2016, 27.7% of *S. aureus* isolates were MRSA, decreasing from 28.0% in 2013 to 23.5% in 2016. Susceptibility of *Streptococcus pneumoniae* isolates was 100% to vancomycin, and > 99.0% to levofloxacin, linezolid and meropenem; 3.0% were penicillin-resistant *S. pneumoniae* (100% susceptibility to vancomycin and linezolid). *Escherichia coli* isolates were highly susceptible (> 98.0%) to meropenem, tigecycline and amikacin. The rate of extended-spectrum β-lactamase (ESBL) positive *E. coli* increased from 2004 (3.0%), but was stable from 2012 (23.1%) to 2016 (19.8%). Susceptibility of *Klebsiella pneumoniae* isolates was 99.4% to meropenem and 96.5% to amikacin. The proportion of ESBL-positive *K. pneumoniae* isolates increased from 2004 (7.5%) to 2012 (33.3%) and was highest in 2016 (43.6%). *A. baumannii* was susceptible to meropenem (81.0%) and amikacin (74.9%); none of the 6.2% of isolates identified as multidrug-resistant (MDR) was susceptible to any agents with breakpoints. *P. aeruginosa* isolates were most susceptible to amikacin (88.5%), and MDR rates were 13.6% in 2013 to 4.0% in 2016; susceptibility of MDR isolates was no higher than 31.4% to amikacin.

(Continued on next page)

* Correspondence: jean-winoc.decousser@aphp.fr
[1]University Hospital Henri Mondor, 9400 Creteil, France

(Continued from previous page)

Conclusions: Rates of MRSA decreased slowly, while rates of ESBL-positive *E. coli* and *K. pneumoniae* increased from 2004 to 2016. Susceptibility of Gram-positive isolates to vancomycin, tigecycline, meropenem and linezolid was well conserved, as was susceptibility of Gram-negative isolates to tigecycline and meropenem. The spread of MDR non-fermentative isolates must be carefully monitored.

Keywords: France, Gram-positive, Gram-negative, Multidrug-resistance, Antimicrobial surveillance, Tigecycline

Background

Despite significant efforts to reduce antibiotic use, France has one of the highest rates of antimicrobial consumption in the community in Europe [1], and has seen considerable changes in trends of antibacterial resistance during recent years [2–5]. In France, resistance to antibiotics has been monitored since 2002 by the French national healthcare-associated infection early warning, investigation and surveillance network (RAISIN), which recently reported a 182% increase in the prevalence of extended-spectrum β-lactamase (ESBL)-producing Enterobacteriaceae during nine years [2]. Extensively drug-resistant bacteria such as vancomycin-resistant enterococci (VRE) and carbapenemase-producing Enterobacteriaceae (CPE) are not endemic in France, although VRE are disseminated in neighbouring countries such as Italy and Germany, and CPE are considered endemic in Italy [6, 7]. Methicillin-resistant *Staphylococcus aureus* (MRSA) rates in France have been considered to be decreasing during the decade from 2000 to 2010 and in subsequent years [3, 8, 9], and this is consistent with reduced MRSA rates reported in Germany since 2007 [3, 10–12] and from 2010 in the UK [3, 13]. The situation regarding antimicrobial resistance in France requires rigorous monitoring, particularly for second-line antimicrobial compounds and clinically relevant bacterial species. To meet the challenge presented by antimicrobial resistance, authorities in France have developed a number of national initiatives that include antibiotic stewardship in hospitals and surveillance of antibiotic use [14].

The broad-spectrum antimicrobial agent tigecycline is indicated for the treatment of complicated skin and soft tissue infections (cSSTIs), excluding diabetic foot infections, and complicated intra-abdominal infections (cIAIs), and, in the USA, community-acquired bacterial pneumonia [15, 16]. The Tigecycline Evaluation and Surveillance Trial (T.E.S.T.) was instigated in 2004 with the intention of global surveillance of antimicrobial activity of tigecycline and a panel of other antimicrobial agents against an array of clinically important Gram-positive and Gram-negative pathogens. In this study, we report an update to that provided by Cattoir and Dowzicky [17] regarding the *in vitro* susceptibility to tigecycline and comparators of isolates collected from community or hospitalized patients in France between 2004 and 2016.

Methods

Materials and methods for isolates collected as part of the T.E.S.T. study in France have been published previously [17], with minimum inhibitory concentrations (MICs) determined locally according to the broth microdilution method described by the Clinical and Laboratory Standards Institute (CLSI) [18, 19].

Isolates were collected if considered to be of clinical significance as the probable causative agent of a hospital- or community-acquired infection. Isolates were accepted from all body sites, including the following sources: samples of body fluids (classified as abdominal, ascites, bile, paracentesis, peritoneal), central nervous system, cardiovascular system, gastrointestinal (GI) sources (abscess, appendix, diverticulum, oesophagus, faeces/stool, gall bladder, large colon, liver, pancreas, rectum, small colon, stomach, general GI or other GI), genito-urinary, head, ears, eyes, nose and throat, integument, lymph, muscular, reproductive, respiratory, skeletal or medical instruments (i.e. catheters, drains, forceps, probes). Duplicate isolates from a single patient were not accepted.

Coordination of isolate collection and transport was carried out by International Health Management Associates (IHMA), Schaumburg, IL, USA. The panel of antimicrobial agents for the T.E.S.T. study included an aminoglycoside (amikacin), agents in the penicillin class (ampicillin, amoxicillin-clavulanate, penicillin, piperacillin-tazobactam), cephalosporins (cefepime, ceftazidime, ceftriaxone) a carbapenem (imipenem), a fluoroquinolone (levofloxacin), an oxazolidinone (linezolid), a tetracycline (minocycline), a glycylcycline (tigecycline) and a glycopeptide (vancomycin). In 2006, meropenem replaced imipenem due to stability issues associated with imipenem testing, and the *S. pneumoniae* test panel was expanded to include three macrolides (azithromycin, clarithromycin, erythromycin) and a lincosamide (clindamycin), with isolates tested retrospectively for susceptibility to these agents wherever possible. Antimicrobial susceptibility of aerobic isolates was performed using the breakpoints established by the European Committee on Antimicrobial Susceptibility Testing (EUCAST) [20]. Susceptibility data are included in the tables only when interpretive breakpoints are available. Methicillin resistance in *S. aureus* and ESBL-production among *E. coli* and *Klebsiella* spp. were determined by IHMA according to CLSI guidelines [19]. As specified in a previous T.E.S.T. study [21], isolates that were resistant to three or more classes of antimicrobial agents were defined as multidrug-resistant (MDR). Classes used to define MDR *A. baumannii* were aminoglycosides (amikacin), β-lactams (cefepime, ceftazidime, ceftriaxone or piperacillin-tazobactam), carbapenems (imipenem/meropenem), fluoroquinolones (levofloxacin) and tetracyclines (minocycline), and the classes used to define MDR *P. aeruginosa* were aminoglycosides (amikacin), β-lactams (cefepime, ceftazidime, or piperacillin-tazobactam), carbapenems (imipenem/meropenem), and fluoroquinolones (levofloxacin) [21].

The Cochran Armitage Trend Test was used to identify statistically significant changes in susceptibility between 2004 and 2016, and results with a p-value of < 0.01 were deemed significant.

Results

A total of 26,486 isolates were collected from 33 centres in France between 2004 and 2016 (eight in 2004, six in 2005, 12 in 2006, 16 in 2007, 21 in 2008, 20 in 2009, 16 in 2010 and 2011, 14 in 2012, 12 in 2013 and 2014, 11 in 2015 and four in 2016).

Gram-positives
Enterococcus spp

All isolates of *E. faecalis* ($N = 1429$) were highly susceptible (≥98.4%) to ampicillin, linezolid, tigecycline and vancomycin (Table 1). All isolates of VRE *E. faecalis* ($N = 11$, 0.8%) were susceptible to tigecycline and 90.9% were susceptible to linezolid. Between 2004 and 2016, 537 isolates of *E. faecium* were collected, which included 410 (76.4%) ampicillin-resistant isolates. All isolates were highly susceptible to tigecycline (100%), linezolid (99.8%) and vancomycin (94.4%) (Table 1). Thirty *E. faecium* isolates (5.6%) were identified as VRE, which were 100% susceptible to linezolid and tigecycline.

S. aureus

All *S. aureus* isolates ($N = 3437$) were susceptible to tigecycline and vancomycin (Table 1). Susceptibility to linezolid was > 99.9%, to minocycline 95.0% and to levofloxacin 73.2%. The proportion of isolates identified as MRSA ($N = 953$) between 2004 to 2016 was 27.7% (range, 18.3–34.3%) and during the period 2013 to 2016 decreased from 28.0 to 23.5% (Table 2). All MRSA isolates were susceptible to linezolid, tigecycline and vancomycin (Table 1), and susceptibility to minocycline was 94.2%. The susceptibility of MRSA isolates collected between 2004 and 2016 to levofloxacin was relatively low, at 16.7%. A vancomycin MIC of > 1 mg/L was observed in 35 (3.7%) of the MRSA isolates, and of these, 2.9% were susceptible to levofloxacin, and 74.3% to minocycline. MRSA isolates that exhibited a vancomycin

MIC that was ≤1 mg/L ($N = 918$) exhibited susceptibility of 17.2% to levofloxacin and 95.0% to minocycline.

S. agalactiae
Susceptibility of *S. agalactiae* isolates ($N = 1348$) was 100% to linezolid, penicillin and vancomycin; isolates were also highly susceptible to tigecycline (99.8%), and to levofloxacin (99.1%).

S. pneumoniae
A total of 1684 isolates of *S. pneumoniae* were collected during the study, and all were susceptible to vancomycin, with > 99.6% of isolates susceptible to levofloxacin, linezolid and meropenem ($N = 1557$ for meropenem). Tigecycline exhibited an *in vitro* MIC_{90} value of 0.06 mg/L against *S. pneumoniae* isolates, and during the study there was a statistically significant increase ($p < 0.0001$) in susceptibility to azithromycin (2004, 50.0%; 2016, 76.2%), clarithromycin (2004, 50.0%; 2016, 78.6%), clindamycin (2004, 52.3%; 2016, 83.3%) and erythromycin (2004, 50.0%; 2016, 78.6%), and also to minocycline ($p < 0.01$; 2004, 52.7%; 2016, 78.6%). A total of 51 (3.0%) penicillin-resistant *S. pneumoniae* isolates were collected between 2004 to 2016 and all of these were susceptible to vancomycin and linezolid. Rates of penicillin-resistant *S. pneumoniae* susceptibility to levofloxacin (98.0%) and meropenem (94.1%) were relatively high and stable; the MIC_{90} of tigecycline was 0.03 mg/L. Penicillin-resistant *S. pneumoniae* isolates collected between 2013 and 2016 and tested for susceptibility to erythromycin ($N = 13$) and minocycline ($N = 14$) showed susceptibility rates of 38.5 and 21.4%, respectively, which were lower compared with all *S. pneumoniae* isolates that were collected during the same period and tested against erythromycin ($N = 473$, 66.4% susceptibility) and minocycline ($N = 496$, 61.7% susceptibility).

Gram-negatives
Enterobacter spp
The agent with the lowest *in vitro* MIC_{90} value against *Enterobacter* spp. isolates ($N = 3424$) was meropenem (MIC_{90} 0.25 mg/L), to which 99.2% of isolates were susceptible (Table 3). Susceptibility to amikacin (96.9%) and tigecycline (86.3%) was stable, and susceptibility to levofloxacin was 71.5%. A lower proportion of isolates were susceptible to the cephalosporins on the T.E.S.T. panel, cefepime (69.5%) and ceftriaxone (50.9%).

E. coli
Isolates of *E. coli* ($N = 3527$) were highly susceptible to meropenem (99.9%), tigecycline (99.4%) and amikacin (98.1%) (Table 3). The susceptibility of *E. coli* isolates to piperacillin-tazobactam (89.6%) was

Table 1 Minimum inhibitory concentrations (MIC$_{90}$, MIC range [mg/L]) and antimicrobial susceptibility (%S) and resistance (%R) of Gram-positive isolates

Organism/ Antimicrobial	2004–2016				2013–2016			
	MIC$_{90}$ (mg/L)	MIC Range (mg/L)	% S	% R	MIC$_{90}$ (mg/L)	MIC Range (mg/L)	% S	% R
E. faecalis	N = 1429				N = 373			
Ampicillin[a]	2	≤0.06 to ≥32	98.4	1.0	1	≤0.06 to ≥32	97.1	2.1
Linezolid	2	≤0.5 to ≥16	99.9	0.1	2	≤0.5 to ≥16	99.7	0.3
Tigecycline	0.25	≤0.008 to 0.5	99.9	0.0	0.12	0.03 to 0.25	100	0.0
Vancomycin	2	0.25 to ≥64	99.2	0.8	2	0.25 to ≥64	99.2	0.8
E. faecalis, VRE	N = 11				N = 3			
Amox-clav	≥16	0.25 to ≥16	81.8	18.2	≥16	0.5 to ≥16	[1]	[2]
Ampicillin	≥32	0.5 to ≥32	81.8	18.2	≥32	1 to ≥32	[1]	[2]
Linezolid	2	1 to ≥16	90.9	9.1	≥16	1 to ≥16	[2]	[1]
Tigecycline	0.25	0.06 to 0.25	100	0.0	0.25	0.06 to 0.25	[3]	[0]
E. faecium	N = 537				N = 159			
Linezolid	2	≤0.5 to 8	99.8	0.2	2	≤0.5 to 8	99.4	0.6
Tigecycline	0.25	0.015 to 0.25	100	0.0	0.12	0.015 to 0.25	100	0.0
Vancomycin	2	0.25 to ≥64	94.4	5.6	1	0.25 to ≥64	98.1	1.9
E. faecium, VRE	N = 30				N = 3			
Linezolid	2	1 to 2	100	0.0	2	1 to 2	[3]	[0]
Tigecycline	0.25	0.03 to 0.25	100	0.0	0.25	0.06 to 0.25	[3]	[0]
S. aureus	N = 3437				N = 947			
Levofloxacin[b]	32	≤0.06 to ≥64	73.2	26.8	16	≤0.06 to ≥64	76.7	23.3
Linezolid	2	≤0.5 to 8	> 99.9	< 0.1	2	≤0.5 to 8	99.9	0.1
Minocycline[b]	0.5	≤0.25 to ≥16	95.0	3.0	≤0.25	≤0.25 to ≥16	97.5	2.1
Penicillin	≥16	≤0.06 to ≥16	15.0	85.0	≥16	≤0.06 to ≥16	16.6	83.4
Tigecycline	0.25	≤0.008 to 0.5	100	0.0	0.12	0.015 to 0.5	100	0.0
Vancomycin	1	≤0.12 to 2	100	0.0	1	0.25 to 2	100	0.0
S. aureus, MRSA	N = 953				N = 234			
Levofloxacin[b]	≥64	≤0.06 to ≥64	16.7	83.3	32	0.12 to ≥64	17.5	82.5
Linezolid	2	≤0.5 to 4	100	0.0	4	≤0.5 to 4	100	0.0
Minocycline[b]	0.5	≤0.25 to ≥16	94.2	4.6	≤0.25	≤0.25 to 8	95.3	3.8
Penicillin	≥16	0.5 to ≥16	0.0	100	≥16	0.25 to ≥16	0.0	100
Tigecycline	0.25	0.015 to 0.25	100	0.0	0.25	0.015 to 0.5	100	0.0
Vancomycin	1	≤0.12 to 2	100	0.0	1	0.25 to 2	100	0.0
S. agalactiae	N = 1348				N = 378			
Levofloxacin	1	≤0.06 to 32	99.1	0.9	1	0.12 to 32	97.9	2.1
Linezolid	1	≤0.5 to 2	100	0.0	1	≤0.5 to 2	100	0.0
Minocycline	≥16	≤0.25 to ≥16	16.1	82.0	≥16	≤0.25 to ≥16	15.6	83.1
Penicillin	0.12	≤0.06 to 0.12	100	0.0	0.12	≤0.06 to 0.12	100	0.0
Tigecycline	0.12	0.015 to 4	99.8	0.1	0.12	0.015 to 4	99.7	0.3
Vancomycin	0.5	≤0.12 to 1	100	0.0	0.5	≤0.12 to 1	100	0.0
S. pneumoniae	N = 1684 (AZM, CLR, CLI, ERY, N = 1500)				N = 496 (AZM, CLR, CLI, ERY, N = 473)			
Azithromycin[b]	≥128	≤0.03 to ≥128	60.5	39.1	≥128	≤0.03 to ≥128	65.8	33.8
Ceftriaxone	1	≤0.03 to 16	80.8	0.5	1	≤0.03 to 2	84.7	0.0
Clarithromycin[b]	≥128	≤0.015 to ≥128	60.9	38.5	≥128	≤0.015 to ≥128	66.4	32.6

Table 1 Minimum inhibitory concentrations (MIC$_{90}$, MIC range [mg/L]) and antimicrobial susceptibility (%S) and resistance (%R) of Gram-positive isolates *(Continued)*

Organism/ Antimicrobial	2004–2016				2013–2016			
	MIC$_{90}$ (mg/L)	MIC Range (mg/L)	% S	% R	MIC$_{90}$ (mg/L)	MIC Range (mg/L)	% S	% R
Clindamycin[b]	≥128	≤0.015 to ≥128	68.5	31.5	≥128	≤0.015 to ≥128	71.9	28.1
Erythromycin[b]	≥128	≤0.015 to ≥128	60.6	38.7	≥128	≤0.015 to ≥128	66.4	33.2
Levofloxacin	1	≤0.06 to ≥64	99.7	0.3	1	≤0.06 to 2	100	0.0
Linezolid	1	≤0.5 to 4	99.9	0.0	1	≤0.5 to 2	100	0.0
Meropenem (N = 1557) [c]	0.5	≤0.12 to ≥32	99.8	0.2	1	≤0.12 to 8	99.8	0.2
Minocycline[b] (*N* = 1683)	8	≤0.25 to ≥16	52.4	38.6	8	≤0.25 to ≥16	61.7	31.9
Penicillin	2	≤0.06 to ≥16	53.0	3.0	2	≤0.06 to 8	53.4	2.8
Tigecycline	0.06	≤0.008 to 0.5	–	–	0.03	≤0.008 to 0.06	–	–
Vancomycin	0.5	≤0.12 to 1	100	0.0	0.5	≤0.12 to 1	100	0.0
S. pneumoniae, PRSP	*N* = 51 (AZM, CLR, CLI, ERY, N = 48)				*N* = 14 (AZM, CLR, CLI, ERY, N = 14)			
Azithromycin	≥128	≤0.03 to ≥128	22.9	77.1	≥128	0.06 to ≥128	38.5	61.5
Ceftriaxone	2	≤0.03 to 8	9.8	9.8	2	≤0.03 to 2	21.4	0
Clarithromycin	≥128	≤0.015 to ≥128	22.9	77.1	≥128	≤0.015 to ≥128	38.5	61.5
Clindamycin	≥128	≤0.015 to ≥128	37.5	62.5	≥128	0.03 to ≥128	46.2	53.8
Erythromycin	≥128	≤0.015 to ≥128	22.9	75.0	≥128	0.03 to ≥128	38.5	61.5
Levofloxacin	1	0.25 to 16	98.0	2.0	1	0.5 to 1	100	0.0
Linezolid	1	≤0.5 to 2	100	0.0	1	≤0.5 to 2	100	0.0
Meropenem[c]	2	≤0.12 to ≥32	94.1	5.9	2	≤0.12 to 8	92.9	7.1
Minocycline	≥16	≤0.25 to ≥16	19.6	70.6	8	≤0.25 to ≥16	21.4	64.3
Tigecycline	0.03	0.015 to 0.12	–	–	0.03	0.015 to 0.03	–	–
Vancomycin	0.5	0.25 to 1	100	0.0	0.5	025 to 1	100	0.0

[a] indicates statistically significant decrease in susceptibility (*p* < 0.01) from 2004 to 2016
[b] indicates statistically significant increase in susceptibility (*p* < 0.01) from 2004 to 2016
[c] Meropenem was introduced to the testing panel in 2006, replacing imipenem; N values of activity against organisms collected from 2006 to 2016 are given
Amox-clav, amoxicillin-clavulanic acid, *AZM*, azithromycin, *CLR*, clarithromycin, *CLI*, clindamycin, *ERY*, erythromycin, *MIC*, minimum inhibitory concentration, *MIC$_{90}$*, minimum inhibitory concentration required to inhibit growth of 90% of isolates (mg/L), *MRSA*, methicillin-resistant *S. aureus*, *Pip-taz*, piperacillin-tazobactam, *PRSP*, Penicillin-resistant *S. pneumoniae*, *R*, resistant, *S*, susceptible, *VRE*, vancomycin-resistant enterococci

relatively stable, but there was a decline in susceptibility to levofloxacin (92.1% in 2004 to 76.2% in 2016) and statistically significant declines in susceptibility to cefepime (97.0% in 2004 to 77.2% in 2016; *p* < 0.0001) and ceftriaxone (96.0% in 2004 to 78.2% in 2016; *p* < 0.0001).

The proportion of *E. coli* isolates identified as ESBL-positive *E. coli* between 2004 and 2016 (*N* = 489) was 13.9%. This is lower than the annual rates between 2013 (14.9%) and 2016 (19.8%), although these were stable (Table 2). Susceptibility of all ESBL-positive *E. coli* isolates was 99.2% to tigecycline, 92.6% to amikacin, and 100% to meropenem for the 472 isolates tested from 2006 onwards. Susceptibility of ESBL-positive *E. coli* to piperacillin-tazobactam (78.3%) was lower compared with all isolates of *E. coli* (89.6%), and only 37.8% of ESBL-positive *E. coli* isolates were susceptible to levofloxacin and 45.8% to amoxicillin-clavulanate; no isolates were susceptible to ceftriaxone and 3.9% were susceptible to cefepime.

Table 2 Percentages of resistant phenotypes among Gram-positive and Gram-negative isolates by year, 2013—2016

	E. coli ESBL-positive		*K. pneumoniae* ESBL-positive		*H. influenzae* BL positive		*P. aeruginosa* MDR		*A. baumannii* MDR		MRSA	
	n	%	n	%	n	%	n	%	n	%	n	%
2013	46	14.9	75	36.1	39	25.3	33	13.6	11	12.2	84	28.0
2014	43	15.6	85	40.7	27	18.9	21	9.8	10	13.5	76	27.9
2015	47	16.8	71	36.4	36	25.7	11	5.3	7	9.1	50	18.3
2016	20	19.8	34	43.6	20	35.1	3	4.0	7	24.1	24	23.5

BL, β-lactamase, *ESBL*, extended-spectrum β-lactamase, *MDR*, multidrug-resistant, *MRSA*, methicillin-resistant *S. aureus*

Table 3 Minimum inhibitory concentrations (MIC$_{90}$, MIC range [mg/L]) and antimicrobial susceptibility (%S) and resistance (%R) of Gram-negative isolates

Organism/ Antimicrobial	2004–2016				2013–2016			
	MIC$_{90}$ (mg/L)	MIC Range (mg/L)	% S	% R	MIC$_{90}$ (mg/L)	MIC Range (mg/L)	% S	% R
Enterobacter spp.	N = 3424				N = 924			
Amikacin	4	≤0.5 to ≥128	96.9	1.1	4	≤0.5 to ≥128	98.4	0.8
Cefepime[a]	16	≤0.5 to ≥64	69.5	15.8	32	≤0.5 to ≥64	67.1	19.8
Ceftriaxone	64	≤0.06 to ≥128	50.9	45.6	64	≤0.06 to 64	49.1	47.3
Levofloxacin[c]	≤16	≤0.008 to ≥16	71.5	25.0	8	≤0.008 to ≥16	75.8	19.7
Meropenem (N = 3113)[b]	0.25	≤0.06 to ≥32	99.2	0.3	0.25	≤0.06 to ≥32	99.4	0.2
Minocycline	16	≤0.5 to ≥32	–	–	8	≤0.5 to ≥32	–	–
Pip-taz[c]	128	≤0.06 to ≥256	60.7	30.5	128	≤0.06 to ≥256	64.7	25.6
Tigecycline	2	0.06 to 16	86.3	5.2	2	0.06 to 16	89.5	3.5
E. coli	N = 3527				N = 965			
Amikacin	4	≤0.5 to ≥128	98.1	0.5	4	≤0.5 to ≥128	98.4	0.2
Amox-clav	32	0.25 to ≥64	72.1	27.9	16	0.5 to ≥64	75.1	24.9
Ampicillin	≥64	≤0.5 to 64	37.9	62.1	≥64	≤0.5 to 64	38.5	61.5
Cefepime[a]	8	≤0.5 to ≥64	82.5	12.4	16	≤0.5 to ≥64	80.7	13.8
Ceftriaxone[a]	64	≤0.06 to ≥128	82.6	16.8	64	≤0.06 to 64	81.3	18.4
Levofloxacin	≥16	≤0.008 to ≥16	78.5	20.2	8	≤0.008 to ≥16	79.6	19.4
Meropenem (N = 3203)[b]	≤0.06	≤0.06 to 8	99.9	0.0	≤0.06	≤0.06 to 8	99.9	0.0
Minocycline	8	≤0.5 to ≥32	–	–	8	≤0.5 to ≥32	–	–
Pip-taz	16	≤0.06 to ≥256	89.6	7.2	8	≤0.06 to ≥256	91.6	6.2
Tigecycline	0.5	≤0.008 to 16	99.4	0.1	0.25	0.03 to 16	99.5	0.1
E. coli, ESBL	N = 489				N = 156			
Amikacin	8	≤0.5 to ≥128	92.6	2.2	8	1 to ≥128	95.5	0.6
Amox-clav[c]	32	2 to ≥64	45.8	54.2	16	2 to ≥64	59.0	41.0
Ampicillin	≥64	32 to ≥64	0.0	100	≥64	64 to ≥64	0.0	100
Cefepime	≥64	≤0.5 to ≥64	3.9	78.3	≥64	1 to ≥64	3.2	79.5
Ceftriaxone	≥128	2 to ≥128	0.0	99.2	64	4 to 64	0.0	100
Levofloxacin	≥16	≤0.008 to ≥16	37.8	59.7	≥16	0.015 to ≥16	42.3	55.1
Meropenem (N = 472)[b]	≤0.06	≤0.06 to 2	100	0.0	≤0.06	≤0.06 to 1	100	0.0
Minocycline	16	≤0.5 to ≥32	–	–	16	≤0.5 to ≥32	–	–
Pip-taz[c]	32	0.25 to ≥256	78.3	12.7	16	0.25 to ≥256	88.5	3.8
Tigecycline	0.5	0.03 to 2	99.2	0.0	0.25	0.03 to 2	99.4	0.0
H. influenzae	N = 1786				N = 494			
Amikacin	8	≤0.5 to 64	–	–	8	≤0.5 to 16	–	–
Amox-clav	1	≤0.12 to 16	99.2	0.8	1	≤0.12 to 4	99.0	1.0
Ampicillin	32	≤0.5 to ≥64	75.4	24.6	32	≤0.5 to ≥64	74.1	25.9
Cefepime	≤0.5	≤0.5 to 2	–	–	≤0.5	≤0.5 to 2	–	–
Ceftriaxone	≤0.06	≤0.06 to 4	98.6	1.4	≤0.06	≤0.06 to 2	99.4	0.4
Levofloxacin	0.015	≤0.008 to 8	98.4	1.6	0.015	≤0.008 to 8	98.6	1.4
Meropenem (N = 1629)[b]	0.12	≤0.06 to 0.5	100	0.0	0.12	≤0.06 to 0.5	100	0.0
Minocycline	1	≤0.5 to 16	91.8	1.6	1	≤0.5 to 4	93.1	0.8
Pip-taz	≤0.06	≤0.06 to 0.5	–	–	≤0.06	≤0.06 to 0.5	–	–
Tigecycline	0.25	≤0.008 to 4	–	–	0.25	≤0.008 to 0.25	–	–

Table 3 Minimum inhibitory concentrations (MIC$_{90}$, MIC range [mg/L]) and antimicrobial susceptibility (%S) and resistance (%R) of Gram-negative isolates *(Continued)*

Organism/ Antimicrobial	2004–2016				2013–2016			
	MIC$_{90}$ (mg/L)	MIC Range (mg/L)	% S	% R	MIC$_{90}$ (mg/L)	MIC Range (mg/L)	% S	% R
H. influenzae, BL Positive	N = 410				N = 122			
Amikacin	8	≤0.5 to 32	–	–	8	≤0.5 to 16	–	–
Amox-clav	2	≤0.12 to 16	97.3	2.7	2	≤0.12 to 4	95.9	4.1
Ampicillin	≥64	≤0.5 to ≥64	0.5	99.5	≥64	≤0.5 to ≥64	0.8	99.2
Cefepime	≤0.5	≤0.5 to 2	–	–	≤0.5	≤0.5 to 2	–	–
Ceftriaxone	≤0.06	≤0.06 to 4	97.8	2.2	≤0.06	≤0.06 to 2	99.2	0.8
Levofloxacin	0.03	≤0.008 to 1	97.8	2.2	0.015	≤0.008 to 0.5	97.5	2.5
Meropenem (N = 378)[b]	0.12	≤0.06 to 0.5	100	0.0	0.12	≤0.06 to 0.5	100	0.0
Minocycline	1	≤0.5 to 16	93.2	0.5	1	≤0.5 to 2	93.4	0.0
Pip-taz	≤0.06	≤0.06 to 0.5	–	–	≤0.06	≤0.06 to 0.5	–	–
Tigecycline	0.25	≤0.008 to 0.5	–	–	0.25	≤0.008 to 0.25	–	–
K. oxytoca	N = 975				N = 225			
Amikacin	4	≤0.5 to ≥128	98.9	0.4	4	≤0.5 to 16	99.1	0.0
Amox-clav	32	0.25 to ≥64	79.8	20.2	16	0.25 to ≥64	82.2	17.8
Cefepime	2	≤0.5 to ≥64	88.4	3.9	2	≤0.5 to ≥64	88.4	4.9
Ceftriaxone	8	≤0.06 to ≥128	83.2	14.5	4	≤0.06 to 64	85.8	12.0
Levofloxacin	1	≤0.008 to ≥16	89.5	8.4	0.25	0.015 to ≥16	94.2	4.4
Meropenem (N = 872)[b]	≤0.06	≤0.06 to ≥32	99.8	0.1	≤0.06	≤0.06 to 1	100	0.0
Minocycline	4	≤0.5 to ≥32	–	–	2	≤0.5 to 16	–	–
Pip-taz	≥256	≤0.06 to ≥256	84.0	15.1	64	0.25 to ≥256	87.6	11.6
Tigecycline	1	0.015 to 8	95.8	1.0	0.5	0.12 to 4	96.9	0.9
K. pneumoniae	N = 2398				N = 690			
Amikacin	4	≤0.5 to ≥128	96.5	1.5	4	≤0.5 to ≥128	96.8	1.7
Amox-clav[a]	32	0.5 to ≥64	68.6	31.4	32	1 to ≥64	61.4	38.6
Cefepime[a]	≥64	≤0.5 to ≥64	72.1	23.4	≥64	≤0.5 to ≥64	59.9	35.5
Ceftriaxone[a]	64	≤0.06 to ≥128	70.3	28.7	64	≤0.06 to 64	58.4	41.4
Levofloxacin[a]	8	≤0.008 to ≥16	76.1	20.0	8	0.015 to ≥16	72.3	23.2
Meropenem[a] (N = 2186)[b]	0.12	≤0.06 to ≥32	99.4	0.4	0.12	≤0.06 to ≥32	98.8	1.0
Minocycline	16	≤0.5 to ≥32	–	–	16	≤0.5 to ≥32	–	–
Pip-taz	64	0.12 to ≥256	81.9	13.1	32	0.12 to ≥256	84.1	10.3
Tigecycline[a]	2	0.06 to 16	87.4	5.0	2	0.06 to 8	86.2	7.0
K. pneumoniae, ESBL	N = 622				N = 265			
Amikacin	8	≤0.5 to ≥128	90.0	4.2	8	≤0.5 to ≥128	94.7	3.8
Amox-clav	32	1 to ≥64	19.0	81.0	32	1 to ≥64	20.8	79.2
Cefepime[a]	≥64	≤0.5 to ≥64	5.0	85.0	≥64	≤0.5 to ≥64	3.8	86.8
Ceftriaxone	≥128	≤0.06 to ≥128	1.3	98.4	64	≤0.06 to 64	1.1	98.9
Levofloxacin[c]	≥16	0.03 to ≥16	30.2	61.1	≥16	0.03 to ≥16	38.9	50.9
Meropenem (N = 603)[b]	0.12	≤0.06 to ≥32	99.0	0.3	0.12	≤0.06 to 16	99.2	0.4
Minocycline	≥32	≤0.5 to ≥32	–	–	≥32	≤0.5 to ≥32	–	–
Pip-taz[c]	≥256	0.25 to ≥256	54.0	32.8	128	0.25 to ≥256	68.7	18.5
Tigecycline	2	0.12 to 8	79.4	7.2	2	0.12 to 8	80.0	7.9
S. marcescens	N = 1345				N = 360			

Table 3 Minimum inhibitory concentrations (MIC$_{90}$, MIC range [mg/L]) and antimicrobial susceptibility (%S) and resistance (%R) of Gram-negative isolates *(Continued)*

Organism/ Antimicrobial	2004–2016				2013–2016			
	MIC$_{90}$ (mg/L)	MIC Range (mg/L)	% S	% R	MIC$_{90}$ (mg/L)	MIC Range (mg/L)	% S	% R
Amikacin	4	≤0.5 to ≥128	97.3	1.1	4	≤0.5 to 64	98.3	0.6
Cefepime	≤0.5	≤0.5 to ≥64	94.5	2.2	≤0.5	≤0.5 to ≥32	94.7	1.9
Ceftriaxone	8	≤0.06 to ≥128	82.2	13.8	2	≤0.06 to 64	86.9	8.9
Levofloxacin[c]	2	≤0.008 to ≥16	84.2	10.6	1	≤0.008 to ≥16	89.4	5.6
Meropenem (N = 1227)[b]	0.12	≤0.06 to ≥32	99.1	0.1	0.12	≤0.06 to 2	100	0.0
Minocycline	8	≤0.5 to ≥32	–	–	4	≤0.5 to ≥32	–	–
Pip-taz	16	≤0.06 to ≥256	89.9	6.2	8	≤0.06 to 128	93.9	3.3
Tigecycline	2	0.015 to 8	80.7	2.6	2	0.03 to 4	80.3	1.1
A. baumannii	N = 1496				N = 270			
Amikacin	≥128	≤0.5 to ≥128	74.9	19.9	≥128	1 to ≥128	73.7	20.4
Cefepime	32	≤0.5 to ≥64	–	–	≥64	≤0.5 to ≥64	–	–
Ceftazidime (N = 1488)	≥64	≤1 to ≥64	–	–	32	≤1 to 32	–	–
Ceftriaxone	≥128	≤0.06 to ≥128	–	–	64	2 to 64	–	–
Levofloxacin	≥16	≤0.008 to ≥16	54.5	43.2	≥16	≤0.008 to ≥16	56.7	42.6
Meropenem[a] (N = 1326)[b]	≥32	≤0.06 to ≥32	81.0	11.8	≥32	0.12 to ≥32	74.1	20
Minocycline	8	≤0.5 to ≥32	–	–	8	≤0.5 to ≥32	–	–
Pip-taz	≥256	≤0.06 to ≥256	–	–	≥256	≤0.06 to ≥256	–	–
Tigecycline	1	≤0.008 to 8	–	–	1	0.03 to 2	–	–
A. baumannii MDR	N = 93				N = 35			
Amikacin	≥128	32 to ≥128	0.0	100	≥128	32 to ≥128	0.0	100
Cefepime	≥64	8 to ≥64	–	–	≥64	8 to ≥64	–	–
Ceftazidime (N = 92)	≥64	≤1 to ≥64	–	–	32	2 to 32	–	–
Ceftriaxone	≥128	64 to ≥128	–	–	64	64 to 64	–	–
Levofloxacin	≥16	2 to ≥16	0.0	100	≥16	2 to ≥16	0.0	100
Meropenem (N = 92)[b]	≥32	16 to ≥32	0.0	100	≥32	16 to ≥32	0.0	100
Minocycline	16	≤0.5 to ≥32	–	–	16	≤0.5 to ≥32	–	–
Pip-taz	≥256	≤0.06 to ≥256	–	–	≥256	64 to ≥256	–	–
Tigecycline	4	0.12 to 4	–	–	2	0.25 to 2	–	–
P. aeruginosa	N = 2734				N = 738			
Amikacin	16	≤0.5 to ≥128	88.5	6.9	8	≤0.5 to ≥128	91.1	5.1
Cefepime	32	≤0.5 to ≥64	77.8	22.2	16	≤0.5 to ≥64	79.8	20.2
Ceftazidime (N = 2730)	32	≤1 to ≥64	77.2	22.8	32	≤1 to 32	80.2	19.8
Levofloxacin[c]	≥16	≤0.008 to ≥16	60.6	39.4	≥16	0.015 to ≥16	65.7	34.3
Meropenem (N = 2474)	8	≤0.06 to ≥32	74.6	8.7	16	≤0.06 to ≥32	75.2	10.0
Pip-taz[c]	128	≤0.06 to ≥256	74.4	25.6	128	≤0.06 to ≥256	78.7	21.3
Tigecycline	16	≤0.008 to ≥32	–	–	16	0.12 to 16	–	–
P. aeruginosa MDR	N = 271				N = 68			
Amikacin	≥128	1 to ≥128	31.4	58.3	≥128	2 to ≥128	38.2	50.0
Cefepime	≥64	2 to ≥64	14.0	86.0	≥64	4 to ≥64	8.8	91.2
Ceftazidime	≥64	2 to ≥64	21.4	78.6	32	4 to 32	23.5	76.5
Levofloxacin	≥16	0.5 to ≥16	1.5	98.5	≥16	2 to ≥16	0.0	100
Meropenem[a] (N = 258)[b]	≥32	≤0.06 to ≥32	17.8	66.7	≥32	0.25 to ≥32	11.8	82.4

Table 3 Minimum inhibitory concentrations (MIC$_{90}$, MIC range [mg/L]) and antimicrobial susceptibility (%S) and resistance (%R) of Gram-negative isolates *(Continued)*

Organism/ Antimicrobial	2004–2016				2013–2016			
	MIC$_{90}$ (mg/L)	MIC Range (mg/L)	% S	% R	MIC$_{90}$ (mg/L)	MIC Range (mg/L)	% S	% R
Pip-taz^c	≥256	0.5 to ≥256	14.0	86.0	≥256	1 to ≥256	20.6	79.4
Tigecycline	≥32	1 to ≥32	–	–	16	2 to 16	–	–

– indicates no susceptibility breakpoints are available for this agent
^{a} indicates statistically significant decrease in susceptibility (p < 0.01) from 2004 to 2016
^{b} Meropenem was introduced to the testing panel in 2006, replacing imipenem; N values of activity against organisms collected from 2006 to 2016 are given
^{c} indicates statistically significant increase in susceptibility (p < 0.01) from 2004 to 2016
Amox-clav, amoxicillin-clavulanic acid, *BL*, β-lactamase, *ESBL*, extended-spectrum β-lactamase, *MDR*, multidrug-resistant, *MIC*, minimum inhibitory concentration, *MIC$_{90}$*, minimum inhibitory concentration required to inhibit growth of 90% of isolates (mg/L), *Pip-taz*, piperacillin-tazobactam, *R*, resistant, *S*, susceptible

H. influenzae

H. influenzae isolates (N = 1786), including β-lactamase positive isolates (N = 410, 23.0%) collected between 2004 to 2016 (Table 3) were susceptible (> 91.0%) to agents in the T.E.S.T. panel with a breakpoint, with the exception of ampicillin, to which 75.4% of all *H. influenzae* isolates and 0.5% of β-lactamase positive isolates were susceptible.

Klebsiella spp

A total of 975 *K. oxytoca* isolates were collected during the study, and susceptibilities were highest to meropenem (N = 872, 99.8%), amikacin (98.9%) and tigecycline (95.8%). Over 80% of isolates were susceptible to cefepime, ceftriaxone, levofloxacin and piperacillin-tazobactam, and 79.8% of isolates were susceptible to amoxicillin-clavulanate.

Susceptibility of *K. pneumoniae* isolates collected between 2004 to 2016 (N = 2398) was highest to meropenem (N = 2186, 99.4%,), amikacin (96.5%) and tigecycline (87.4%) (Table 3). There was a significant (p < 0.0001) decline in susceptibilities to amoxicillin-clavulanate from 85.1% in 2004 to 46.2% in 2016, cefepime (95.5% in 2004 to 48.7% in 2016), ceftriaxone (91.0% in 2004 to 47.4% in 2016), levofloxacin (92.5% in 2004 to 66.7% in 2016) and meropenem (100% in 2004 to 92.3% in 2016).

The proportion of *K. pneumoniae* isolates identified as ESBL-positive between 2004 and 2016 (N = 622) was highest during 2016 (43.6%) (Table 2), an increase from 36.1% in 2013 and from 7.5% in 2004. Susceptibility was highest to meropenem (N = 603, 99.0%), amikacin (90.0%) and tigecycline (79.4%). Six *K. pneumoniae* isolates collected from one centre in 2016 were resistant to meropenem and these isolates were not ESBL-producers. Very few ESBL-positive isolates were susceptible to cefepime (5.0%) and ceftriaxone (1.3%) during the study, although susceptibility to levofloxacin improved to its highest level in 2016 (47.1%), and the susceptibility to piperacillin-tazobactam was 79.4% in 2016, a similar value compared with 80.0% susceptibility in 2004.

S. marcescens

Between 2004 and 2016, 1345 isolates of *S. marcescens* were collected, and susceptibility was highest to meropenem (N = 1227, 99.1%), amikacin (97.3%) and cefepime (94.5%).

A. baumannii

Few agents showed *in vitro* activity against *A. baumannii* isolates (N = 1496) (Table 3), with tigecycline and minocycline the two agents with relatively low MIC$_{90}$ values (1 mg/L and 8 mg/L respectively); clinical breakpoints for these two agents are not available. Susceptibility to meropenem (N = 1326) was 81.0% and to amikacin 74.9%. There was a significant decrease (p < 0.0001) in the proportion of isolates that were susceptible to meropenem, from 84.8% in 2006 to 65.5% in 2016. None of the *A. baumannii* MDR isolates was susceptible to amikacin, levofloxacin (both N = 93) and meropenem (N = 92), the three agents with breakpoints. Antimicrobial activity of tigecycline against *A. baumannii* MDR isolates appeared reduced (MIC$_{90}$ 4 mg/L) compared with all *A. baumannii* isolates. The proportion of *A. baumannii* MDR isolates increased from zero in 2004 to a high of 24.1% in 2016 (Table 2).

P. aeruginosa

A total of 2734 *P. aeruginosa* isolates were collected during the study and susceptibility to antimicrobial agents was stable. Susceptibility was 88.5% to amikacin, whilst 77.8% of isolates were susceptible to cefepime, 77.2% to ceftazidime, 74.6% to meropenem and 74.4% to piperacillin-tazobactam. The proportion of *P. aeruginosa* isolates (N = 271) that were identified as MDR declined during the study from a high of 13.6% in 2013 to 4.0% in 2016, and susceptibility of these isolates was highest to amikacin (31.4%).

Discussion

This report is an update to data previously presented by Cattoir and Dowzicky [17] for France, and includes data from isolates that were collected between 2004 and 2016. Data presented by Cattoir and Dowzicky that were based on isolates collected in France from 2004 to 2012 are included in the dataset we describe in this update.

The proportion of isolates identified as MRSA in our study was stable between 2004 and 2016, and averaged 27.7% compared with an average of 28.3% between 2004 and 2012 [17]. During the last four years of our study, there appeared to be a slight decline in MRSA rates from 28.0% to 23.5%. Rates of MRSA in France were reported to be decreasing from 2003 to 2010 according to data from the RAISIN network published in 2013 by Carbonne et al. [2], and more recently the ECDC surveillance report identified an MRSA rate in France of 17.1% of invasive *S. aureus* isolates in 2013, 17.4% in 2014, 15.7% in 2015 and 13.8% in 2016 [3]. The use of control measures including isolation of patients with MRSA, the use of alcohol-based hand-rub, and screening of high-risk patients [9], have resulted in improved control of MRSA transmission in French hospitals [9, 22]. Consequently the proportion of *S. aureus* isolates identified as MRSA in France is showing a downward trend, and similar trends have been observed in Germany and the UK by the ECDC, which reported MRSA rates in 2016 of 10.3 and 6.7%, respectively [3]. Much higher MRSA rates have been reported in France's neighbouring countries of Spain (25.8% in 2016) and Italy (33.6% in 2016) [3].

Susceptibilities of *S. aureus* isolates collected in our study were stable to tigecycline, vancomycin, linezolid and minocycline, including MRSA isolates, which showed susceptibility rates between 2013 and 2016 of 100% to tigecycline, vancomycin and linezolid and 95.3% to minocycline. The same values were reported by Cattoir and Dowzicky [17] for MRSA isolates collected between 2004 and 2012 ($N = 631$) for tigecycline, vancomycin and linezolid, with minocycline susceptibility similar at 93.5%. MRSA isolates collected in our study between 2013 to 2016 did not show any meaningful improvement in *in vitro* susceptibility to levofloxacin (17.5%) compared with 2004 to 2012 (13.2%) [17]. Beyond these favourable data, the spread of MRSA strains exhibiting a vancomycin MIC superior to 1 mg/L should be carefully monitored, according to their putative role in clinical therapeutic failure and additional associated resistance [23].

Susceptibility to vancomycin amongst Gram-positive isolates was 100% amongst *S. aureus, S. agalactiae* and *S. pneumoniae*, including resistant phenotypes. The proportion of *Enterococcus* spp. that were identified as vancomycin-resistant isolates from 2004 to 2012 by Cattoir and Dowzicky [17] was low (*E. faecalis* VRE 0.7%, *E. faecium* VRE 5.4%) and we report a similar observation after a further four years of study (2004 to 2016: *E. faecalis* VRE 0.8%; *E. faecium* VRE 5.6%).

There was a considerable reduction in the susceptibility of penicillin-resistant *S. pneumoniae* isolates to macrolides compared with all *S. pneumoniae* isolates in our study. However, susceptibility of penicillin-resistant *S. pneumoniae* was appreciably higher to erythromycin amongst isolates that were collected in our study between 2013 and 2016 (38.5%), compared with 19.4% susceptibility amongst isolates collected between 2004 and 2012 and reported by Cattoir and Dowzicky [17].

In our study, the proportion of ESBL-producers among *E. coli* (16.2%) between 2013 and 2016 represented a small increase compared with the 2004 to 2012 period reported by Cattoir and Dowzicky (12.0%) [17]. A study in France by Carbonne et al. on behalf of the RAISIN network reported a threefold increase in *E. coli* ESBL-producers identified from isolates collected from patients in participating healthcare facilities between 2003 and 2010 [2]. The increasing prevalence of ESBL-positive Enterobacteriaceae reported in healthcare settings is compounded by an increasingly frequent distribution in community settings. A recent study investigating risk factors of *E. coli* ST131 in children in the community found a doubling of ESBL-positive Enterobacteriaceae between 2010 and 2015 that was mainly attributed to the *E. coli* ST131 clonal group [24]. The spread of ESBL-positive Enterobacteriaceae in France appears to be due to CTX-M-type enzymes encoded in plasmids playing a major role, with three ESBLs (CTX-M-15, CTX-M-1, CTX-M-14) accounting for > 75% of isolates in a recent study of 200 clinical ESBL-positive samples collected from 18 French hospitals [4].

In our study, the *in vitro* susceptibility of tigecycline (99.5%), amikacin (98.4%) and meropenem (99.9%) observed against all *E. coli* isolates between 2013 and 2016 was retained among ESBL-positive isolates (99.4, 95.5 and 100%, respectively), and was similar to values for ESBL-positive *E. coli* reported by Cattoir and Dowzicky for the period 2004 to 2012 (tigecycline, 98.9%, amikacin 90.5%, meropenem 100%) [17]. Further comparison with the 2004 to 2012 dataset reveals an improvement in susceptibility of ESBL-positive *E. coli* isolates to amoxicillin-clavulanate (from 36.7% between 2004 to 2012 to 59.0% between 2013 to 2016) and to piperacillin-tazobactam (from 72.4% between 2004 to 2012 to 88.5% between 2013 and 2016). Susceptibility trends similar to those observed for *E. coli* isolates were observed amongst *K. pneumoniae* and ESBL-positive *K. pneumoniae* isolates for tigecycline, amikacin and meropenem. The sustained decline in susceptibility of *K. pneumoniae* to ceftriaxone during our study appears to be attributable to the increase in the proportion of ESBL-positive *K. pneumoniae* isolates that was observed as the study progressed, reaching its highest value of 43.6% in 2016. The high prevalence of *K. pneumoniae* isolates with antibiotic resistance has also been reported by the ECDC, which observed that 28.9% of *K. pneumonia* isolates from France in 2016 were resistant to third-generation cephalosporins, and the majority of these were ESBL-positive [3].

A recent study of infections caused by carbapenemases that were notified by local healthcare facilities to the French Institute for Public Health in France between 2004 and 2011 reported a sharp increase in annual reported episodes of CPE from three or less from 2004 to 2008, then six in 2009, 26 in 2010 and 13 in 2011 [5]. A total of 53 episodes were reported in all, and 42 were associated with cross-border transfers, suggesting that CPE were not endemic in France by 2011. Most CPE were mainly K. pneumoniae or E. coli, with the majority of carbapenemases identified as OXA-48 or a K. pneumoniae carbapenemase (KPC). A further study, by Dortet et al. [25], identified a more than twofold increase in Enterobacteriaceae isolates with decreased susceptibility to carbapenems that were received at the French Associated National Reference Centre from 2012 to 2014. The predominant carbapenemases identified in their study were OXA-48 variants. Despite apparent increases in the numbers of carbapenemases reported in France, the proportion of Enterobacteriaceae isolates with non-susceptibility to carbapenems would appear to remain very low; a rate of 0.63% was identified amongst 133,244 clinical isolates collected from 71 laboratories across France by Robert et al. [26], and 0.4% of K. pneumoniae isolates collected across France as part of the ECDC antimicrobial surveillance in Europe were identified as carbapenemase-resistant [3]. These findings are consistent with our study, in which almost all ESBL-positive isolates were susceptible to meropenem.

The proportion of A. baumannii isolates identified as MDR between 2004 and 2012 by Cattoir and Dowzicky was 4.7% [17], and although the proportion of MDR isolates increased considerably during the four further years of our study, increasing to 24.1% in 2016, the number of MDR isolates (n = 7) was low. A recent study in France of A. baumannii carbapenem non-susceptible isolates noted that the proportion of carbapenem non-susceptible strains amongst all A. baumannii isolates was low during 2001 and 2002, increased to 2.6% in 2003 and remained at ≤3.2% until 2009, when it increased to 5.0% of isolates or higher until the study concluded in 2011 [27]. The clinical threat presented by the increasing frequency of A. baumannii isolates that harbour carbapenemases is likely to be limited by the relatively low proportion of infections caused by A. baumannii, which were reported to account for just 0.02% of infections per 100 patients in French healthcare facilities in the 2012 French Point Prevalence Survey [28]. During our study, A. baumannii MDR isolates accounted for just 0.4% of all isolates collected between 2004 and 2016, suggesting that MDR A. baumannii is rare in France. Despite this, we report a notable fall in the in vitro susceptibility of MDR A. baumannii isolates to amikacin, levofloxacin and meropenem to the extent that none of the isolates was susceptible. Furthermore, the

increase in the MIC$_{90}$ value of tigecycline to 4 mg/L against MDR A. baumannii isolates from 1 mg/L against all A. baumannii isolates suggests a reduction in its antimicrobial activity, and underlines the paucity of effective antimicrobial agents that are available to physicians when treating infections caused by MDR A. baumannii.

Limitations of this study include a reduction in the number of centres in 2016 to four, which has the potential to magnify resistance rates should a single site experience a clonal outbreak or a resistant phenotype. There was one occurrence of this during 2016, when six ESBL-negative K. pneumoniae isolates from one centre were identified as resistant to meropenem. The source of one of these isolates was body fluids, and the remaining five were from faeces/stools. This outbreak was unlikely to significantly affect the antimicrobial susceptibility trends that we report, however there is the possibility of clonal outbreaks at a single site influencing the reported rates of resistant pathogens in our study. A further possible limitation might arise from the collection of isolates. The T.E.S.T. protocol specifies that each submitted isolate must be considered by the contributing centre to be the probable causative agent of an infection. Between 2004 and 2016, 36.4% (N = 772) of isolates from GI sources originated from faeces/stool (1.1% of the total number of isolates collected in the study), and it is conceivable that organisms identified from these isolates may not have been the probable causative agent of infection, a fact that has probably very slightly overestimated the resistance rates in Enterobacteriaceae. However, we would suggest that given the very low proportion of isolates obtained from this source, the overall trends we have observed in antimicrobial activity and rates of resistant phenotypes remain valid. Finally, although the report of global resistance rate is relevant, more accurate data according to the origin of the infection (i.e. community-associated or healthcare-associated) or the clinical context (e.g. bacteraemia, urinary tract infection, respiratory tract infection) should be of interest.

Conclusions

During this study, nearly all (> 90.0%) Gram-positive isolates collected between 2004 and 2016 were susceptible in vitro to tigecycline, meropenem and linezolid, including MRSA and VRE phenotypes. Tigecycline and meropenem were also active in vitro against most Gram-negative isolates, including ESBL producers. The rates of MRSA and VRE we observed are stable, however there were notable increases in the rates of ESBL producers in E. coli and K. pneumoniae, accompanied by an increase in the proportion of A. baumannii isolates that were identified as MDR. These trends highlight the continued importance of surveillance studies for monitoring antimicrobial resistance and demonstrate the need for effective strategies to control the spread of resistant pathogens in hospital- and community-acquired infections in France.

Abbreviations
cIAIs: Complicated intra-abdominal infections; CLSI: Clinical and Laboratory Standards Institute; CPE: Carbapenemase-producing Enterobacteriaceae; cSSTIs: Complicated skin and soft tissue infections; ECDC: European Centre for Disease Prevention and Control; ESBL: Extended-spectrum β-lactamase; EUCAST: European Committee on Antimicrobial Susceptibility Testing; GI: Gastrointestinal; IHMA: International Health Management Associates; KPC: *Klebsiella pneumonia* carbapenemase; MDR: Multidrug-resistant; MIC: Minimum inhibitory concentration; MIC_{90}: MIC required to inhibit growth of 90% of isolates; MRSA: Methicillin-resistant *Staphylococcus aureus*; RAISIN: French national healthcare-associated infection early warning, investigation and surveillance network [Réseau d'alerte, d'investigation et de surveillance des infections nosocomiales]; T.E.S.T.: Tigecycline Evaluation and Surveillance Trial; VRE: Vancomycin-resistant enterococci

Acknowledgements
The authors would like to thank all T.E.S.T. investigators and laboratories in France for their participation in the study and would also like to thank the staff at IHMA for their coordination of T.E.S.T.

Funding
T.E.S.T. is funded by Pfizer. Medical writing support was provided by Dr. Neera Hobson, Dr. Wendy Hartley and Mike Leedham, employees of Micron Research Ltd., Ely, UK, and was funded by Pfizer. Micron Research Ltd. also provided data management services which were funded by Pfizer.

Authors' contributions
C-JS, J-WD, P-LW and MF-G all participated in data collection and interpretation as well as drafting and reviewing the manuscript. MJD was involved in the study design and participated in data interpretation and drafting and review of the manuscript. All authors read and approved the final manuscript.

Competing interests
C-J.S., J-W.D., P-L.W. and M.F-G have no competing interests relating to this paper. M.J.D. is an employee of Pfizer, Inc.

Author details
[1]University Hospital Henri Mondor, 9400 Creteil, France. [2]Caen University Hospital, 14033 Caen, Cedex 9, France. [3]Pfizer Inc, Collegeville, PA, USA.

References
1. European Centre for Disease Prevention and Control (ECDC). Summary of the latest data on antibiotic consumption in EU: 2016. Available at: https://ecdc.europa.eu/en/publications-data/summary-latest-data-antibiotic-consumption-eu-2016. Accessed 12 Oct 2017.
2. Carbonne A, Arnaud I, Maugat S, Marty N, Dumartin C, Bertrand X, on behalf of the MDRB National Steering Group (BMR-Raisin), et al. National multidrug-resistant bacteria (MDRB) surveillance in France through the RAISIN network: a 9 year experience. J Antimicrob Chemother. 2013;68:954–9.
3. European Centre for Disease Prevention and Control. Surveillance of antimicrobial resistance in Europe 2016. Annual Report of the European Antimicrobial Resistance Network (EARS-Net). Stockholm: ECDC; 2017. https://ecdc.europa.eu/en/publications-data/antimicrobial-resistance-surveillance-europe-2016. Accessed 05 Jan 2018.
4. Robin F, Beyrouthy R, Bonacorsi S, Aissa N, Bret L, Brieu N, et al. Inventory of extended-spectrum-β-lactamase-producing Enterobacteriaceae in France as assessed by a multicenter study. Antimicrob Agents Chemother. 2017;61:e01911 6.
5. Vaux S, Carbonne A, Thiolet JM, Jarlier V, Coignard B, RAISIN and Expert Laboratories Groups. Emergence of carbapenemase-producing Enterobacteriaceae in France, 2004 to 2011. Euro Surveill. 2011;16(22):19880.
6. Albiger B, Glasner C, Strueiens MJ, Monnet DL, the European Survey of Carbapenemase-Producing Enterobacteriaceae (EuSCAPE) working group. Carbapenemase-producing Enterobacteriaceae in Europe: assessment by national experts from 38 countries, May 2015. Euro Surveill. 2015;20(45):30062.
7. Lepelletier D, Berthelot P, Lucet JC, Fournier S, Jarlier V, Grandbastien B, et al. French recommendations for the prevention of 'emerging extensively drug-resistant bacteria' (eXDR) cross-transmission. J Hosp Infect. 2015;90(3):186–95.
8. European Centre for Disease Prevention and Control. Antimicrobial resistance surveillance in Europe 2010. Annual Report of the European Antimicrobial Resistance Network (EARS-net). Stockholm: ECDC;2011. https://ecdc.europa.eu/en/publications-data/antimicrobial-resistance-surveillance-europe-2010. Accessed 05 Jan 2018.
9. Jarlier V, Trystram D, Brun-Buisson C, Fournier S, Carbonne A, Marty L, et al. Curbing methicillin-resistant Staphylococcus aureus in 38 French hospitals through a 15-year institutional control program. Arch Intern Med. 2010; 170(6):552–9.
10. Meyer E, Schroder C, Gastmeier P, Geffers C. The reduction of nosocomial MRSA infection in Germany: an analysis of data from the hospital infection surveillance system (KISS) between 2007 and 2012. Dtsch Arztebl Int. 2014; 111(19):331–6.
11. Walter J, Haller S, Blank HP, Eckmanns T, Abu Sin M, Hermes J. Incidence of invasive methicillin-resistant Staphylococcus aureus infections in Germany, 2010 to 2014. Euro Surveill. 2015;20(46):30067.
12. Walter J, Noll I, Weiss B, Claus H, Werner G, Eckmanns T, et al. Decline in the proportion of methicillin resistance among Staphylococcus aureus isolates from non-invasive samples and in outpatient settings, and changes in the co-resistance profiles; an analysis of data collected within the antimicrobial resistance surveillance network, Germany 2010 to 2015. BMC Infect Dis. 2017;17:169.
13. Guy R, Geoghegan L, Heginbotham M, Howe R, Muller-Pebody B, Reilly JS, et al. Non-susceptibility of Escherichia coli, Klebsiella spp., Pseudomonas spp., Streptococcus pneumoniae and Staphylococcus aureus in the UK: temporal trends in England, Northern Ireland, Scotland and Wales. J Antimicrob Chemother. 2016;71:1564–9.
14. Touraine M. Tackling antimicrobial resistance in France. Lancet. 2016; 387(10034):2177–9. https://doi.org/10.1016/S0140-6736(16)30356-7.
15. Pfizer Limited. Tygacil summary of product characteristics. Sandwich, Kent; February, 2016.
16. Pfizer Inc. Wyeth Pharmaceuticals. Philadelphia: Tygacil® Product Insert; 2016. http://labeling.pfizer.com/showlabeling.aspx?id=491&pagename=tygacil_fly.
17. Cattoir V, Dowzicky MJ. A longitudinal assessment of antimicrobial susceptibility among important pathogens collected as part of the Tigecycline Evaluation and Surveillance Trial (T.E.S.T.) in France between 2004 and 2012. Antimicrob Resist Infect Control. 2014;3:36. https://doi.org/10.1186/2047-2994-3-36.
18. Clinical and Laboratory Standards Institute (CLSI). Methods for Dilution Antimicrobial Susceptibility Tests for Bacteria That Grow Aerobically; Approved standards – Tenth edition. CLSI Document M07-A10. Wayne, PA: CLSI; 2015.
19. Clinical and Laboratory Standards Institute (CLSI). Performance Standards for Antimicrobial Susceptibility Testing – Twenty-Sixth Informational Supplement. CLSI Document M100-S26. Wayne, PA: CLSI; 2016.
20. The European Committee on Antimicrobial Susceptibility Testing. Breakpoint tables for interpretation of MICs and zone diameters. Version 7.1, 2017. http://www.eucast.org. Accessed 04 Oct 2017.
21. Stefani S, Dowzicky MJ. Longitudinal assessment of antimicrobial susceptibility among gram-negative and gram-positive organisms collected from Italy as part of the Tigecycline evaluation and surveillance trial between 2004 and 2011. Pharmaceuticals. 2013;6:1381–406.
22. Chalfine A, Kitzis M-D, Bezie Y, Benali A, Perniceni L, Nguyen J-C, et al. Ten-year decrease of acquired methicillin-resistant Staphylococcus aureus (MRSA) bacteremia at a single institution: the result of a multifaceted program combining cross-transmission prevention and antimicrobial stewardship. Antimicrob Resist Infect Control. 2012;1(1):18. https://doi.org/10.1186/2047-2994-1-18

23. Gould IM. Treatment of bacteraemia: methicillin-resistant Staphylococcus aureus (MRSA) to vancomycin-resistant S. Aureus (VRSA). Int J Antimicrob Agents. 2013;42 Suppl:S17–21.

24. Birgy A, Levy C, Bidet P, Thollot F, Derkx V, Béchet S, et al. ESBL-producing *Escherichia coli* ST131 versus non-ST131: evolution and risk factors of carriage among French children in the community between 2010 and 2015. J Antimicrob Chemother. 2016;71:2949–56.

25. Dortet L, Cuzon G, Ponties V, Nordmann P. Trends in carbapenemase-producing Enterobacteriaceae, France, 2012 to 2014. Euro Surveill. 2017; 22(6) https://doi.org/10.2807/1560-7917.

26. Robert J, Pantel A, Mérens A, Lavigne J-P, Nicolas-Chanoine M-H. On behalf of ONERBA's carbapenem resistance study group. Incidence rates of carbapenemase-producing Enterobacteriaceae clinical isolates in France: a prospective nationwide study in 2011–12. J Antimicrob Chemother. 2014;69:2706–12.

27. Jeannot K, Diancourt L, Vaux S, Thouverez M, Ribeiro A, Coignard B, et al. Molecular epidemiology of carbapenem non-susceptible *Acinetobacter baumannii* in France. PLoS One. 2014;9(12):e115452. https://doi.org/10.1371/journal.pone.0115452.

28. Anonymous (2013). Réseau d'alerte, d'investigation et de surveillance des infections nosocomiales (Raisin). Enquête nationale de prévalence des infections nosocomiales et des traitements anti-infectieux en établissements de santé, France, mai-juin 2012. Résultats. Saint-Maurice: InVS; 2013. p. 181.

18

Should antibiotic prophylaxis before orthopedic implant surgery depend on the duration of pre-surgical hospital stay?

Marie Davat[1], Lydia Wuarin[1], Dimitrios Stafylakis[1], Mohamed Abbas[2], Stephan Harbarth[2], Didier Hannouche[1] and Ilker Uçkay[3]* (iD)

Abstract

Background: Prolonged hospital stay before surgery is a risk for colonization with antibiotic-resistant microorganisms and possible antibiotic-resistant surgical site infections (SSI), which lacks acknowledgement in international guidelines for perioperative antibiotic prophylaxis.

Method: Retrospective cohort study focusing on prophylaxis-resistant SSI in adult orthopedic implant patients; with emphasis on length of hospital stay prior to the index surgery.

Results: We enrolled 611 cases of SSI (median age, 65 years; 241 females and 161 immune-suppressed) in four large implant groups: arthroplasties ($n = 309$), plates ($n = 127$), spondylodeses ($n = 31$), and nails ($n = 46$). The causative pathogen was resistant to the perioperative antibiotic prophylaxis regimen in 307 cases (307/611; 50%), but the length of pre-surgical hospitalization did not influence the incidences of prophylaxis-resistant SSIs. These incidences were (107/211;51%) for the admission day, (170/345;49%) within 10 days of delay, (19/35;54%) between 10 and 20 days, and (11/20; 55%) beyond 20 days of hospital stay before surgery. The corresponding incidences of methicillin-resistant staphylococci were 13%, 14%, 17%, and 5%, respectively. In adjusted group comparisons, the length of prior hospital stay was equally unrelated to future prophylaxis-resistant SSI (odds ratio 1.0, 95% confidence interval 0.99–1.01).

Conclusions: In our retrospective cohort of orthopedic implant SSI, the length of pre-surgical hospital stay was unrelated to the incidence of prophylaxis-resistant pathogens.

Keywords: Perioperative antibiotic prophylaxis, Implant orthopedic surgery, Length of hospital stay, Surgical site infections

Background

Prolonged hospital stay before orthopedic surgery is a potential risk for acquisition of antibiotic-resistant microorganisms [1]. Thus in case of delayed surgery and surgical site infections (SSI) [2], the SSI might be multi-resistant or resistant to the perioperative antibiotic prophylaxis that was administered during the index operation. For example in our hospital, lengthening of hospital stay by one additional day was associated with a 5% increment of new MRSA carriage [1]. Moreover,

prophylaxis-resistant germs may remain undetected except for outbreak situations or scientific studies [3]. This possible threat not only concerns methicillin-resistant *Staphylococcus aureus* (MRSA) [2, 3], but also methicillin-resistant coagulase-negative staphylococci [4], cephalosporin-resistant enterococci [5], non-fermenting Gram-negative rods [6] or extended-spectrum β-lactamase (ESBL) producing rods [7]. These pathogen groups all escape to standard prophylaxis with first-and second generation cephalosporins [2]. Especially, implant-related orthopedic surgery [8] is prone to SSI by methicillin-resistant staphylococci [4].

Many colleagues administer vancomycin or other broad-spectrum agents as prophylaxis, alone or in combination, for patients with long hospital stays (*personal*

---
* Correspondence: ilker.uckay@balgrist.ch
[3]Infectiology, Balgrist University Hospital, Forchstrasse 340, 8008 Zürich, Switzerland

communication). There are no data supporting this practice. National [9] and international [10] guidelines and consensus meetings [11] do not provide robust evidence on the choice of the prophylactic agent upon the length of pre-surgical stay. Indeed, international experts unanimously advocate single-dose cephalosporins or vancomycin for any orthopedic procedures [9–12].

In this retrospective cohort analysis, we specifically link the duration of pre-surgical hospital stay to the antibiotic resistance profile of orthopedic implant-related SSIs. We do not compute SSI risks or report treatment successes that we already have published elsewhere [13–15].

Methods

The Geneva University Hospitals is a tertiary center with a long tradition of clinical research regarding prevention of orthopedic implant-related infections [8]. The most recent prevalence of methicillin-resistant *Staphylococcus aureus* (MRSA) and methicillin-resistant coagulase-negative staphylococci among the clinical isolates in the orthopedic service were1% [13] and 75% [4, 16], respectively. The hospital recommends a single intravenous dose of pre-operative cefuroxime 1.5 g as standard prophylaxis in orthopedic surgery and traumatology. Only for cases with convincing history of penicillin allergy [17] or past/present MRSA carriage [3], we recommend one dose of vancomycin 1 g intravenously. Discipline regarding these recommendations is very good, with only maximal 5–10% deviations according to the last control assessments. We currently lack a univ ersal policy for searching and decolonizing *S. aureus* body carriage before surgery. Positive urinary or anal carriage of ESBL [7] does not alter our recommendations for orthopedic surgery. If surgery lasts for more than 4 h, prophylaxis is repeated. In selected cases, surgeons may continue it up to 24 h; except for open fractures with longer durations of preemptive treatment [18]. Since 2016, the standard dose was doubled for obese patients with more than 100 kg weight [19]. In selected cases, surgeons also implement arthroplasties with or without aminoglycoside-containing cement.

For the actual study, we used a composite database (Ethical Committee no. 13–178, 08–057 [13], 08–061 [20], and 14–198), including all adult patients with orthopedic implant SSI [8] and a minimal follow-up of two years [1]. We excluded cases that were amputated [21], orthopedic surgery cases without implants, community-acquired infections, recurrent episodes of the same infection and all patients necessitating actual or recent systemic antibiotic administration during the last 2 weeks. Our SSI definitions were based on the Center of Disease Control standards [22]. Basically, any infection within 1 year of implantation was a SSI, unless proven otherwise; e.g. by clear evidence of a hematogenous [23] or lymphogenous origins [24]. We defined hospital stay as a hospitalization in acute care settings. Consequently, we considered long-term care facilities not as hospitals. We collected several microbiological samples from pus or deep intraoperative tissues, and ignored results of superficial specimens or of a sinus tract. The microbiology laboratory processed all specimens according to Clinical and Laboratory Standard's Institute recommendations [25], before switching to the EUCAST criteria (European Committee) in 2014 [26].

Statistical analyses

Our primary objective was to assess the association between the length of prior hospital stay to future SSIs that were resistant to standard antibiotic prophylaxis (cefuroxime or vancomycin). We performed group comparisons using the Pearson-χ^2 or the Wilcoxon-ranksum-test. An unmatched multivariate logistic regression analysis determined associations with the outcome "SSI resistant to standard prophylaxis". We introduced independent variables with a p value ≤ 0.05 in the univariate analysis stepwise into the multivariate analysis, except for length of prior hospital stay, which we forced into the final model. We arbitrarily categorized the length of hospital stay individually for the days 0, 1, 2, 3, 4, for the groups between 5 and 9 days, 10–20 days, and more than 20 days; and plotted them against the occurrence of resistant SSIs. We used STATA software (9.0, STATA™, USA) and considered p values ≤ 0.05 (two-tailed) as significant.

Results

We included 611 orthopedic SSI cases meeting our study criteria (among 611 patients, 241 females (39%) and including 161 immune-suppressed persons (27%): diabetes mellitus ($n = 73$), active cancer (40), severe chronic alcoholism (25), medicamentous immune-suppression (20), cirrhosis CHILD C (11), dialysis (4), solid organ transplantation (1), or a combination of different immune-suppressed states. Upon diagnosis, the median age of the patients was 65 years and the median serum C-reactive protein levels were 83 mg/L. The presence of soft-tissue abscesses and bacteremia complicated the infections in 73 (12%) and 98 (16%) episodes, respectively. The infected implants were: arthroplasties ($n = 309$), plates (127), spondylodeses (31) [27], nails (46) [15], and various others (98). In 25 episodes, the infection occurred in the foot. Our laboratory detected 84 different microbiological constellations with the five most frequently identified pathogens being *Staphylococcus aureus* ($n = 166$), streptococci (46), Gram-negatives [6] (140; with 80 non-fermenters including 42 *Pseudomonas aeruginosa* cases, and 24 anaerobes [28]), enterococci [5] (33), *S. lugdunenssis* [16] (9), and skin commensals (134). In 100 cases, SSI were polymicrobial and in 35 cases culture-negative [29].

Associations with previous hospital stay

Overall, 556 (90%) implant surgeries with subsequent SSI were performed within 10 days after admission, 35 between 10 to 20 days, and 20 after 20 days since admission. Formally, the study population was already hospitalized during a median delay of 1 day (range, 0–178 d, interquartile range, 0–3 d) before the index surgery, and 44 patients had previously known MRSA carriage [3]. The prophylactic regimens followed the institutional standards for the majority of cases, but we detected the following deviations: several doses of cefuroxime ($n = 30$), use of ciprofloxacin (1), amoxicillin/clavulanic acid (1), clindamycin (1), and cefazolin (1). Overall, 36 patients received vancomycin, of which 28 episodes because of previous positive MRSA carriage in the past, and 8 probably because of presumed betalactam allergy or betalactam intolerance of various nature. In contrast, 16 former MRSA carriers lacked vancomycin for which the reasons were unknown. In 33 episodes (5%), we ignored the agent of prophylaxis, which was classified as "usual" according to the records.

Overall, the causative pathogen of future SSI was resistant to prior prophylaxis in 307 cases (307/611; 50%) (Table 1), but lacked association to previous length of pre-surgical hospitalization. The incidences of resistant pathogens were (107/211; 51%) for surgeries performed on the day of admission, (89/200; 45%) on Day 1, (24/41; 59%) on Day 2, (25/40; 63%) on Day 3, (9/17; 53%) on Day 4, (18/39; 46%) between 5 and 9 days since admission, (24/43; 56%) between 10 and 20 days, and (11/20; 55%) beyond 20 days after admission. The corresponding incidences of SSI due to methicillin-resistant staphylococci were 13% (27/211), 10% (19/200), 24% (10/41), 20% (8/40), 24% (4/17), 13% (5/39), 21% (9/43) and 5% (1/20), respectively. Figure 1 display the proportion graphically and denies the existent of a threshold in the number of days of hospital stay prior to surgery and subsequent prophylaxis-resistant and methicillin-resistant SSIs. The proportion of aminoglycoside-resistant SSI (that we computed because of possible cemented arthroplasty) was very low (3 of 611 cases; 1%). A (past) history of MRSA and lack of vancomycin prophylaxis was the only variable related to multi-resistant SSI.

Multivariate adjustment

In view of the considerable case-mix, we performed an adjusted logistic regression analysis. Here, the length of prior hospital stay was equally unrelated to prophylaxis-resistant SSI as a continuous variable (odds ratio 1.0, 95% confidence interval 0.99–1.01) or when breaking down to various stratifications (Table 2). Also, in this regression analysis, and unlike the former crude group comparison, immune-suppression lacked associations with prophylaxis-resistant SSI. The goodness-of-fit testing of our final model was non-significant ($p = 0.31$).

Discussion

In our cohort of orthopedic implant infections among adult patients, the length of hospital stay before the index surgery (implantation) was unrelated to the risk of future SSI due to prophylaxis-resistant pathogens such as methicillin-resistant staphylococci [4, 13]. Therefore, we argue against the broadening of the antibiotic prophylaxis with second-generation cephalosporins towards combinations that include more Gram-positive or

Table 1 Comparisons of demographic and clinical variables of adult orthopaedic implant patients with future surgical site infections resistant to the prophylactic regimen of the index surgery versus prophylaxis-susceptible surgical site implant infections

	Susceptible to prior prophylaxis		Resistant to prior prophylaxis
Total $n = 611$	$n = 304$	p value*	$n = 307$
Female sex	118 (39%)	0.752	123 (40%)
Age (median)	67 years	0.097	62 years
Past history of MRSA[b] body carriage	12 (4%)	*0.002*	32 (10%)
Immune suppression[a]	91 (30%)	*0.030*	70 (23%)
- diabetes mellitus	45 (15%)	*0.045*	28 (9%)
Shoulder implants	12 (4%)	0.235	7 (2%)
Arthroplasties	147 (48%)	0.275	162 (53%)
Spondylodeses	14 (5%)	0.600	17 (6%)
Plates	66 (22%)	0.575	61 (20%)
Intramedullary nails	20 (7%)	0.376	26 (8%)
Foot osteosyntheses	15 (5%)	0.295	10 (3%)
Duration of prior hospital stay (median)	1 day (range, 0–178 d)	0.408	1 day (range, 0–68 d)

*Significant p values ≤0.05 are displayed **in bold and italic**
[a]Immune suppression = diabetes mellitus, corticosteroid medication, organ transplantation, cirrhosis CHILD C, dialysis, or active cancer
[b]Methicillin-resistant *Staphylococcus aureus*

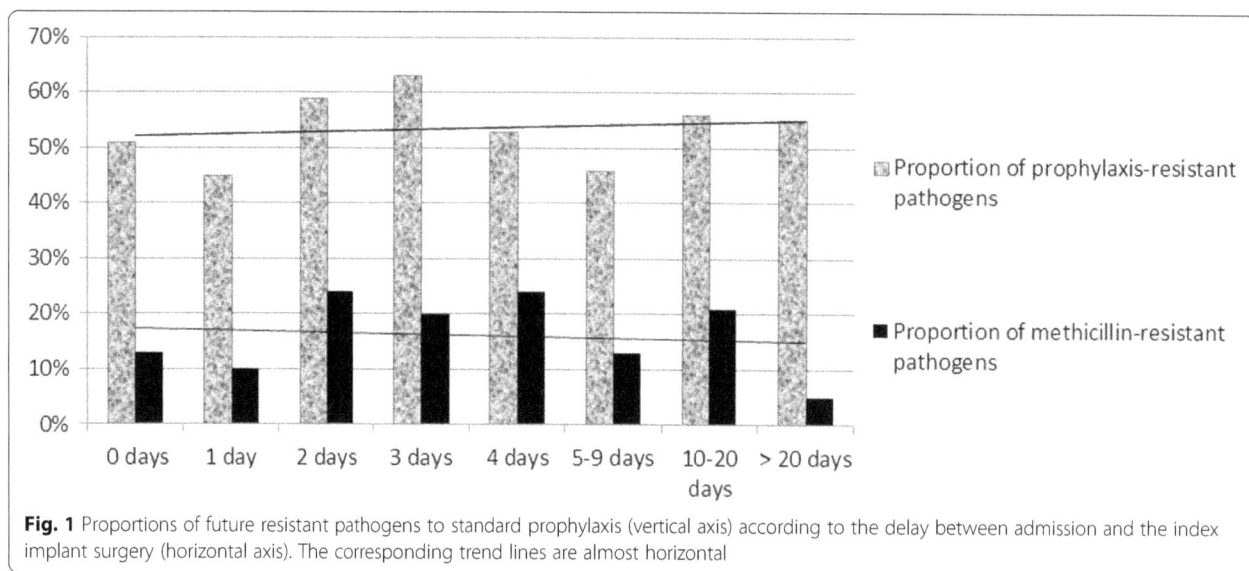

Fig. 1 Proportions of future resistant pathogens to standard prophylaxis (vertical axis) according to the delay between admission and the index implant surgery (horizontal axis). The corresponding trend lines are almost horizontal

Gram-negative coverage. One might argue, whether the study question is of importance. International recommendations are clear and do not recommend this [1, 2]. And yet, according to our experience, many surgeons or physicians often broaden the prophylaxis against official recommendations. Regarding prophylactic issues, our center shows high compliance and the study population is homogenous. Hence, we could easily perform tour study by avoiding major confounding and substantial interactions, making the interpretations more difficult.

In the literature, many research groups investigated the influence of a delay between admission and surgery with the occurrence of subsequent infection and its pathogen profile. However, these studies concerned open fractures, with time delays ranging from 0 to 24 h [18]. We found only one study specifically linking longer hospitalization delays with healthcare-associated infections [30]. In this study from Brazil, patients with nosocomial infections due to MSSA (not only orthopedic implants) revealed a median delay of prior hospital stay of 9 days, compared to MRSA infections with a past median delay of 18 days [30].

Table 2 Univariate and multivariate analyses of factors potentially related to antibiotic prophylaxis-resistant surgical site infections (*Logistic regression analysis; results expressed as odds ratios with 95% confidence intervals*)

Total n = 611	Univariate analysis	Multivariate analysis
Female sex	1.0, 0.7–1.4	n.d.
Age	1.0, 1.0–1.0	1.0, 1.0–1.0
Past history of MRSA[b] body carriage	*1.3, 1.1–2.9*	*1.4, 1.1–3.3*
Immune suppression[a]	0.7, 0.5–1.1	n.d.
- Diabetes mellitus	0.7, 0.4–1.2	n.d.
Shoulder implants	0.5, 0.2–1.5	n.d.
Arthroplasties	1.1, 0.8–1.8	1.2, 0.8–1.9
Spondylodeses	1.4, 0.7–2.9	1.4, 0.6–3.1
Plates	1.0, 0.6–1.5	n.d.
Intramedullary nails	1.2, 0.6–2.3	1.3, 0.6–2.6
Foot osteosyntheses	0.7, 0.3–1.6	0.8, 0.3–1.9
Duration of prior hospital stay	1.0, 1.0–1.0	1.0, 1.0–1.0
- 10–20 days compared to ≤10 days	1.1, 0.5–2.4	1.2, 0.5–2.5
- ≥ 20 days compared to ≤10 days	1.0, 0.6–1.7	1.1, 0.4–3.3

n d. = not done
*Statistically significant results are displayed *in bold and italic*
[a]Immune suppression = diabetes mellitus, corticosteroid medication, organ transplantation, cirrhosis CHILD C, dialysis, or active cancer
[b]Methicillin-resistant *Staphylococcus aureus*

In contrast, the literature is full of opinion papers and retrospective studies investigating the possibility of better outcomes with broader prophylaxis. The propositions of the authors differ from one paper to another and focus on different strategies which are: continuing the prophylaxis beyond a single dose [31, 32], augmenting of doses [19], combining with local prophylaxis [33, 34] (especially local vancomycin in spine surgery [35]), double prophylaxis [36] against Gram-negative [37], Gram-positive [38, 39], methicillin-resistant strains [4] and anaerobes [28], or by investigating the performance of universal glycopeptid prophylaxis [40–42]. In summary, the majority of these enhancements failed to reduce SSI risk, at least not in orthopedic surgery [34, 39–42]. Exceptions remain rare [32, 37], very specific and often not reproducible by other research groups [12, 31, 36]. Branch-Elliman et al. estimated that the number of orthopedic cases needed to prevent one Gram-positive SSI with vancomycin would be 1:53 for known MRSA carriers, compared to 1:176 for unknown carriers [39]. Also, concomitant colonization with MRSA does not always protect from colonization by susceptible *S. aureus* (MSSA) strains [1].

Broader antibiotic prophylaxis can be harmful, especially with prophylactic aminoglycosides against Gram-negative pathogens [38, 39]. Numerous studies reported transient kidney injuries by aminoglycosides [39] or combined vancomycin prophylaxis [12] in orthopedic surgery. The risk for antibiotic-resistant organisms seems to be negligible [35]. Walker et al. reported that following a change in prophylaxis (from floxacillin & gentamycin to amoxicillin/clavulanic acid), they witnessed a 63% decrease in postoperative renal insufficiencies [43]. In 2009, Scotland issued a target to reduce *Clostridium difficile* outbreaks. Consequently, hospitals changed prophylaxis from a cephalosporin to gentamicin-containing regimens (4 mg/kg), resulting in a 94% increase in kidney injuries [38].

Besides the fact that our study is retrospective, it has several limitations. First, we excluded already infected cases. Hence, we can only address the risk of prophylaxis-resistant SSI, but we cannot compare between infected and non-infected populations, or with patients who were under systemic antibiotic selection for any reason. Second, our orthopedic service has no policy of pre-surgical *S. aureus* [2] decolonization. Such a strategy might alter the association between the length of hospital stay and the patterns of subsequent SSI. Third, we assume like many other colleagues that most SSIs origin in the operating theatre [2], and that the length of hospital stay is a surrogate of nosocomial acquisitions of resistant pathogens. In our daily clinical practice, we usually neglect to assess individual colonization throughout the hospital stay. This assumption might not be granted. Studies from Sweden suggest a mounting colonization pressure by methicillin-resistant staphylococci after two to three days

[4] post-admission, and ESBL acquisitions in orthopedic wards has also been demonstrated [7], i.e. during wound care or wound breakdowns. Regarding these ward-born SSIs, the perioperative antibiotic prophylaxis during the index surgery would naturally lack influence; which we equally cannot control for in our retrospective analysis. Fourth, in our tertiary center, we use cefuroxime as standard antibiotic prophylaxis for many surgical disciplines, instead of cefazolin, which is another recommended agent in most guidelines for orthopedic surgeries. Most experts would agree that the difference and ecological impact between the two second-generation cephalosporins would be minimal, as they are close molecules in terms of clinical spectrum and efficacy. Although we cannot formally pronounce on the hypothetical results of our study performed under cefazolin, we nevertheless would expect the same results. Fifth, most of our patients had surgery within few days since admission, with a median delay of only 1 day. From a microbiological point of view, it seems rather unlikely that such a short hospitalization changes colonization with antibiotic-resistant germs. Nevertheless, we intended to study real-life conditions without selection biases. Theoretically, we could have performed a study only with those patients operated after 1 week of hospital stay or longer. This would, however, introduce a major bias and a very small and too specific study population, which we avoided. Sixth, many our implant infections were due to coagulase-negative staphylococci and other skin commensals. Usually, these bacteria are often regarded as contaminants. In our study, all bacterial results stem from several deep intraoperative tissue specimens, making contamination unlikely. Moreover, skin commensals, including coagulase-negative staphylococci and especially *S. epidermidis*, are frequent pathogens of low-grade orthopedic implants [8, 14–16] due to their ability to perform biofilms [44]. Lastly, we cannot retrospectively enumerate the individual reasons for a delayed surgery. As simple as it seems, in a retrospective study this question is very difficult to be answered. The reasons may vary between lack of operation slots, triage issues, lack of patient's and family's consent, nosocomial fractures occurring during a hospital stay for another reason, availability of the individual surgeon, week-ends and holidays, non-availability of the specific osteosynthesis material, or a panoply of combined reasons. However, we do not think that the individual reason for delay would have influenced our findings in this large epidemiological study.

Conclusions

According to our retrospective cohort analysis, a long pre-surgical hospital stay was not associated with more prophylaxis-resistant SSIs, in 611 adult patients undergoing orthopedic implant surgery, when compared to those with prophylaxis-susceptible pathogens. We keep our antibiotic perioperative prophylaxis policy as it is, regardless of the duration of pre-surgical length of hospital stay.

Acknowledgements
We thank the teams of the Laboratory of Bacteriology and the Orthopedic Service for support.

Funding
None.

Authors' contributions
MD, LW, DH, and IU conceived and designed the study. DH and SH were major contributors in writing and supervising the manuscript. MD, LW, DS treated most patients and supervised the study. MD and IU performed the data analysis. All authors read and approved the final manuscript.

Consent for publication
No applicable.

Competing interests
The authors declare that they have no competing interests.

Author details
[1]Orthopedic Surgery Service, Geneva University Hospitals, Geneva, Switzerland. [2]Infection Control Program, Geneva University Hospitals, Geneva, Switzerland. [3]Infectiology, Balgrist University Hospital, Forchstrasse 340, 8008 Zürich, Switzerland.

References
1. Landelle C, Iten A, Uçkay I, Sax H, Camus V, Cohen G, Renzi G, et al. Does colonization with methicillin-susceptible *Staphylococcus aureus* protect against nosocomial acquisition of methicillin-resistant *S. aureus*? Infect Control Hosp Epidemiol. 2014;35:527–33.
2. Uçkay I, Hoffmeyer P, Lew D, Pittet D. Prevention of surgical site infections in orthopaedic surgery and bone trauma: state-of-the-art update. J Hosp Infect. 2013;84:5–12.
3. Uçkay I, Sax H, Iten A, Camus V, Renzi G, Schrenzel J, et al. Effect of screening for methicillin-resistant *Staphylococcus aureus* carriage by polymerase chain reaction on the duration of unnecessary preemptive contact isolation. Infect Control Hosp Epidemiol. 2008;29:1077–9.
4. Uçkay I, Harbarth S, Ferry T, Lübbeke A, Emonet S, Hoffmeyer P, et al. Methicillin-resistance in orthopaedic coagulase-negative staphylococcal infections. J Hosp Infect. 2011;79:248–53.
5. Uçkay I, Pires D, Agostinho A, Guanziroli N, Öztürk M, Bartolone P, et al. Enterococci in orthopaedic infections: who is at risk getting infected? J Inf Secur. 2017;75:309–14.
6. Jamei O, Gjoni S, Zenelaj B, Kressmann B, Belaieff W, Hannouche D, et al. Which Orthopaedic patients are infected with gram-negative non-fermenting rods? J Bone Jt Infect. 2017;2:73–6.
7. Agostinho A, Renzi G, Haustein T, Jourdan G, Bonfillon C, Rougemont M, et al. Epidemiology and acquisition of extended-spectrum beta-lactamase-producing *Enterobacteriaceae* in a septic orthopedic ward. SpringerPlus. 2013;2:91.
8. Cuérel C, Abrassart S, Billières J, Andrey D, Suvà D, Dubois-Ferrière V, et al. Clinical and epidemiological differences between implant-associated and implant-free orthopaedic infections. Eur J Orthop Surg Traumatol. 2017;27:229–31.
9. Bratzler DW, Dellinger EP, Olsen KM, Perl TM, Auwaerter PG, Maureen K, Bolon MK, et al. Clinical practice guidelines for antimicrobial prophylaxis in surgery. Am J Health Syst Pharm. 2013;70:195–283.
10. WHO Global guidelines for the prevention of surgical site infections. WHO. In: Geneva; 2016.
11. Parvizi J, Gehrke T, Chen AF. Proceedings of the international consensus meeting on Periprosthetic joint infection. Bone Joint J. 2013;95-B:1450 2.
12. Courtney PM, Melnic CM, Zimmer Z, Anari J, Lee GC. Addition of Vancomycin to Cefazolin prophylaxis is associated with acute kidney injury after primary joint Arthroplasty. Clin Orthop Relat Res. 2015;473:2197–203.
13. Uçkay I, Lübbeke A, Harbarth S, Emonet S, Tovmirzaeva L, Agostinho A, et al. Low risk despite high endemicity of methicillin-resistant *Staphylococcus aureus* infections following elective total joint arthroplasty: a 12-year experience. Ann Med. 2012;44:360–8.
14. Teterycz D, Ferry T, Lew D, Stern R, Assal M, Hoffmeyer P, et al. Outcome of orthopedic implant infections due to different staphylococci. Int J Infect Dis. 2010;14:913–8.
15. Al-Mayahi M, Betz M, Müller DA, Stern R, Tahintzi P, Bernard L, et al. Remission rate of implant-related infections following revision surgery after fractures. Int Orthop. 2013;37:2253–8.
16. Mohamad M, Uçkay I, Hannouche D, Miozzari H. Particularities of *Staphylococcus lugdunensis* in orthopaedic infections. Infect Dis (Lond). 2018;50:223–5.
17. Tan TL, Springer BD, Ruder JA, Ruffolo MR, Chen AF. Is Vancomycin-only prophylaxis for patients with penicillin allergy associated with increased risk of infection after Arthroplasty? Clin Orthop Relat Res. 2016;474:1601–6.
18. Gonzalez A, Suvà D, Dunkel N, Nicodème JD, Lomessy A, Lauper N, et al. Are there clinical variables determining antibiotic prophylaxis-susceptible versus resistant infection in open fractures? Int Orthop. 2014;38:2323–7.
19. Lübbeke A, Zingg M, Vu D, Miozzari HH, Christofilopoulos P, Uçkay I, et al. Body mass and weight thresholds for increased prosthetic joint infection rates after primary total joint arthroplasty. Acta Orthop. 2016;87:132–8.
20. Jugun K, Vaudaux P, Garbino J, Pagani L, Hoffmeyer P, Lew D, et al. The safety and efficacy of high-dose daptomycin combined with rifampicin for the treatment of gram-positive osteoarticular infections. Int Orthop. 2013;37:1375–80.
21. Dunkel N, Belaieff W, Assal M, Corni V, Karaca Ş, Lacraz A, et al. Wound dehiscence and stump infection after lower limb amputation: risk factors and association with antibiotic use. J Orthop Sci. 2012;17:588–94.
22. Mangram AJ, Horan TC, Pearson ML, Silver LC, Jarvis WR. Guideline for prevention of surgical site infection, 1999. Centers for Disease Control and Prevention (CDC) Hospital Infection Control Practices Advisory Committee. Am J Infect Control. 1999;27:97–132.
23. Uçkay I, Lübbeke A, Emonet S, Tovmirzaeva L, Stern R, Ferry T, et al. Low incidence of haematogenous seeding to total hip and knee prostheses in patients with remote infections. J Inf Secur. 2009;59:337–45.
24. Sendi P, Christensson B, Uçkay I, Trampuz A, Achermann Y, Boggian K, et al. Group B streptococcus in prosthetic hip and knee joint-associated infections. J Hosp Infect. 2011;79:64–9.
25. Performance Standards for Antimicrobial Susceptibility Testing; 17th Informational Supplement. Clinical and Laboratory Standards Institute. Pennsylvania; USA: Wayne; 2007.
26. European Committee on Antimicrobial Susceptibility Testing. Breakpoint tables for interpretation of MICs. Version. 2014:4 http://www.eucast.org/clinical_breakpoints.
27. Billières J, Uçkay I, Faundez A, Douissard J, Kuczma P, Suvà D, et al. Variables associated with remission in spinal surgical site infections. J Spine Surg. 2016;2:128–34.
28. Lebowitz D, Kressmann B, Gjoni S, Zenelaj B, Grosgurin O, Marti C, et al. Clinical features of anaerobic orthopaedic infections. Infect Dis (Lond). 2017;49:137–40.
29. Al-Mayahi M, Cian A, Lipsky BA, Suvà D, Müller C, Landelle C, et al. Administration of antibiotic agents before intraoperative sampling in orthopedic infections alters culture results. J Inf Secur. 2015;71:518–25.
30. Baraboutis IG, Tsagalou EP, Papakonstantinou I, Marangos MN, Gogos C, Skoutelis AT, et al. Length of exposure to the hospital environment is more important than antibiotic exposure in healthcare associated infections by methicillin-resistant *Staphylococcus aureus*: a comparative study. Braz J Infect Dis. 2011;15:426–35.
31. Nadeem RD, Akhtar M, Cheema OI, Hashmi AR, Nadeem MJ, Nadeem A. Antibiotic prophylaxis in hip surgery: a comparison of two vs. three doses of cefuroxime. J Pak Med Assoc. 2015;65:136–41.
32. Engesaeter LB, Lie SA, Espehaug B, Furnes O, Vollset SE, Havelin LI. Antibiotic prophylaxis in total hip arthroplasty: effects of antibiotic prophylaxis systemically and in bone cement on the revision rate of 22,170 primary hip replacements followed 0-14 years in the Norwegian Arthroplasty register. Acta Orthop Scand. 2003;74:644–51.
33. O'Toole RV, Joshi M, Carlini AR, Murray CK, Allen LE, Scharfstein DO, et al. Local antibiotic therapy to reduce infection after operative treatment of fractures at high risk of infection: a multicenter, randomized, controlled trial (VANCO study). J Orthop Trauma. 2017;31:18 24.

34. Westberg M, Frihagen F, Brun OC, Figved W, Grøgaard B, Valland H, et al. Effectiveness of gentamicin-containing collagen sponges for prevention of surgical site infection after hip arthroplasty: a multicenter randomized trial. Clin Infect Dis. 2015;60:1752–9.

35. Chotai S, Wright PW, Hale AT, Jones WA, McGirt MJ, Patt JC, et al. Does Intrawound Vancomycin application during spine surgery create Vancomycin-resistant organism? Neurosurgery. 2017;80:746–53.

36. Burger JR, Hansen BJ, Leary EV, Aggarwal A, Keeney JA. Dual-agent antibiotic prophylaxis using a single preoperative Vancomycin dose effectively reduces prosthetic joint infection rates with minimal renal toxicity risk. J Arthroplast. 2018;33:213–8.

37. Bosco JA, Tejada PRR, Catanzano AJ, Stachel AG, Phillips MS. Expanded gram-negative antimicrobial prophylaxis reduces surgical site infections in hip Arthroplasty. J Arthroplast. 2016;31:616–21.

38. Bell S, Davey P, Nathwani D, Marwick C, Vadiveloo T, Sneddon J, et al. Risk of AKI with gentamicin as surgical prophylaxis. J Am Soc Nephrol. 2014;25:2625–32.

39. Branch-Elliman W, Ripollone JE, O'Brien WJ, Itani KMF, Schweizer ML, Perencevich E, et al. Risk of surgical site infection, acute kidney injury, and *Clostridium difficile* infection following antibiotic prophylaxis with vancomycin plus a beta-lactam versus either drug alone: a national propensity-score-adjusted retrospective cohort study. PLoS Med. 2017;14: 1002340.

40. Cranny G, Elliott R, Weatherly H, Chambers D, Hawkins N, Myers L, et al. A systematic review and economic model of switching from non-glycopeptide to glycopeptide antibiotic prophylaxis for surgery. Health Technol Assess. 2008;12:1–147.

41. Mini E, Nobili S, Periti P. Methicillin-resistant staphylococci in clean surgery. Is there a role for prophylaxis? Drugs. 1997;54:39–52.

42. Crawford T, Rodvold KA, Solomkin JS. Vancomycin for surgical prophylaxis? Clin Infect Dis. 2012;54:1474–9.

43. Walker H, Patton A, Bayne G, Marwick C, Sneddon J, Davey P, et al. Reduction in post-operative acute kidney injury following a change in antibiotic prophylaxis policy for orthopaedic surgery: an observational study. J Antimicrob Chemother. 2016;71:2598–605.

44. Uçkay I, Pittet D, Vaudaux P, Sax H, Lew D, Waldvogel F. Foreign body infections due to *Staphylococcus epidermidis*. Ann Med. 2008;14:1–11.

19

Implementing an infection control and prevention program decreases the incidence of healthcare-associated infections and antibiotic resistance in a Russian neuro-ICU

Ksenia Ershova[1]* [iD], Ivan Savin[2], Nataliya Kurdyumova[2], Darren Wong[3], Gleb Danilov[4], Michael Shifrin[5], Irina Alexandrova[6], Ekaterina Sokolova[2], Nadezhda Fursova[7], Vladimir Zelman[1,8] and Olga Ershova[9]

Abstract

Background: The impact of infection prevention and control (IPC) programs in limited resource countries such as Russia are largely unknown due to a lack of reliable data. The aim of this study is to evaluate the effect of an IPC program with respect to healthcare associated infection (HAI) prevention and to define the incidence of HAIs in a Russian ICU.

Methods: A pioneering IPC program was implemented in a neuro-ICU at Burdenko Neurosurgery Institute in 2010 and included hand hygiene, surveillance, contact precautions, patient isolation, and environmental cleaning measures. This prospective observational cohort study lasted from 2011 to 2016, included high-risk ICU patients, and evaluated the dynamics of incidence, etiological spectrum, and resistance profile of four types of HAIs, including subgroup analysis of device-associated infections. Survival analysis compared patients with and without HAIs.

Results: We included 2038 high-risk patients. By 2016, HAI cumulative incidence decreased significantly for respiratory HAIs (36.1% vs. 24.5%, *p*-value = 0.0003), urinary-tract HAIs (29.1% vs. 21.3%, p-value = 0.0006), and healthcare-associated ventriculitis and meningitis (HAVM) (16% vs. 7.8%, p-value = 0.004). The incidence rate of EVD-related HAVM dropped from 22.2 to 13.5 cases per 1000 EVD-days. The proportion of invasive isolates of *Klebsiella pneumoniae* and *Acinetobacter baumannii* resistant to carbapenems decreased 1.7 and 2 fold, respectively. HAVM significantly impaired survival and independently increasing the probability of death by 1.43.

Conclusions: The implementation of an evidence-based IPC program in a middle-income country (Russia) was highly effective in HAI prevention with meaningful reductions in antibiotic resistance.

Keywords: Cross infection, Intensive care unit, Infection control, Drug resistance, Survival analysis

* Correspondence: ksenia.ershova@skolkovotech.ru
Center for Data-Intensive Biotechnology and Biomedicine, Skolkovo Institute of Science and Technology, Moscow, Russia

Background

Infection prevention and control (IPC) programs have been repeatedly shown to be effective at decreasing the incidence of healthcare-associated infections (HAIs). A landmark paper on this topic in 1985 showed a 32% decrease in the hospital infection rate after 5 years of an ongoing IPC program [1]. In 1999 the CDC identified seven key evidence-based elements of an effective IPC strategy including voluntary participation of all hospitals, standardized case definitions and protocols, targeted interventions for high risk patient populations, risk adjusted comparisons of infection rates across hospitals, education and adequacy of resources, and feedback to healthcare providers [2]. The elements of an IPC program have since been significantly updated, forming the concept of "multimodal strategy" [3].

To prevent HAIs, the WHO recommends implementing an IPC program in every acute healthcare facility [4]. However, according to the most-recent survey, only 29% of 133 countries surveyed have IPC programs in all tertiary hospitals [3]. In Russia, IPC programs are also not widely used. The rate of HAIs in Russia has been heavily underestimated for decades. In 2016 it was reported to be approximately 0.08% (24,771 [5] cases per 31.3 million hospitalized patients [6]) yet a concurrent meta-analysis which included Russia reported the prevalence of HAIs at 15.5% [7]. According to the latest World Bank report, Russia has a gross national income per capita of US $9720, corresponding to a middle-income country [8].

Besides significant underreporting of HAIs, Russia faces other challenges in establishing IPC programs, such as lack of commitment, punishment-based HAI reporting systems, lack of expertise, and inadequate allocation of resources [9]. Since the dissolution of the Soviet Union, Russia has made some progress in adopting the IPC programs [10]. A pioneering Russian hospital where an evidence-based IPC program was implemented in 2010 is Burdenko National Medical Research Center of Neurosurgery (NSI) in Moscow. Herein we report the results of our study which aimed to evaluate the impact of this program on HAI prevention in the ICU.

Methods

Study design and healthcare facility

This study was a prospective observational cohort study with annual interim data analyses. The study was done in the neuro-ICU department at NSI in Moscow, Russia. NSI is a specialized neurosurgical hospital with 300 beds that cares for approximately 8000 patients per year, 95% of whom undergo surgery. The NSI ICU has 38 single-bed rooms with a flow of approximately 3000 patients per year.

Infection prevention and control program

In September 2010, an IPC program was first set up in the neuro-ICU, inspired by the results of the European HELICS-ICU program [11]. The protocols for our IPC program were adopted from the 2007 CDC guidelines [12] and included three key components: education, infection prevention measures, and surveillance (Fig. 1). The surveillance software was designed in-house and integrated in the NSI electronic health record system [13]. At the time of initiation of this program, an antibiotic stewardship program was in existence at our facility. However, during the study period there were refinements to this program and coordination of antibiotic stewardship initiatives with the infection control program.

Patients

We studied a high-risk patient population, which we defined as patients who required > 48 h of care in the neurosurgical ICU. All of these patients were qualified to participate in the study until discharge or death. Enrollment period was between January 1st, 2011 and December 31st, 2016. Following ICU discharge, the parameters of total length of stay and outcome were collected.

To identify cases of HAIs, we used the 2008 CDC definition [14]. Four types of HAIs were surveilled: bloodstream, respiratory and urinary-tract infections, and healthcare-associated ventriculitis and meningitis (HAVM). We specifically focused on the subgroup of device-related infections, such as central line-associated bloodstream infections (CLABSI), ventilator-associated pneumonia (VAP), catheter-associated urinary-tract infections (CAUTI), and external ventricular drain (EVD)-associated HAVM. In accordance with the CDC case definitions, an infection was considered device-related if the patient had a device in place for > 48 h prior to developing the HAI [12].

In addition to HAIs, we monitored superficial surgical-site infections (SSSI) after neurosurgery, and ICU-acquired intestinal dysfunction. The latter was clinically defined by the presence of one or more of the following gastrointestinal symptoms, as delineated in the literature [15]: vomiting, diarrhea, absence or abnormality of bowel sounds, bowel dilation, gastrointestinal bleeding, or increased nasogastric aspirate volume (> 500 ml/day).

Data collection and preprocessing

Data was collected prospectively on a daily basis and incorporated 54 different characteristics (Additional file 1: Table S1). The spectrum and susceptibility profile of identified organisms causing the HAIs was built for each infection type. In January of each year, interim analysis was performed, and the results were then disseminated to NSI staff to encourage compliance with IPC measures.

Microbiological analysis

Clinical samples were collected form patients with HAIs and delivered to the microbiological laboratory without

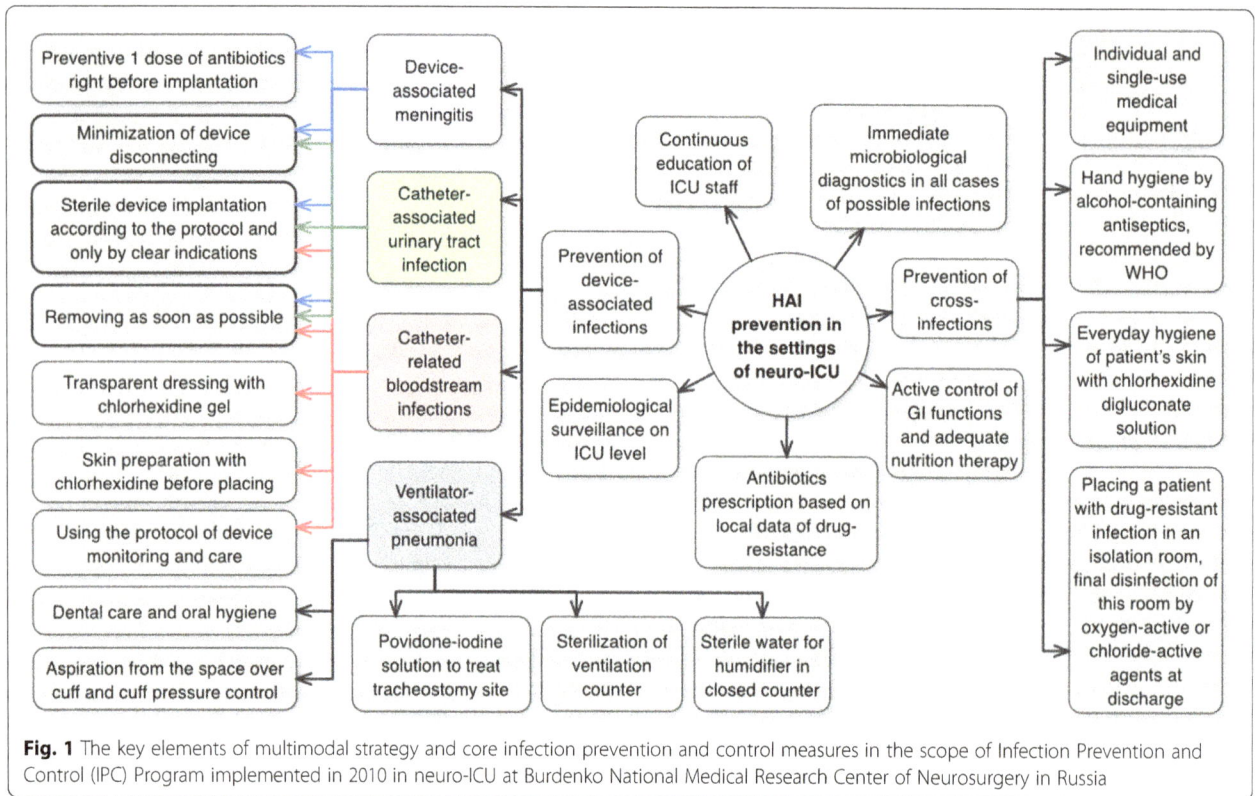

Fig. 1 The key elements of multimodal strategy and core infection prevention and control measures in the scope of Infection Prevention and Control (IPC) Program implemented in 2010 in neuro-ICU at Burdenko National Medical Research Center of Neurosurgery in Russia

delay. Blood and CSF samples were processed using BD BACTEC (Becton, Dickinson and Company, USA). All samples of pure bacterial cultures underwent automated identification by VITEK®2 (Biomerieux, France) with standard AST Cards. Selected samples of pure bacterial cultures were subsequently identified by MALDI-TOF MS, MALDI Biotyper® (Bruker Daltonik GmbH, Germany). Minimal inhibitory concentrations obtained from VITEK®2 were interpreted in accordance with the current CLSI guidelines [16]. A profile of antibiotic resistance for each strain was built using the WHONET software [17].

Statistical analysis

Statistical analysis was performed in Python3.6 using StatsModels [18] and Scipy [19]. Categorical variables for dichotomous events were reported as number of events of one category with percentage and 95% confidence interval (CI) for binomial distribution. Continuous variables were reported as a median value with first and third quartiles (Q1; Q3). Incidence of HAIs was calculated as a number of cases per 100 high-risk patients or as a number of cases per 1000 patient-days. DA-HAIs were measured as cases per 1000 device-days. Device utilization ratio (DUR) was calculated as proportion of device-days to patient-days. We used Chi-square test to compare binary and categorical variables and linear regression analysis to compare continuous variables over years. In survival analysis we

used Cox regression, including HAIs, diagnosis, surgeries, and preexisting characteristics. Log-rank test was used to compare survival curves. *P*-values below 0.05 were considered statistically significant.

Results

A total of 2038 patients of all ages and both genders were included in the study during 6 years (the study data set is available at https://doi.org/10.5281/zenodo.1021503). The code for data analysis is available at https://github.com/KseniaErshova/IPC_paper.git.

Study population included 50% males, 16.9% children under 18 years, and a patient median age of 46 [Q1;Q3: 26.0; 59.0] years. The patients were uniformly distributed across the years by disease types, surgery types, and patient features. However, the number of lethal outcomes and the length of stay in the ICU decreased from 2011 to 2016. The baseline characteristics of the study population for each year and averaged over the 6 years are shown in Table 1.

HAIs and patients' stay in the ICU

A median number of 344 [Q1;Q3: 330; 349] patients per year accounted for a median 6998 [Q1;Q3: 6678; 7399] patient-days per year (Additional file 1: Table S2). Since the number of patients increased from 2011 to 2016 by an average of 2.3% annually and the number of patient-days gradually decreased simultaneously by 2.7%

Table 1 Baseline characteristics of the study population by years

	Parameters	Total	2011	2012	2013	2014	2015	2016	p-value
			No of pts. (%)	No of pts. (%)	No of pts. (%)	No of pts. (%)	No of pts. (%)	No of pts. (%)	
	Patients, total	2038	313 (100%)	350 (100%)	361 (100%)	341 (100%)	326 (100%)	347 (100%)	1.000
	Children	345 (16.9%)	52 (16.6%)	57 (16.3%)	58 (16.1%)	65 (19.1%)	42 (12.9%)	71 (20.5%)	0.315
	Male gender	1020 (50%)	154 (49.2%)	184 (52.6%)	186 (51.5%)	168 (49.3%)	164 (50.3%)	164 (47.3%)	0.976
Diagnosis	Brain trauma	255 (12.5%)	43 (13.7%)	54 (15.4%)	51 (14.1%)	41 (12.0%)	28 (8.6%)	38 (11.0%)	0.192
	Brain tumor	1271 (62.4%)	185 (59.1%)	221 (63.1%)	240 (66.5%)	200 (58.7%)	209 (64.1%)	216 (62.2%)	0.911
	Congenital disorders	23 (1.1%)	4 (1.3%)	5 (1.4%)	3 (0.8%)	7 (2.1%)	2 (0.6%)	2 (0.6%)	0.436
	Vascular brain diseases	454 (22.3%)	77 (24.6%)	60 (17.1%)	63 (17.5%)	89 (26.1%)	80 (24.5%)	85 (24.5%)	0.066
	Other diseases	29 (1.4%)	3 (1.0%)	10 (2.9%)	4 (1.1%)	4 (1.2%)	4 (1.2%)	4 (1.2%)	0.302
Surgeries	Craniotomy	1537 (75.4%)	230 (73.5%)	261 (74.6%)	279 (77.3%)	262 (76.8%)	245 (75.2%)	260 (74.9%)	0.998
	INSD	650 (31.9%)	101 (32.3%)	130 (37.1%)	124 (34.3%)	112 (32.8%)	94 (28.8%)	89 (25.6%)	0.227
	Endovascular surgery	194 (9.5%)	31 (9.9%)	37 (10.6%)	26 (7.2%)	40 (11.7%)	25 (7.7%)	35 (10.1%)	0.407
	EETS	87 (4.3%)	13 (4.2%)	15 (4.3%)	15 (4.2%)	14 (4.1%)	15 (4.6%)	15 (4.3%)	1.000
	Spinal surgery	4 (0.2%)	1 (0.3%)	0 (0.0%)	0 (0.0%)	0 (0.0%)	2 (0.6%)	1 (0.3%)	0.377
	Other surgeries	873 (42.8%)	151 (48.2%)	161 (46.0%)	156 (43.2%)	146 (42.8%)	127 (39.0%)	132 (38.0%)	0.523
Outcomes	Recovery	80 (3.9%)	15 (4.8%)	14 (4.0%)	14 (3.9%)	19 (5.6%)	9 (2.8%)	9 (2.6%)	0.365
	Positive dynamics	934 (45.8%)	133 (42.5%)	153 (43.7%)	170 (47.1%)	159 (46.6%)	150 (46.0%)	169 (48.7%)	0.934
	No dynamics	210 (10.3%)	34 (10.9%)	41 (11.7%)	37 (10.2%)	30 (8.8%)	29 (8.9%)	39 (11.2%)	0.818
	Negative dynamics	505 (24.8%)	81 (25.9%)	67 (19.1%)	78 (21.6%)	92 (27.0%)	96 (29.4%)	91 (26.2%)	0.153
	Death	307 (15%)	50 (16.0%)	75 (21.4%)	62 (17.2%)	41 (12.0%)	41 (12.6%)	38 (11.0%)	0.009
		Median [Q1;Q3]	Median [Q1;Q3]	Median [Q1;Q3]	Median [Q1;Q3]	Median [Q1;Q3]	Median [Q1;Q3]	Median [Q1;Q3]	p-value
	Age, years	46 [26.0; 59.0]	44 [25.0; 57.0]	44 [25.0; 58.0]	47 [26.0; 60.0]	44 [25.0; 57.0]	50 [30.0; 59.75]	48 [24.5; 60.5]	0.099
	CCI score	3 [2.0; 5.0]	3 [2.0; 4.0]	3 [2.0; 5.0]	3 [2.0; 5.0]	3 [2.0; 4.0]	3 [2.0; 5.0]	3 [2.0; 4.0]	1.000
	Length of stay in ICU, days	10 [6.0; 22.0]	13 [7.0; 27.0]	12 [6.0; 25.0]	10 [6.0; 24.0]	8 [6.0; 22.0]	9 [6.0; 22.0]	8 [5.0; 17.0]	0.010

Abbreviations: *INSD* Implantation of neurosurgical devices, *EETS* Endoscopic endonasal transsphenoidal surgery, *CCI* Charlson comorbidity index

per year (from 6778 to 5809), an average patient spent less time in the ICU, from the median of 13 days [Q1;Q3: 7.0; 27.0] in 2011 to 8 days [Q1;Q3: 5.0; 17.0] in 2016, p-value = 0.01 (Table 1). We found that over the six-year study, the lowest percentage of DA-HAIs was in the HAVM group: 40.4% [95% CI 33.6–47.1]. The highest percentage of DA-HAIs was in healthcare-associated bloodstream infections: 86.6% [95% CI 80.4–92.7]. Thus, most healthcare-associated bloodstream infections were CLABSI, whereas less than half of HAVM cases were EVD-associated (Additional file 1: Table S3, Fig. 2).

DUR was relatively high for mechanical ventilation (0.65 [Q1;Q3: 0.65; 0.69]), central line (0.70 [Q1;Q3: 0.66; 0.76]), and urinary catheter (0.70 [Q1;Q3: 0.67; 0.72]), but low for EVD (0.12 [Q1;Q3: 0.12; 0.13]) (Additional file 1: Table S2, Fig. 2). Although, DURs varied slightly over time, we observed a significant decrease in the number of days with respiratory HAIs: from 1643 days in 2011 to 690 in 2016 (mean annual reduction rate 11.9%, p-value = 0.038), while the number of

days with VAP remained unchanged (Fig. 2a). The number of patients with HAVM and with DA-HAVM decreased significantly from 2011 to 2016 (Fig. 2d).

Incidence of healthcare-associated infections

The incidence of all-cause HAIs and DA-HAIs was analyzed. The cumulative incidence of all-cause HAIs decreased significantly for respiratory infections (from 36.1% [95% CI 30.8–41.4] in 2011 to 24.5% [95% CI 20.0–29.0] in 2016, p-value = 0.0003), urinary tract infections (from 29.07% [95% CI 24.0–34.1] in 2011 to 21.33% [95% CI 17.0–25.6], p-value = 0.0006), and HAVM (from 15.97% [95% CI 11.9–20.0] in 2011 to 7.78% [95% CI 5.0–10.6] in 2016, p-value = 0.004) (Fig. 3a, Additional file 1: Table S4). Time-adjusted incidence rate of all-cause HAIs identified a declining trend for all four types of HAIs (Fig. 3c). In the group of DA-HAIs, only the cumulative incidence of CAUTI decreased significantly, from 28.04 [95% CI 22.7–33.4] per

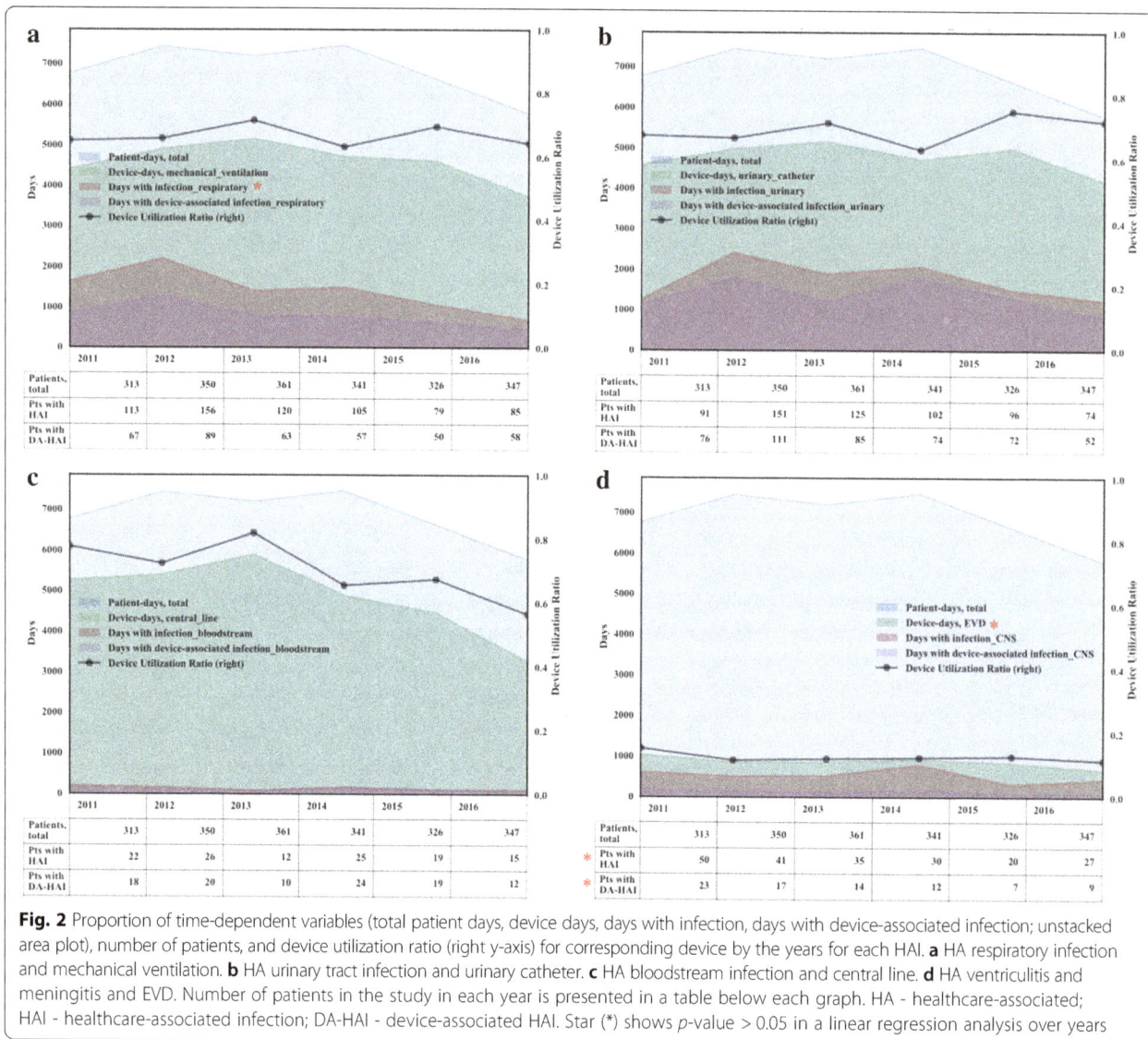

Fig. 2 Proportion of time-dependent variables (total patient days, device days, days with infection, days with device-associated infection; unstacked area plot), number of patients, and device utilization ratio (right y-axis) for corresponding device by the years for each HAI. **a** HA respiratory infection and mechanical ventilation. **b** HA urinary tract infection and urinary catheter. **c** HA bloodstream infection and central line. **d** HA ventriculitis and meningitis and EVD. Number of patients in the study in each year is presented in a table below each graph. HA - healthcare-associated; HAI - healthcare-associated infection; DA-HAI - device-associated HAI. Star (*) shows p-value > 0.05 in a linear regression analysis over years

100 patients with a urinary catheter in 2011 to 18.31 [95% CI 13.8–22.8] in 2016, p-value = 0.026 (Fig. 3b, Additional file 1: Table S4). However, once we adjusted incidence to the device-days at risk, EVD-associated HAVM demonstrated a significant drop from 2011 to 2016 (22.2 vs. 13.5 cases per 1000 EVD-days, respectively) (Fig. 3d, Additional file 1: Table S2). Risk-adjusted incidence of VAP and CAUTI also trended toward a decrease. The incidence rate of CLABSI did not change and remained at the median level of 3.7 [Q1;Q3: 3.5; 4.1] per 1000 central line-days (Fig. 3d, Additional file 1: Table S2). Of note, in 2012 the rates of respiratory and urinary HAIs as well as VAP and CAUTI spiked increasing 4–14% compare to 2011 (Additional file 1: Table S4). Therefore, the reduction in infection rate at the end of the study period in 2016 was more pronounced when compared to peak rates seen in 2012.

Microbiological profile of HAIs

We observed that in 2011–2012 approximately half of bloodstream HAIs were caused by *Klebsiella pneumoniae* and *Acinetobacter baumannii*. However, in 2016 the proportion of *K. pneumoniae* decreased to 14% from a high of 47% in 2012 and *A. baumannii* did not appear on the profile for the first time (Fig. 4a). There was a tendency for Gram-negative species to be replaced by Gram-positive species (Fig. 4a). For other HAIs, the etiological spectrum remained relatively stable over time (Additional file 1: Figures S1–S3).

By 2016 *K. pneumoniae* became more susceptible to the most-tested antibiotics: there were significantly fewer isolates resistant to cephalosporins, ciprofloxacin, and imipenem as compared to 2011 (Additional file 1: Figure S4). The proportion of imipenem-resistant *K. pneumoniae* decreased from 34.5% [95% CI 29.9–39.1] in 2011 to 20.2% [95% CI 15.6–24.8], p-value < 0.001 (Fig. 4b).

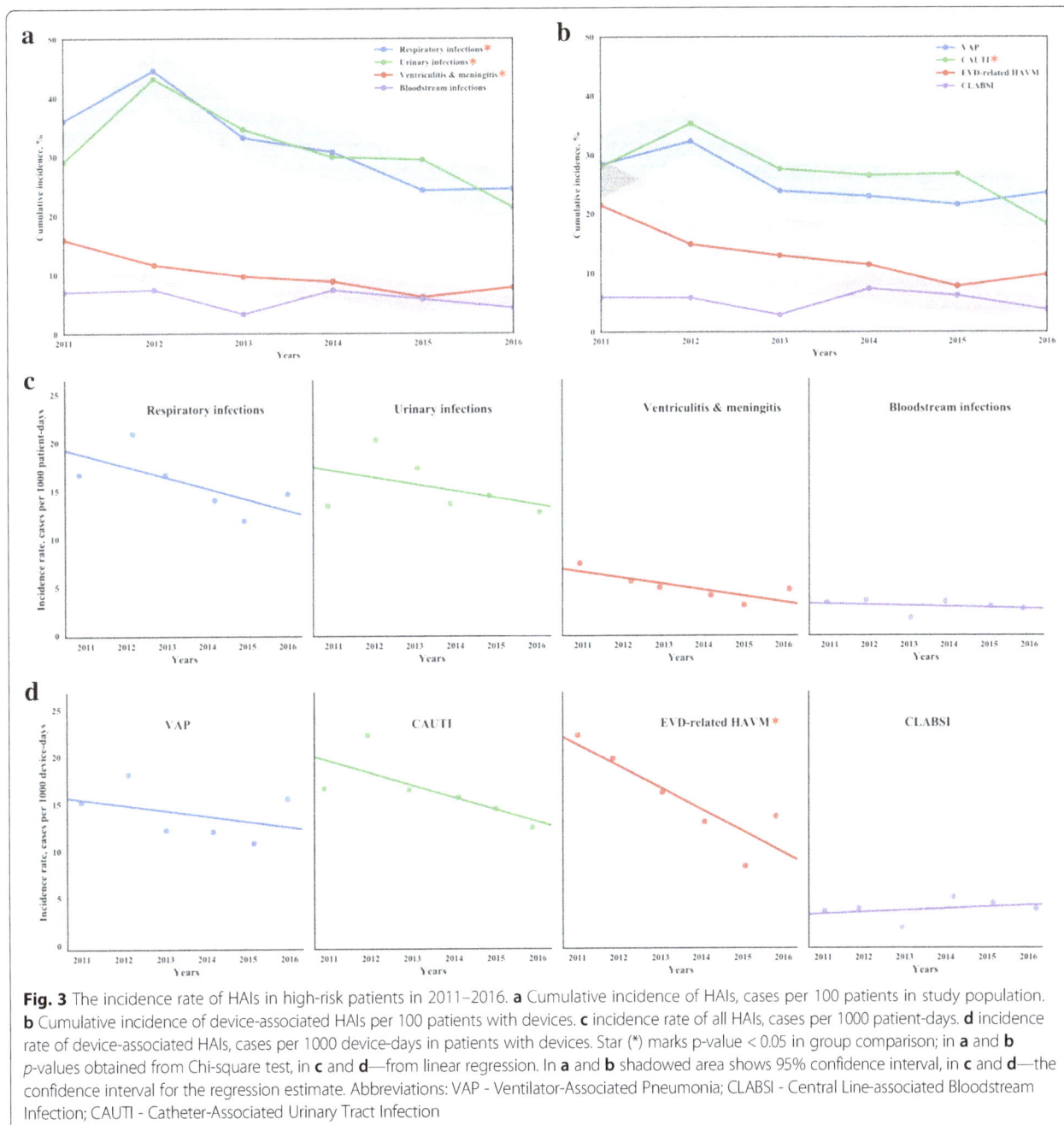

Fig. 3 The incidence rate of HAIs in high-risk patients in 2011–2016. **a** Cumulative incidence of HAIs, cases per 100 patients in study population. **b** Cumulative incidence of device-associated HAIs per 100 patients with devices. **c** incidence rate of all HAIs, cases per 1000 patient-days. **d** incidence rate of device-associated HAIs, cases per 1000 device-days in patients with devices. Star (*) marks p-value < 0.05 in group comparison; in **a** and **b** p-values obtained from Chi-square test, in **c** and **d**—from linear regression. In **a** and **b** shadowed area shows 95% confidence interval, in **c** and **d**—the confidence interval for the regression estimate. Abbreviations: VAP - Ventilator-Associated Pneumonia; CLABSI - Central Line-associated Bloodstream Infection; CAUTI - Catheter-Associated Urinary Tract Infection

Dramatic changes were found in cephalosporin resistance, e.g. in 2011 there were 90.3% isolates resistant to cefepime [95% CI 87.4–93.1] vs. 45.6% [95% CI 39.9–51.4] in 2016, p-value < 0.001 (Additional file 1: Figure S4).

The number of imipenem-resistant isolates of *A. baumannii* decreased from 77.7% [95% CI 72.3–83.0] in 2011 to 38% [95% CI 30.9–45.1] in 2016, p-value < 0.001 (Fig. 4b). While the proportion of ampicillin/sulbactam-resistant isolates increased from 48.1% [95% CI 34.8–61.5] in 2011 to 82% [95% CI 76.2–87.9] in 2016, p-value < 0.001, the resistance to the rest of tested antibiotics

remained virtually unchanged (Additional file 1: Figure S5). These changes in resistance occurred with a concurrent reduction in antibiotic utilization over the study period. Antibiotic use was measured as antibiotic-days per 1000 patient-days. The rate of antibiotic utilization was initially 1066 antibiotic days per 1000 patient-days in 2011. This highlights that multiple antibiotics were administered in many patients and a high overall usage rate was in effect. Over the six-year study period the utilization rate consistently declined. In 2016 the utilization rate was 807 antibiotic days per 1000 patient-days.

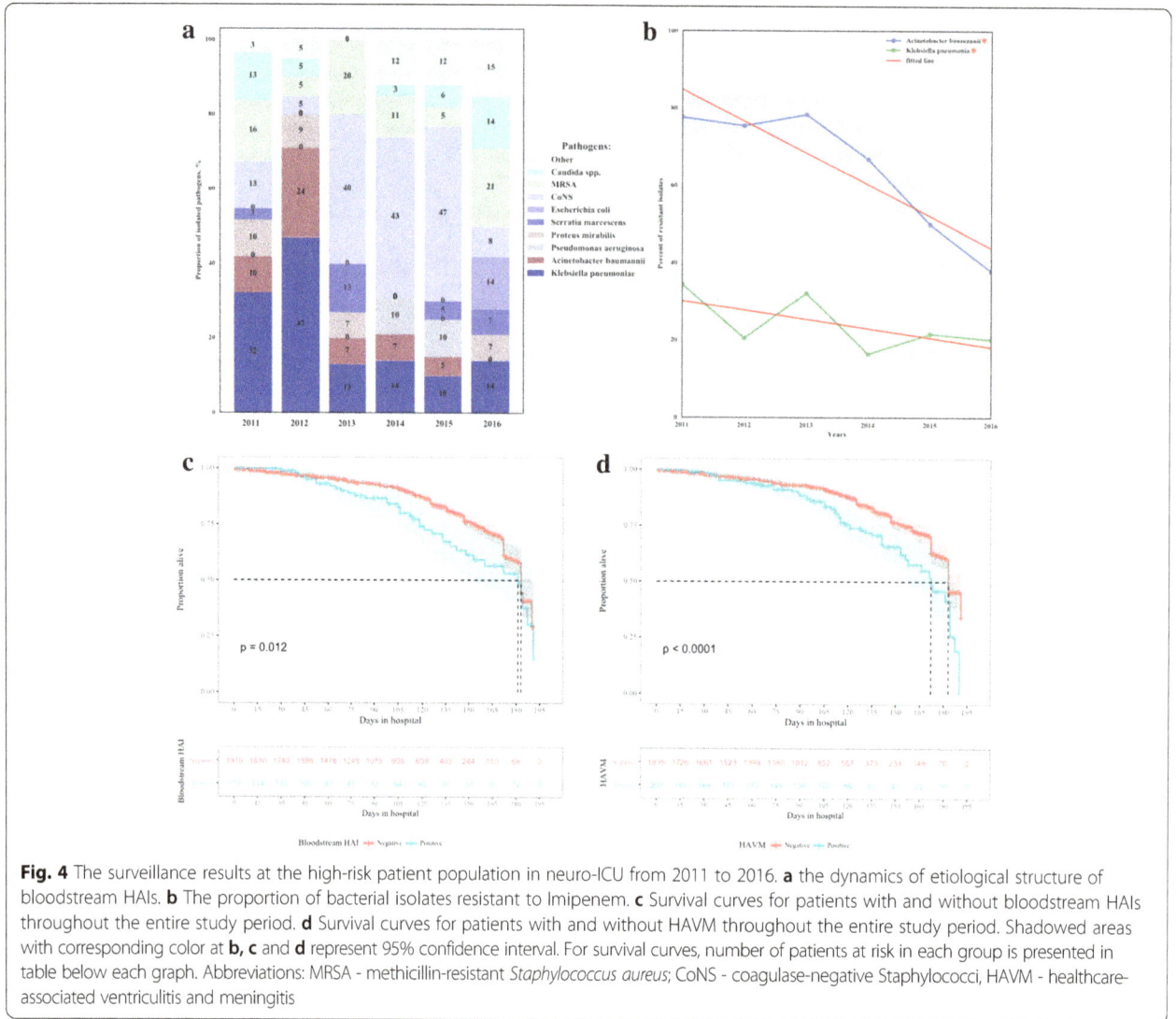

Fig. 4 The surveillance results at the high-risk patient population in neuro-ICU from 2011 to 2016. **a** the dynamics of etiological structure of bloodstream HAIs. **b** The proportion of bacterial isolates resistant to Imipenem. **c** Survival curves for patients with and without bloodstream HAIs throughout the entire study period. **d** Survival curves for patients with and without HAVM throughout the entire study period. Shadowed areas with corresponding color at **b, c** and **d** represent 95% confidence interval. For survival curves, number of patients at risk in each group is presented in table below each graph. Abbreviations: MRSA - methicillin-resistant *Staphylococcus aureus*; CoNS - coagulase-negative Staphylococci, HAVM - healthcare-associated ventriculitis and meningitis

Survival analysis in patients with HAIs

Bloodstream HAIs and HAVM significantly impair survival (log-rank *p*-values = 0.012 and < 0.0001, respectively), Fig. 4c and 4d. In order to confirm their influence on mortality, multifactorial survival analyses were done by Cox regression (Additional file 1: Table S5). We confirmed that only HAVM affected survival independently from other factors, increasing the probability of death 1.43 times (95% CI 1.03–1.98, p-value = 0.034). Other types of HAIs did not influence survival (Additional file 1: Figure S6). Besides HAIs, other factors were shown to independently affect survival. While brain tumor (HR = 1.57 [95% CI 1.1–2.24], p-value = 0.012) and implantation of neurosurgical devices (HR = 1.59 [95% CI 1.24–2.03], p-value = 0.0002) enhanced mortality, craniotomy decreased mortality: HR = 0.64 [95% CI 0.48–0.87], p-value = 0.0037 (Additional file 1: Figure S7).

ICU-acquired intestinal dysfunction

The cumulative incidence of overall intestinal dysfunctions dropped from 54.9% [95% CI 49.4–60.5] in 2011 to 23.9% [95% CI 19.4–28.4] in 2016, p-value < 0.001 (Additional file 1: Figure S8A, Additional file 1: Table S6). Intestinal dysfunction impaired survival independently increasing the probability of death 1.46 times [95% CI 1.11–1.93], p-value = 0.0069; log-rank test p-value = 0.019 (Additional file 1: Figure S8D).

Discussion

A comprehensive IPC program with a focus on hand hygiene and patient isolation was started in NSI's ICU in 2010 (Fig. 1a). By that time, the use of our IPC program to prevent HAIs in the ICU became a paradigm-shifting solution across Russia as HAI prevention strategies had previously remained unchanged for years and had become outdated [20].

The importance of HAI prevention programs is clearly indicated by the observation that HAIs directly deteriorate patient survival. It was found that HAIs increased the probability of death by 1.4–1.5 [21] and odds of mortality increased 1.5 to 1.9-fold [22]. In our study, we found that HAVM decreased the probability of survival by 1.43, while other HAIs did not significantly influence survival. It has been previously reported that HAVM increased mortality rate approximately three times [23]. Although the exact mechanism is not yet understood, prospective studies have found that in ICU patients, gastrointestinal dysfunction is also an independent risk factor for increased mortality [15]. We can postulate that the intestinal microbiome serves an important role in immune function and consequently, is a well described reservoir for antibiotic resistance [24]. Additionally, in critically ill patients intestinal dysbiosis could be postulated as a potential contributor to gut translocation of pathogens and may play a role in enteric absorption. In our study, ICU-acquired intestinal dysfunction decreased the probability of survival by 1.46, which is consistent with earlier studies. The implementation of IPC initiatives and the accompanying reduction in the incidence of infections, thereby reducing the requirement for antibiotics, can be assumed to at least in part account for reduction in gastrointestinal dysbiosis. This finding further highlights the potential unseen morbidity impact of IPC beyond simple measures of antibiotic utilization and resistance rates.

The implementation of the IPC program was followed by significant reduction of HAIs in the ICU. In fact, the impact of this program may actually be under-estimated. Our IPC program was implemented in 9/2010 whereas study data collection began 1/2011. Therefore, although adherence to IPC protocols would be expected to improve with greater time and familiarity, the totality of impact of this program may be under-estimated. Key initiatives, such as early removal of indwelling catheters, would be expected to have an immediate impact in the reduction of nosocomial infections. Even discounting the IPC impact in the initial months after implementation, the fact that a sustained and continued reduction in HAI rate occurred is both meaningful and serves as a reinforcement of overall utility. In high-risk ICU patients we observed a substantial decrease in HAI incidence: cumulative incidence of respiratory HAIs declined by 1.47 (from 36.1 to 24.5%), urinary tract HAIs by 1.4-fold (from 29.1 to 21.3%), HAVM by twofold (from 16 to 7.8%), CAUTI by 1.93 (from 35.4 to 18.3%) (Fig. 3), and ICU-acquired intestinal dysfunction by 2.3 fold. These results are consistent with previously reported evidence, demonstrating a reduction of HAI prevalence by approximately 1.7 fold (from 11.7 to 6.8%) [25].

We also found that the risk-adjusted incidence of EVD-related HAVM reduced 1.64 fold (from 22.2 to 13.5 cases per 1000 EVD-days) over the six-year study period. The impact of an IPC program on decreasing DA-HAI incidence has been previously reported. For example, one publication reported a 2.7-fold decrease in CAUTI episodes per 100 patients within a year after IPC implementation [26]. However, for some HAIs, like HAVM, such statistics are absent. In addition, the changes in the incidence of intestinal dysfunction could be confounded by the implementation of an advanced nutritional protocol in 2012 at the ICU.

We did find that in 2012 the rates of several infection subcategories did increase in comparison to 2011. The rate of respiratory and urinary HAIs had increases ranging from 4 to 14% compared to 2011. The reason for this increase is unclear, but we postulate that this may be related to several factors. One contributor may be that staff were educated on the appropriate identification of HAIs and utilized clear standardized case definitions. As staff became more familiar with these definitions, they may have been able to better identify cases leading to an apparent increase in infection rates. Additionally, during initial implementation of IPC protocols, staff underwent in-service training and consequently there was a specific focus on the strict adherence to protocols. However, adherence to infection control practices may wane with time, and that probably what happened in 2012. Therefore, continued reinforcement of best practices along with feedback to healthcare teams is necessary for sustained adherence to IPC initiatives. Following the re-education of staff, a renewed attention to IPC may have contributed to reductions seen in 2013 HAI rate.

Additionally, both the length of patients' stays in the ICU and the incidence of patient mortality did decrease over the study period. Although a direct causality cannot be determined, it would be fair to postulate that the associated decrease in HAI incidence may at least have been a partial contributor for this reduction. Thus, a reduction in the rate of HAIs may result in a meaningful reduction in healthcare cost, and potential benefit in overall mortality. However, we did not monitor all other parameters that could have influenced the mortality and the length of stay, thus other explanations should be investigated. Additionally, we admit that the overall approach in patient treatment did not change much, and the DUR did not change for any of the devices we monitored.

The prevention of the spread of carbapenem-resistant, Gram-negative bacteria was named the first priority of IPC efforts by the latest WHO guidelines because these strains pose significant threat to global health [27]. We found firstly that the proportion of such Gram-negatives as K. pneumoniae and A. baumannii in the spectrum of bloodstream HAIs decreased and secondly that the resistance of both pathogens to carbapenems was significantly reduced. In our study the initial percentage of isolates resistant to imipenem was 34.5% for *K. pneumonia* and 77.7% for *A. baumannii*. By the end of the study, the percentage decreased 1.7- and 2-fold, respectively (Fig. 4b). The initial prevalence of carbapenem-resistant isolates in the NSI neuro-ICU was shown to be higher than the mean prevalence in Europe (8.1% for *K. pneumoniae* and 50% for *A. baumannii*), and in the U.S. (7.9% for *K. pneumoniae* and 49.5% for *A. baumannii*) [27]. This finding could partly be explained by the study population because we analyzed only intensive care unit patients which may be a higher risk population. However, we postulate these initial rates of carbapenem resistance were at least in part due to nosocomial cross-infection of patients.

Our hypothesis is that the implementation of IPC protocols acted in a two-fold manner with an initial reduction in nosocomial patient-to-patient transmission which consequently lead to a reduction in nosocomial infection rate. Our most critical interventions involved implementation of contact precautions utilizing gloves, gown, and mask, isolation of patients identified with carbapenemase resistance genes, and cohorting of patients with *Acinetobacter* or *Klebsiella* (Fig. 1). These efforts were paired with intensive environmental disinfection measures, skin antisepsis for indwelling devices, as well as initiates focused on hand hygiene as a multi-modal strategy (Fig. 1).

Of note, hand hygiene compliance was particularly difficult to implement with a compliance rate of 27% in 2011. Compliance with hand hygiene in the subsequent years 2012 through 2016 were 40, 69, 63, 68, and 81% respectively. The reduction in infection rate over time could reasonably be postulated to result in a secondary reduction in the necessity of broad spectrum antibiotic therapy. This reduction in antibiotic utilization is underscored by the dramatic decline in the rate of antibiotic utilization over the study period. It must be noted that an antibiotic stewardship program was in existence prior to IPC implementation. Antibiotic stewardship involved institutional protocols for perioperative antibiotic prophylaxis and for empiric antibiotic therapy. However, integration of IPC protocols, including surveillance measures may have enhanced the effectiveness of antibiotic stewardship interventions. The ultimate result was that within the study period, our observed resistance rates decreased to the level of global and regional estimations.

This improvement in susceptibility rates, is in contrast to the global trend of increasing carbapenem resistance over the past decade [27], indicating that in limited-resource settings IPC programs can be highly effective. The programs may be especially significant in healthcare settings with high levels of resistance where they can serve as a cost-effective intervention leading to a substantial clinical impact. The substantial diminution in carbapenem resistance supports the notion that implemented IPC strategies contain effective measures to prevent and control the resistance to carbapenems (Fig. 1). Moreover, this is supported by the recent WHO guidelines which affirmed that the core components of multimodal IPC strategy can help to prevent carbapenem resistance.

This paper reports a prospective study of the impact of an infection control program in a high acuity limited resource setting with regard to the reduction in HAI risk. Such studies are limited to date but have been identified by the WHO as particularly needed [27]. Thus, this study can help to fill this research gap providing insight regarding an approach to implantation of these programs and highlighting the most essential IPC components. Our results suggest that a focus on robust surveillance paired with isolation/infection control measures can promote a sustainable and meaningful reduction in HAI incidence and antibiotic resistance.

The current study has certain limitations. It is a single-center study in a highly specialized ICU facility. Thus, one should be careful when generalizing these results to other hospitals and other wards. In addition, we only studied a cohort of high-risk patients, those staying in the dedicated neuro-ICU for > 48 h—not the entire ICU population. Thus, reported HAI incidences are higher than those calculated for the entire ICU population. However, the underlying principles of our IPC program leading to the reduction of CAUTI, CLABSI, and VAP would be expected to be generalizable to other hospitalized settings with a similar expected impact.

One aspect that was not able to be fully evaluated were *Clostridium difficile* infections (CDI). The prevalence of CDI, identified by a positive PCR stool assay and compatible symptoms, was measured quarterly. However, the quarterly rate included all patients in the ICU at the time of a positive diagnosis and included patients that did not meet the defined criteria for high-risk population that were studied. Additionally, the incidence rate was low throughout the six-year period with a peak rate of 1.5% in 2011 and a nadir of 0.9% in 2015. Notably, patients who were transferred out of the ICU and subsequently developed CDI would not have been identified. Therefore, we can postulate that IPC initiatives may result in a reduction in CDI as the rate did decline from 2011; however, the low overall incidence of CDI and aforementioned limitations do not allow for definitive conclusions.

By design, the study did not include a control group (i.e. a group treated in the ICU before the IPC program had been implemented), because HAI rates without surveillance are unknown. Moreover, the decrease of HAI incidence and length of stay in the ICU could be explained by modification of clinical practices and by regression to the mean. It should be mentioned that survival analysis in our study suffers from immortal time bias. Patients in the HAI group are "immortal" until they get the infection, that favors the HAI group by lowering mortality rate in this group. Thus, HAIs have a stronger influence on survival, posing a higher risk of death in patients once they get HAIs.

Conclusion

Implementation of an evidence-based IPC program was strongly associated with a significant reduction in HAIs in the neuro-ICU. Over a six-year period, there was a decreasing HAI incidence, reduction in the prevalence of carbapenem-resistant invasive bacterial isolates, and consequently improved patient outcomes. Our study supports the finding that an IPC program can be highly effective in a middle-income country (Russia) despite the lack of a national surveillance system and limited resources. Expansion of IPC initiatives, potentially paired with a robust antimicrobial stewardship program, should be considered in resource limited settings as a feasible cost-effective opportunity to achieve meaningful reductions in antibiotic resistance and HAI incidence.

Abbreviations
CAUTI: Catheter-associated urinary tract infection; CDC: Centers for Disease Control and Prevention; CI: Confidence interval; CLABSI: Central line-associated bloodstream infections; DA-HAI: Device-associated HAI; DUR: Device utilization ratio; EVD: External ventricular drain; HAI: Healthcare-associated infection; HAVM: Healthcare-associated ventriculitis and meningitis; HR: Hazard ratio; ICU: Intensive care unit; IPC: Infection prevention and control; NSI: Burdenko National Medical Research Center of Neurosurgery; Q1; Q3: First and third quartiles; SSSI: Superficial surgical site infection; VAP: Ventilator-associated pneumonia; WHO: World Health Organization

Acknowledgements
The authors gratefully acknowledge the contributions of many people who helped to develop, support, implement, and guide this study. Special thanks to all NSI clinicians, nurses, and administrators who patiently accepted and complied with the IPC program, and helped to collect data. We'd like to acknowledge the contribution of Dr. Yulia Savochkina and Dr. Svetlana Sazykina who helped with the microbiological assay. We are grateful for the help with data analysis to Dr. Anton Barchuk (Saint Petersburg Cancer Center), Dr. Rashied Amini (NASA-JPL), and Oleg Khomenko (Skoltech). We thank for providing language help and proofreading to Michael Saint-Onge (Los Angeles Public Library), also Travis Nielsen (University of Southern California).

Authors' contributions
KE and DW analyzed data and wrote the manuscript; OE and IS developed, implemented and maintained IPC program in the ICU; NK, GD, and ES collected data, evaluated and treated study subjects; MS developed and supported electronic surveillance protocol; NF and IA performed microbiological testing; VZ consulted with study design and promoted the IPC program implementation. All authors read and approved the final manuscript.

Consent for publication
All authors they have seen and approved the manuscript and granted the consent for its publication.

Competing interests
The authors declare that they have no competing interests.

Author details
[1]Center for Data-Intensive Biotechnology and Biomedicine, Skolkovo Institute of Science and Technology, Moscow, Russia. [2]Department of Intensive Care, Burdenko National Medical Research Center of Neurosurgery, Moscow, Russia. [3]Division of Infectious Diseases, Keck School of Medicine, University of Southern California, Los Angeles, USA. [4]Laboratory of Biomedical Informatics, Burdenko National Medical Research Center of Neurosurgery, Moscow, Russia. [5]IT Department, Burdenko National Medical Research Center of Neurosurgery, Moscow, Russia. [6]Department of Microbiology, Burdenko National Medical Research Center of Neurosurgery, Moscow, Russia. [7]Federal Budget Institution of Science "State Research Center for Applied Microbiology & Biotechnology" (SRCAMB), Moscow, Russia. [8]Department of Anesthesiology, Keck School of Medicine, University of Southern California, Los Angeles, USA. [9]Department of Epidemiology and Infection Control, Burdenko National Medical Research Center of Neurosurgery, Moscow, Russia.

References
1. Haley R, Culver D, White J, Morgan W, Emori T, Munn V, Hooton T. The efficacy of infection surveillance and control programs in preventing nosocomial infections in US hospitals. Am J Epidemiol. 1985;121(2):182–205. https://www.ncbi.nlm.nih.gov/pubmed/4014115.
2. Centers for Disease Control and Prevention (CDC). Monitoring hospital-acquired infections to promote patient safety, United States, 1990-1999. MMWR Morb Mortal Wkly Rep. 2000;49(8):149–53. https://www.ncbi.nlm.nih.gov/pubmed/10737441.
3. Storr J, Twyman A, Zingg W, Damani N, Kilpatrick C, Reilly J, Price L, et al. Core components for effective infection prevention and control Programmes: new WHO evidence-based recommendations. Antimicrob Resist Infect Control. 2017;6(January):6. https://doi.org/10.1186/s13756-016-0149-9.
4. Guidelines on core components of infection prevention and control programmes at the national and acute health care facility level. Geneva: World Health Organization; 2016. https://www.ncbi.nlm.nih.gov/pubmed/27977095.
5. State report "On the state of sanitary and epidemiological well-being of the population in Russian federation in 2016". Moscow: Federal Service for Surveillance on Consumer Rights Protection and Human Well-being; 2017 128–131. Accessed 16 Aug 2017. http://www.rospotrebnadzor.ru/upload/iblock/0b3/gosudarstvennyy-doklad-2016.pdf.
6. Official report "Health care in Russia in 2015". Moscow: Federal State Statistics Service; 2016. Accessed 16 Sept 2017. http://www.gks.ru/wps/wcm/connect/rosstat_main/rosstat/ru/statistics/publications/catalog/doc_1139919134734. Pages 18 and 97.
7. Allegranzi B, Bagheri Nejad S, Combescure C, Graafmans W, Attar H, Donaldson L, Pittet D. Burden of endemic health-care-associated infection in developing countries: systematic review and meta-analysis. Lancet. 2011; 377(9761):228–41. https://doi.org/10.1016/S0140-6736(10)61458-4.
8. "World Development Indicators." World development indicators data. Accessed 22 Nov 2017. https://data.worldbank.org/data-catalog/world-development-indicators.
9. Ider B-E, Adams J, Morton A, Whitby M, Clements A. Infection control Systems in Transition: the challenges for post-soviet bloc countries. J Hosp Infect. 2012;80(4):277–87. https://doi.org/10.1016/j.jhin.2012.01.012.
10. Stratchounski L, Dekhnitch A, Kozlov R. Infection control system in Russia. J Hosp Infect. 2001;49(3):163–6. https://doi.org/10.1053/jhin.2001.1042.
11. Suetens C, Morales I, Savey A, Palomar M, Hiesmayr M, Lepape A, Gastmeier P, Schmit JC, Valinteliene R, Fabry J. European surveillance of ICU-acquired infections (HELICS-ICU): methods and main results. J Hosp Infect. 2007; 65(Suppl 2):171–3. https://doi.org/10.1016/S0195-6701(07)60038-3.
12. Siegel J, Rhinehart E, Cic R, Jackson M, Chiarello L, Ms RN. Guideline for isolation precautions: preventing transmission of infectious agents in healthcare settings. HICPAC. 2007; https://stacks.cdc.gov/view/cdc/6878.
13. Shifrin M, Kurdumova N, Danilov G, Ershova O, Savin I, Alexandrova I, Sokolova E, Tabasaranskiy T. Electronic patient records system as a monitoring tool. Stud Health Technol Inform. 2015;210:236–8. https://www.ncbi.nlm.nih.gov/pubmed/25991140.
14. Horan T, Andrus M, Dudeck M. CDC/NHSN surveillance definition of health care-associated infection and criteria for specific types of infections in the acute care setting. Am J Infect Control. 2008;36(5):309–32. https://doi.org/10.1016/j.ajic.2008.03.002.
15. Reintam A, Parm P, Kitus R, Kern H, Starkopf J. Gastrointestinal symptoms in intensive care patients. Acta Anaesthesiol Scand. 2009;53(3):318–24. https://doi.org/10.1111/j.1399-6576.2008.01860.x.

16. Clinical and Laboratory Standard Institute. M100: performance standards for antimicrobial susceptibility testing. 26th ed; 2016. 1–56238–804–5.

17. Agarwal A, Kapila K, Kumar S. WHONET software for the surveillance of antimicrobial susceptibility. Med J Armed Forces India. 2009;65(3):264–6. https://doi.org/10.1016/S0377-1237(09)80020-8.

18. Seabold S, Perktold J. Statsmodels: econometric and statistical modeling with python. In: Proceedings of the 9th python in science conference; 2010.

19. E. Jones, T. Oliphant, and P. Peterson. 2001. "SciPy: open source scientific tools for python." http://www.scipy.org.

20. Shestopalov N, Akimkin V, Panteleeva L, Fedorova L, Abramova I. Measures for disinfection and sterilization as the most significant concept in health care infection control system in Russia. Antimicrob Resist Infect Control. 2015;4(1):P47. https://doi.org/10.1186/2047-2994-4-S1-P47.

21. Koch A, Nilsen R, Eriksen H, Cox R, Harthug S. Mortality related to hospital-associated infections in a tertiary hospital; repeated cross-sectional studies between 2004-2011. Antimicrob Resist Infect Control. 2015;4:57. https://doi.org/10.1186/s13756-015-0097-9.

22. Glance L, Stone P, Mukamel D, Dick A. Increases in mortality, length of stay, and cost associated with hospital-acquired infections in trauma patients. Arch Surg. 2011;146(7):794–801. https://doi.org/10.1001/archsurg.2011.41.

23. Korinek A-M, Baugnon T, Golmard J-L, van Effenterre R, Coriat P, Puybasset L. Risk factors for adult nosocomial meningitis after craniotomy: role of antibiotic prophylaxis. Neurosurgery. 2008;62(Suppl 2):532–9. https://doi.org/10.1227/01.neu.0000316256.44349.b1.

24. O'Fallon E, Gautam S, D'Agata E. Colonization with multidrug-resistant gram-negative bacteria: prolonged duration and frequent cocolonization. Clin Infect Dis. 2009;48(10):1375–81. Oxford University Press. https://doi.org/10.1086/598194.

25. Ebnöther C, Tanner B, Schmid F, La Rocca V, Heinzer I, Bregenzer T. Impact of an infection control program on the prevalence of nosocomial infections at a tertiary Care Center in Switzerland. Infect Control Hosp Epidemiol. 2008;29(1):38–43. https://doi.org/10.1086/524330.

26. Stéphan F, Sax H, Wachsmuth M, Hoffmeyer P, Clergue F, Pittet D. Reduction of urinary tract infection and antibiotic use after surgery: a controlled, prospective, before-after intervention study. Clin Infect Dis. 2006; 42(11):1544–51. https://doi.org/10.1086/503837.

27. World Health Organization. "Guidelines for the prevention and control of carbapenem-resistant Enterobacteriaceae, Acinetobacter baumannii and Pseudomonas aeruginosa in health care facilities." Geneva: World Health Organization; 2017. http://www.who.int/infection-prevention/publications/guidelines-cre/en/.

20

A multi-center nested case-control study on hospitalization costs and length of stay due to healthcare-associated infection

Yu Lü, Min Hong Cai, Jian Cheng, Kun Zou, Qian Xiang[*], Jia Yu Wu, Dao Qiong Wei, Zhong Hua Zhou, Hui Wang, Chen Wang and Jing Chen

Abstract

Background: In 2018, the Chinese government demanded nationwide implementation of medical insurance payment methods based on Single-Disease Payment (SDP), but during the operation process the medical insurance system did not fully consider the extra economic burden caused by healthcare-associated infection (HAI). HAIs can prolong the length of stay and increase the hospitalization costs, but only a few studies have been conducted in Sichuan province, China. We evaluated the hospitalization costs and length of stay due to HAI in Sichuan province based on the prevalence survey, and provided data reference for China's medical insurance reform.

Methods: In the hospitals surveyed on the prevalence of HAI, a multi-center nested case-control study was performed by a paired method. The study period was from 6 September 2016 to 30 November 2016. Binary outcomes were tested using χ^2 test, continuous outcomes were tested using Wilcoxon matched-pairs signed rank test, intra-group comparisons were tested using multiple linear regression analysis.

Results: A total of 225 pairs/450 patients were selected in 51 hospitals, and 170 pairs/350 patients were successfully matched. The case fatality rate was 5.14% for the HAIs patients and 3.43% for non-HAs patients, there was no significant difference ($\chi^2 = 0.627$, $P = 0.429$); the median length of stay in patients with HAIs was 21 days, longer than that of patients with non-HAI 16 days, the median of the difference between matched-pairs was 5 days, the difference was statistically significant ($Z = 4.896$, $P = 0.000$). The median hospitalization costs of patients with HAI were €1732.83, higher than that of patients with non-HAI €1095.29, the median of the difference between matched-pairs were €431.34, the difference was statistically significant ($Z = 6.413$, $P = 0.000$). Multiple linear regression results showed that HAIs at different sites have caused different economic burdens, but in different economic regions, the difference was not statistically significant.

Conclusions: In Sichuan, the hospitalization costs and length of stay caused by HAI should be given special attention in the current medical insurance reform. The proportion and scope of medical payment for patients with HAI at different sites should be different. Efforts need to be taken to incentivize reduction of HAI rates which will reduce hospitalization costs and length of stay.

Keywords: Healthcare-associated infections, Hospitalization costs, Length of stay, Multi-center, Nested case-control study

* Correspondence: 3all@163.com
Healthcare-associated Infection Management Office, Sichuan Academy of
Medical Sciences and Sichuan People's Hospital, Chengdu 610072, Sichuan,
People's Republic of China

Background

In 2018, the Chinese government demanded nationwide implementation of medical insurance payment methods based on Single-Disease Payment (SDP) [1], but during the operation process the medical insurance system did not fully consider the extra economic burden caused by complications such as healthcare-associated infections (HAIs). After implementing SDP, most of the extra economic burden will be borne by the hospitals. This situation may lead to the risk that reimbursement cannot cover costs, so that hospitals have the motivation to reduce the quality of medical care, such as refusing patients with certain diseases to be admitted, reducing necessary treatments, or allowing patients to repeat hospital admissions [2, 3]. In order to make the reform successful, it is necessary to study the extra economic burden caused by HAI.

HAIs can bring a serious burden to patients [4], and the situation is in worse year by year [5]. HAIs can prolong the length of hospitalization stay, increase the hospitalization costs, and reduce the turnover rate of hospital beds [6, 7], which seriously affected the quality of medical care. There were many studies in this area, but less in Sichuan province, China. A total of 16.54 million hospitalizations were reported in Sichuan province in 2016 [8], and the prevalence rate of HAI was 2.30% [9]. It is important to understand and assess the hospitalization economic burden due to HAI in order to strengthen the management of HAI. The prevalence survey of HAI in Sichuan was designed by the HAIs quality control center established by Health and Family Planning Commission of Sichuan Province, using a unified questionnaire to complete within the prescribed time period. It has been conducted annually since 2011, and 6 rounds have been completed. Because of the support of the health administration department and the current prevalence survey had been included hospital grade review, the survey data in Sichuan became more accurate and large. This study was based on the prevalence survey, so that the accuracy and completeness of the data were reliable.

Since 2003, the outbreak of atypical pneumonia [severe acute respiratory syndromes (SARS)]has rapidly promoted a series of regulations and standards for HAI management in China, such as the Regulations of Healthcare Associated Infection Management and Accreditation Guideline of Control and Prevention of Healthcare Associated Infection in Hospital, etc. With the implementation of laws and regulations, the current basic measures for prevention and control of HAI in China were basically consistent with the general international standards [10]. The measures for prevention and control in our study were carried out in accordance with the requirements of the Action Plan for Prevention

and Control of Healthcare Associated Infection in Sichuan Province (2012–2015) issued by the Health and Family Planning Commission of Sichuan Province in 2012. The contents of this action include departmental organization and management, education and training, surveillance, hospital layout and workflow, isolation, disinfection and sterilization, hand hygiene, occupational exposure protection, high-risk department management, intubation-associated infection management, disposable sterile medical supplies and disinfection equipment management, medical waste and wastewater management [11], and these measures were not significantly different from other provinces in China. The HAIs Quality Control Center of Sichuan Province organized quality control supervision once a year. Supervising team members conducted quality supervision on the implementation of measures for prevention and control of HAI. After the results of the inspection were reported to the Health and Family Planning Commission of Sichuan Province, they were notified and required to be rectified within the prescribed time.

Methods

Setting

This was a matched-pairs nested case-control study. All the subjects were followed up until they were discharged.

Objects

Fifty one hospitals from 21 prefectures (municipality) were included in the prevalence survey of HAI in Sichuanin 2016.

Selection of cases

The case was defined as those who had definite exposure to HAI during the hospitalization from 6 September 2016 to 30 November 2016. The HAI diagnostic criteria used in this work were issued by the Health and Family Planning Commission of China in 2001 [12]. A total of 10 cases were randomly selected from all patients with HAI in each of the hospital sunder the prevalence survey, and in hospitals with less than 10 HAI cases, all the cases were included.

Systematic sampling steps:

Step 1: Encode all HAI cases obtained from the current prevalence survey;
Step 2: Divide the total number of HAI cases by 10 to get the sampling interval;
Step 3: Use the last few digits of a randomly drawn RMB currency to determine the first case. The selection principle of these digits was that the number to be taken was the maximum number but not greater than the sampling interval;

Step 4: Select the second case by taking the number of first case plus the sampling interval; and so on, select all cases of HAI.

Selection of controls

Controls were the non-HAI patients who met the matching criteria.

Controls were patients that did not yet acquire infection on the 'matching day' but that still can acquire infection later on during their stay. So controls were matched by department of discharge, age, sex, the total length of stay before infection, community-acquired infections, immune function, repeated hospitalization.

Matching criteria:

① Select patients in the same ward with HAI cases;
② In the present prevalence survey, the patients without HAI were selected;
③ It was necessary to eliminate the confounding bias of pre-infection time. So the total length of hospitalization stay before 'matching day' (Interval between the 'matching day' and the admission date) of the selected controls should be longer than or equal that of the HAI cases before infection (Interval between the infections date and admission date);
④ Select the patient with the same gender and in the same age group as the cases, and the age difference should be within 5 years as far as possible; The control of infant case aged <1 year should be the infant aged <1 year;
⑤ The following status of control need to be consistent with the case: whether there was community acquired infections at the time of admission, whether to be hospitalized for 2 times in a year, whether there were tumors, AIDS, malnutrition and other low immune function.
⑥ The classification score of the controls needed to be consistent with that of HAI cases. (Scoring method in the standard of nosocomial infections monitoring in China [13] Table 1).

Confounders

In confounding factors, we considered the hospital scale-sand local economic development index -GDP. The areas were classified by GDP, the hospital scales were classified by the number of beds, and the assignment was shown in Table 2.

Calculation of costs

Hospitalization costs: For each case and each control, the total bill for the entire hospital stay was obtained through the medical records. It was calculated as the sum of the cost of general medical service and general treatment operation, nursing costs, pathological diagnosis costs, laboratory diagnostic costs, imaging diagnostic costs, clinical diagnostic item costs, non-surgical clinical physiotherapy expenses, surgery treatment costs, rehabilitation costs, medicine costs, antibacterial drugs fees, Chinese herbal medicines fees, and the costs of disposable medical materials for examination, treatment or surgery.

Statistical analysis

Binary outcomes were tested using χ^2 test, continuous outcomes were tested using Wilcoxon matched-pairs signed rank test, intra-group comparisons were tested using multiple linear regression analysis, and the test level was $\alpha = 0.05$. Analyses were stratified by the scale of hospital (number of hospital beds), local economic development (GDP) and the different sites of HAIs. All the analyses were conducted using software SPSS 23.0.

Results

Patient inclusion

A total of 225 pairs were enrolled in the study, in which 175 pairs were matched. Due to the different hospitalization time, 48 pairs and 96 patients were not matched successfully.

Data were cleared up by matching, and pairs that did not meet the matching criteria were excluded, and finally 175 pairs were included in the analysis. See Fig. 1 for details.

Table 1 Classification score of disease conditions

Score	Classification basis
1	Routine observation was required and care and treatment were not required (including patients who need to be observed after surgery).
2	Stable condition, but preventive observation is needed, it is not necessary to strengthen care and treatment of patients, for example, some patients for whom myocarditis, myocardial infarction need to be excluded and overnight observation is needed after taking medicine.
3	Stable condition, but care and/or guardianship of patients need to be strengthened, such as coma patients or patients with chronic renal failure.
4	Unstable conditions, increased care and treatment are needed, and regular evaluation and adjustment of treatment programmes are needed, such as arrhythmia, diabetic ketoacidosis patients (but no coma, shock, DIC).
5	Unstable conditions, in a coma or shock state, cardiopulmonary resuscitation is needed or nursing care needs to be strengthened, and the care and treatment of patients need to be evaluated.

Table 2 Variable assignment

Variable	Value
Area (classified by GDP)	
Chengdu	1
Mianyang, Deyang, Yibin, Nanchong, Luzhou, Dazhou, Leshan, Liangshan	2
Panzhihua, Suining, Meishan, Guang' an, Neijiang, Zigong	3
Ziyang, Guangyuan, Ya' an,Bazhong, Aba, Ganzi	4
Number of hospital beds	
< 300	1
300 ≤ and < 500	2
500 ≤ and < 800	3
≥ 800	4

Table 3 Pairs characteristics

Variable	Number of Hospitals (n = 51)	Number of Pairs (n = 175)	Ratio of composition
Classification of GDP			
1	4	19	10.86%
2	23	71	40.57%
3	11	37	21.14%
4	13	48	27.43%
Classification of the number of hospital beds			
1	19	29	16.57%
2	11	47	26.86%
3	13	49	28.00%
4	8	50	28.57%

Characteristics of patients

The study included a total of 175 pairs of cases and controls in 51 hospitals, as showed in Table 3 and Table 4.

Overall analysis

The case fatality rate of HAI group was 5.14% (9/175), the case fatality rate of non-HAI group was 3.43%(6/175), there was no significant difference (χ^2 = 0.627, P = 0.429). The median length of hospitalization stay of HAI patients was 21 days, longer than that of non-HAI patients 16 days, the median of the difference between matched-pairs was 5 days, the difference was statistically significant (Z = 4.896, P = 0.000). The median hospitalization costs of HAI patients were €1732.83, longer than that of non-HAI patients €1095.29, the median of the difference between matched-pairs were €431.34, the difference was statistically significant (Z = 6.413, P = 0.000).

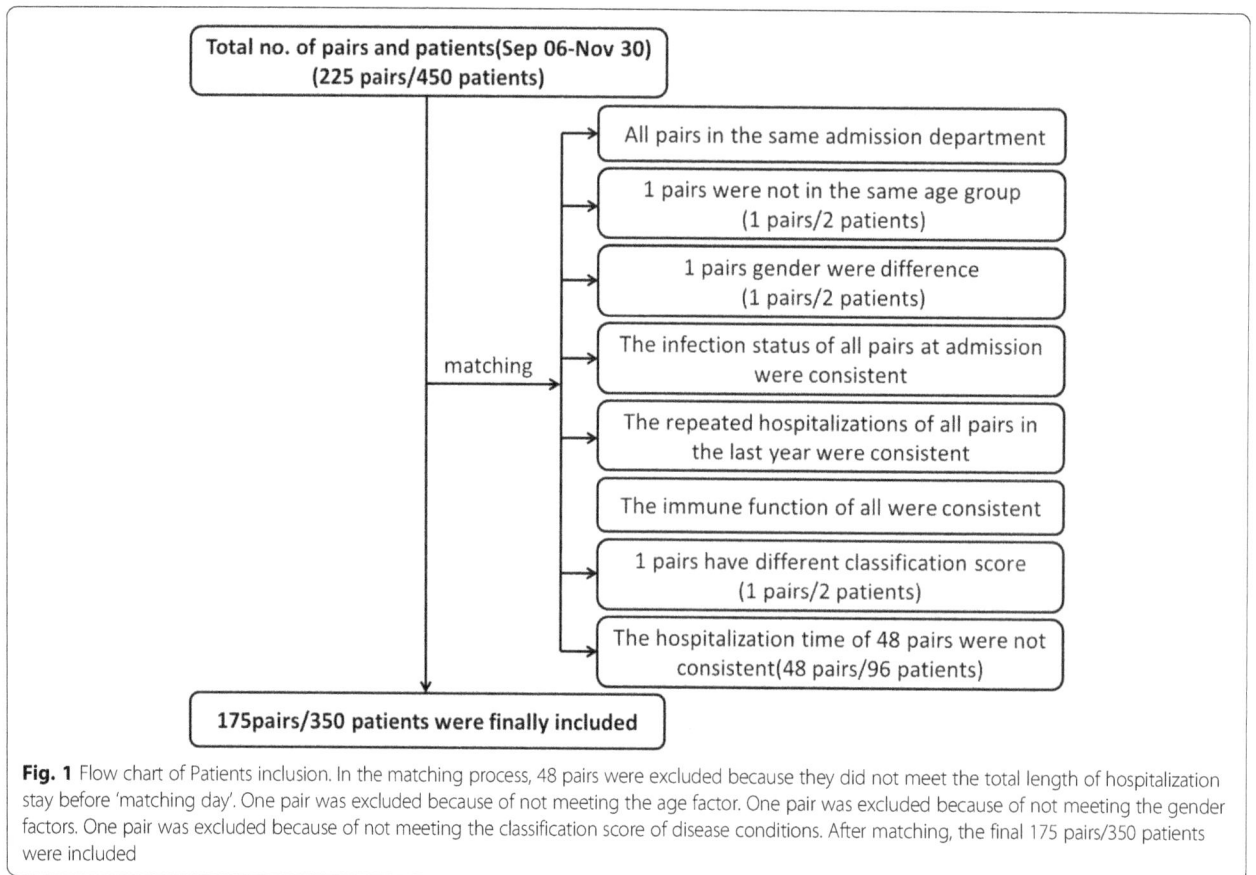

Fig. 1 Flow chart of Patients inclusion. In the matching process, 48 pairs were excluded because they did not meet the total length of hospitalization stay before 'matching day'. One pair was excluded because of not meeting the age factor. One pair was excluded because of not meeting the gender factors. One pair was excluded because of not meeting the classification score of disease conditions. After matching, the final 175 pairs/350 patients were included

Table 4 Patient characteristics: cases and controls

Variable	Cases($n = 175$)	Controls($n = 175$)
Mean age ± SD	58.15 ± 20.56	57.76 ± 20.09
Classification score of disease conditions		
1	40(22.9%)	40(22.9%)
2	63(36.0%)	63(36.0%)
3	42(24.0%)	42(24.0%)
4	26(14.9%)	26(14.9%)
5	4(2.3%)	4(2.3%)
Gender		
Male	99(56.6%)	99(56.6%)
Female	76(43.4%)	76(43.4%)
Community infections	39(22.3%)	39(22.3%)
Repeated hospitalization	41(23.4%)	41(23.4%)
Low immune function	29(16.6%)	29(16.6%)

Stratified analysis

No matter the number of hospital beds, the length of additional hospitalization stay was higher in patients with HAI than in patients without HAI and the difference was statistically significant. Except for GDP level 2, in other economic regions the differences in length of stay were statistically significant.

The results at different sites of HAI showed that there were statistically significant differences in length of stay for upper respiratory infections, superficial incision infections, urinary infections, and lower respiratory infections. See Table 5 for details.

Regardless of the number of hospital beds, or the economic conditions in the area, hospitalization costs caused by HAI were higher in patients with HAI, and the differences were statistically significant. The results at different sites of HAI showed that there were statistically significant differences in hospitalization costs for blood related infections, superficial incision infections, deep incision infections, urinary infections, lower respiratory infections, and gastrointestinal infections. See Table 6 for details.

Multiple linear regression analysis

The hospitalization costs and length of stay might have significant differences in different sites of HAIs. Multiple linear regression methods were used to analyze whether the differences were statistically significant. The cost was skewed data, so logarithmic conversion was performed

Table 5 Comparison of length of stay between the matched pairs (Days)

Variable	Number of Pairs ($n = 175$)	Difference of length of stay in pairs Median (range)	Statistics (Z)	P
Classification of the number of hospital beds				
1	29	4.0(−8~ 107)	3.136	0.002
2	47	4.0(−30~ 52)	2.131	0.033
3	49	6.0(−56~ 134)	2.716	0.005
4	50	6.0(−94~ 52)	2.045	0.041
Classification of GDP				
1	19	5.0(−23~ 69)	2.439	0.015
2	71	3.0(−94~ 134)	1.712	0.087
3	37	4.0(−30~ 88)	2.106	0.035
4	48	7.0(−39~ 107)	3.847	0.000
HAIs sites				
Upper respiratory	23	3.0(−21~ 14)	− 2.236	0.026
Blood related	5	6.0(−22~ 20)	−0.135	0.893
Superficial incision	20	10.0(−3~ 107)	−3.680	0.000
Organ lacunar	2	4.5(3~ 6)	−1.342	0.180
Deep incision	6	12.0(−10~ 52)	− 1.802	0.072
Intra-abdominal tissue	1	5.0(5~ 5)	/	/
Urinary	23	6.0(−13~ 88)	−2.480	0.013
Skin soft-tissue	12	1.0(−14~ 32)	0.157	0.875
Lower respiratory	76	5.0(−94~ 134)	−2.439	0.015
Gastrointestinal	6	1.0(−22~ 54)	−0.674	0.500
Other	1	11.0(11~ 11)	/	/

Table 6 Comparison of hospitalization costs between the matched pairs (€)

Variable	Number of Pairs (n = 175)	Difference of costs in pairs Median (range)	Statistics (Z)	P
Classification of the number of hospital beds				
1	29	133.06(− 986.46~ 7891.43)	2.983	0.003
2	47	194.23(− 1163.39~ 8198.11)	2.106	0.035
3	49	748.94(− 2815.11~ 25,447.11)	4.491	0.000
4	50	572.45(− 6589.03~ 31,153.30)	2.106	0.035
Classification of GDP				
1	19	1362.03(− 270.13~ 25,447.11)	3.662	0.000
2	71	477.72(− 1632.29~ 31,153.30)	4.111	0.000
3	37	230.68(−6589.03~ 6712.01)	2.195	0.028
4	48	253.22(−2815.11~ 9800.81)	2.913	0.004
HAIs sites				
Upper respiratory	23	69.08(−986.46~ 761.57)	−1.186	0.236
Blood related	5	1163.39(390.33~ 1578.86)	−2.023	0.043
Superficial incision	20	574.77(− 1117.95~ 25,447.11)	−3.136	0.002
Organ lacunar	2	685.30(283.52~ 1087.09)	−1.342	0.180
Deep incision	6	1406.22(399.98~ 3431.36)	−2.201	0.028
Intra-abdominal tissue	1	2086.92(2086.92~ 2086.92)	/	/
Urinary	23	330.14(−6589.03~ 6712.01)	−2.201	0.043
Skin soft-tissue	12	39.06(−789.99~ 4542.83)	−0.078	0.937
Lower respiratory	76	993.88(− 6064.87~ 31,153.30)	−5.486	0.000
Gastrointestinal	6	51.63(−12.32~ 5168.36)	− 1.992	0.046
Other	1	335.81(335.81~ 335.81)	/	/

on it. After conversion the Skewness was 0.164, Std. Error of Skewness was 0.184, and Kurtosis was 0.362, Std. Error of Kurtosis was 0.366, which satisfied the normal distribution. The Q-Q chart was showed in Fig. 2.

The F value of the ANOVA test for linear regression was 4.995, $P = 0.000$. The regression results showed that compared with upper respiratory infections, patients with these infections have higher extra hospitalization costs, such as blood related infections, superficial incision infections, organ lacunar infections, deep incision infections, urinary infections and skin soft-tissue infections, and the differences were statistically significant. See the Table 7 for details.

The length of stay was skewed data, so logarithmic conversion was performed on it. After conversion the Skewness was 0.479, Std. Error of Skewness was 0.186; and Kurtosis was 0.544, Std. Error of Kurtosis was 0.369, which satisfied the normal distribution. The Q-Q chart was showed in Fig. 3.

The F value of the ANOVA test for linear regression was 3.083, $P = 0.000$. The results showed that compared with upper respiratory infections, patients with these infections have longer extra hospitalization stays, such as blood related infections, superficial incision infections,

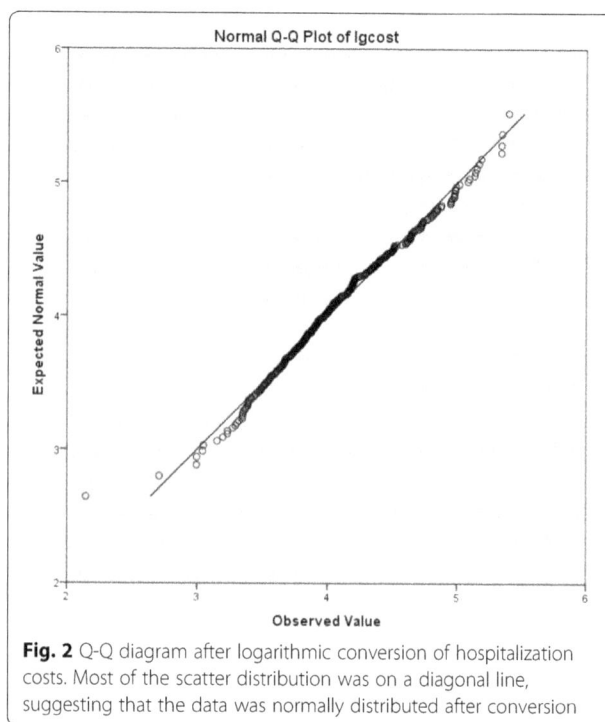

Fig. 2 Q-Q diagram after logarithmic conversion of hospitalization costs. Most of the scatter distribution was on a diagonal line, suggesting that the data was normally distributed after conversion

Table 7 Covariate and equation parameters for linear regression of hospitalization costs

Variable	Unstandardized Coefficients	Std. Error	Standardized Coefficients	Statistics (t)	P
Constant	3.820	.120		31.944	.000
HAIs sites					
Blood related	.762	.208	.265	3.661	.000
Superficial incision	.482	.128	.320	3.760	.000
Organ lacunar	.673	.308	.149	2.184	.030
Deep incision	.774	.195	.294	3.961	.000
Intra-abdominal tissue	.695	.435	.109	1.595	.113
Urinary	.511	.124	.360	4.120	.000
Skin soft-tissue	.422	.151	.222	2.789	.006
Lower respiratory	.606	.104	.625	5.820	.000
Gastrointestinal	.060	.190	.023	.315	.753
Other	−.049	.429	−.008	−.114	.909
Classification of GDP					
1	.088	.124	.057	.710	.479
2	−.052	.081	−.053	−.649	.517
3	−.076	.096	−.064	−.784	.434
Classification of the number of hospital beds					
1	−.241	.102	−.184	−2.367	.019
2	−.162	.090	−.149	−1.795	.075
3	.013	.097	.012	.138	.890

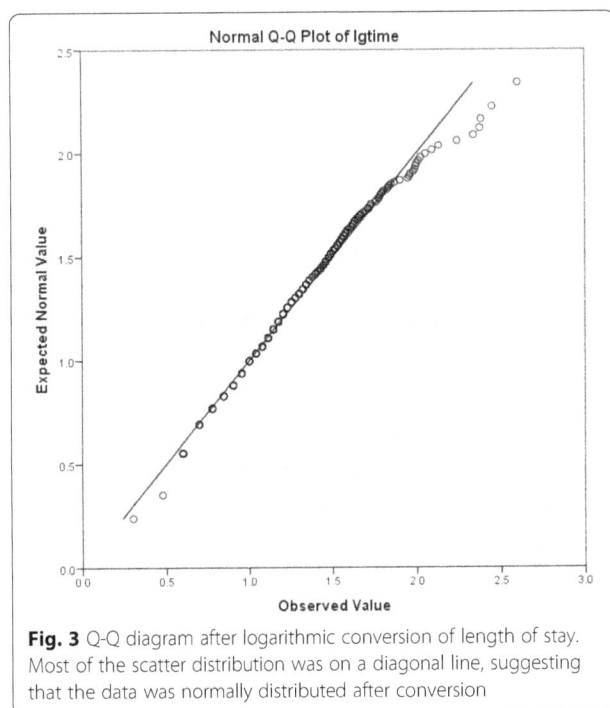

Fig. 3 Q-Q diagram after logarithmic conversion of length of stay. Most of the scatter distribution was on a diagonal line, suggesting that the data was normally distributed after conversion

deep incision infections, urinary infections, and lower respiratory infections, and the differences were statistically significant; the differences may not be statistically significant due to the small sample size, such as organ lacunar infections and intra-abdominal tissue infections. See the Table 8 for details.

Discussion

Our study was a prospective nested case-control study, using a paired method to exclude the effects of confounding factors. The results showed that HAI increased the length of stay and hospitalization costs, with an average of 5 days (increased by 31.25%), and an increase of inpatient costs of €431.34 (increased by 39.38%). We did not classify pathogens, and previous studies had shown that multi-drug resistant nosocomial infections could worsen the financial burden of patients [14–16]. A propensity matched case control study from Singapore, showed that the median per day costs of laboratory tests and antibiotics of patients with HAI were 1.5–2 times higher than that of patients without gram negative bacilli (GNB) infection [17]. A retrospective study from Spain, showed that the total hospital costs of patients with resistant and multidrug resistant *Pseudomonas aeruginosa* infection were 1.4 times and 1.7

Table 8 Covariate and equation parameters for linear regression of length of stay

Variable	Unstandardized Coefficients	Std. Error	Standardized Coefficients	Statistics (t)	P
Constant	1.269	.087		14.533	.000
HAIs sites					
Blood related	.315	.152	.162	2.077	.039
Superficial incision	.305	.093	.299	3.261	.001
Organ lacunar	.070	.224	.023	.314	.754
Deep incision	.579	.142	.326	4.066	.000
Intra-abdominal tissue	.184	.317	.043	.580	.563
Urinary	.288	.090	.301	3.198	.002
Skin soft-tissue	.135	.117	.097	1.153	.251
Lower respiratory	.211	.076	.319	2.769	.006
Gastrointestinal	.041	.138	.023	.298	.766
Other	.278	.312	.065	.891	.374
Classification of GDP					
1	−.028	.090	−.027	−.314	.754
2	−.094	.059	−.140	−1.586	.115
3	−.083	.070	−.104	−1.181	.239
Classification of the number of hospital beds					
1	−.120	.074	−.136	−1.620	.107
2	−.196	.067	−.262	−2.934	.004
3	.038	.070	.052	.535	.593

times higher than those of patients with non-resistant *P.aeruginosa* infectio [18].

Although in the regions with different GDP levels, the relative number of extra economic burdens caused by HAI was quite different, the regression analysis results in our study showed that the difference was not statistically significant. In the previous studies, the extra economic burden caused by HAI varied greatly, such as Wu Anhua's review suggests that the economic costs caused by HAI were related to the size of the survey hospital and the economic level of the hospital's location [19]. but such differences still need to be further elaborated by more rigorous epidemiological methods. Our study found statistically significant differences only between hospitals of different sizes.

Because HAIs were considered to be preventable, the additional costs associated with HAI were avoidable, the SDP currently being tried by China in 2018 could stimulate hospitals to strengthen the management of HAI. However, our study found that the difference in extra economic burden caused by HAI at different sites was statistically significant. In the implementation of SDP, this situation should be regarded, and set different reimbursement ranges and proportions for HAI at different sites. For example, the Centers for Medicare and Medicaid Services (CMS) policy in the United States had done a good

job, it covered 3 types of common infections: (1) selected surgical site infections, (2) vascular catheter-associated infections, and, (3) catheter-associated urinary infections [20]. In China, the management of HAI is not involved in the current medical insurance system. Incentives for HAI management are usually based on quality control reviews of clinical departments or medical staff [21], it is difficult to guarantee the effectiveness. However, it is worth noting that government leaders have also realized that HAI management can be motivated through better allocation of resources [22]. So the economic evaluation data in our study can provide reference for government decision-making in the future.

It was significant to match the hospitalization stay before 'matching day'. Previous studies have shown that if the study did not consider the "risk time" before the infections occurred, it would result in a "time bias", 2 times over estimation [23]. The study by Barnett AG reported that the additional hospitalization stay fell from 11.2 days to 1.4 days after adjusting the length of hospitalization stay before HAI [24]. Our study avoided the "time bias" by matching the period before the infections occurred between matched-pairs.

The data quality of our study was warranted because it was designed and completed within the framework of the prevalence survey, but simultaneously the sample size was limited and only 51 hospitals in 21 municipalities were investigated. Larger multi-center studies should be conducted to validate our findings.

Limitations

The limitations of our study: the proportion of inpatient medical expense reimbursement was not considered, and the personal economic burden, the hospital economic burden and social burden caused by HAI were not differentiated.

Conclusion

Our research shows that HAI significantly increase the length of stay and hospitalization costs, suggesting that efforts need to be taken to incentivize reduction of HAI rates which will reduce hospitalization costs and length of stay. Furthermore, the differences in extra hospitalization costs and length of stay caused by HAI at different sites were statistically significant. Thus, we suggest that when China focuses on the nationwide implementation of SDP policy reforms, in addition to paying more attention to the hospitalization costs and length of stay caused by HAI, the proportion and scope of medical payment for patients with HAI at different sites should be different.

Acknowledgements

We are grateful to the following hospitals for participating in this work. Hospitals list: Yibin County People's Hospital, Yibin Orthopaedic Hospital, Leshan City Shawan District People's Hospital, Langzhong City Chinese Medicine Hospital, Guangyuan City Lizhou District Chinese Medicine Hospital, Leshan Psychiatric Hospital, Longmatan District People's Hospital, Leshan City Wutongqiao District Psychiatric Hospital, Jiuzhaigou County People's Hospital, Chinese and Western Medicine Hospital, Jiangyou City People's Hospital, Wangcang County People's Hospital, Hongya County Chinese Medicine Hospital, Baihua Town Center Health Center, Sichuan Nanchong Mental Health Center, Gaoxian Maternal and Child Health Hospital, Panzhihua City Fourth People Hospital, Renshou Zhongxin Hospital, Enyang District People's Hospital, Tibet Autonomous Region Office in Chengdu, Yanting County People's Hospital, Ziyang Psychiatric Hospital, Ya'an Hospital of Traditional Chinese Medicine, Fushun County People's Hospital, Fushun County Maternal and Child Health Hospital, Ancient Temple County People's Hospital, Dazhou People's Hospital, Ziyang Yanjiang District Chinese Medicine Hospital, Meishan Orthopedic Hospital, Fushun County Traditional Chinese Medicine Hospital, Chinese Medicine Hospital, Mianyang Third People's Hospital, Neijiang Sixth People's Hospital, Zigong 764 Hospital, Guangyuan Third People's Hospital, Anyue County Rehabilitation Hospital, Ziyang City Yanjiang Women and Children Health Care Meter Fertility Service Center, Deyang Sixth People's Hospital, Ya'an Yucheng District People's Hospital, Ya'an Second People's Hospital, Meishan Maternal and Child Health Hospital, Pingshan County Traditional Chinese Medicine Hospital, Anyue County Tongxian Town Center Health Center, Zigong First People's Hospital, Shehong County Jinhua Central Hospital, Zitong County People's Hospital, Gaoxian Chinese Medicine Hospital, Meigu County Hospital, Songpan County People's Hospital, Mianyang City Anzhou District People's Hospital, Luojiang County Chinese Medicine Hospital, Zigong Sixth People's Hospital, Fushun County Chenguang Hospital, Ziyang Orthopaedic Hospital, Sichuan Demobilized Veterans' Hospital, Sichuan Provincial Prison Administration Central Hospital, Cangxi County People's Hospital, Mianyang Maternal and Child Health Hospital, Sichuan Petroleum Administration General Hospital, Zigong City Traditional Chinese Medicine Hospital, Guangyuan First People's Hospital, Sichuan Great Wall Kidney Disease Hospital, Yibin Second People's Hospital, Mianyang Central Hospital, Shifang People's Hospital, Chengdu Zizi infertility hospital, Jianyang City Chinese Medicine Hospital, Pengzhou City, MCH Health Planned Parenthood Service Center, Changning County People's Hospital, Chengdu Shuangliu District First People's Hospital, Qingchuan County Traditional Chinese Medicine Hospital, Chengdu Dekang Hospital (Chengdu Mental Hospital), Wenjiang District People's Hospital, Jianyang Fourth People's Hospital, Linshui County Hospital of Traditional Chinese Medicine, Chengdu Kangfu Nephrology Hospital, Daxian Xinqiao Hospital, Guangyuan Chaotian District Traditional Chinese Medicine Hospital, Hejiang County People's Hospital, Southwestern Ordnance Chengdu Hospital, Santai County Liuying Town Central Health Center, Dayi County Second People's Hospital, Chengdu Xindu Westbridge Hospital, Luzhou City Longmatan District Luhua Hospital, Chaotian District People's Hospital, Jianyang Center Hospital, Chengdu City Longquanyi District First People's Hospital, Qingchuan County People's Hospital, Bazhong Central Hospital, Chengdu Yumei Hospital, Jianyang City Sichuan Air People's Hospital, Mianyang Orthopedic Hospital, Nanchong City Shunqing District Yingxi Central Hospital, Chengdu Ma Shite Tumor Hospital, Renshou County TCM Hospital, Qionglai Medical Center Hospital, Neijiang TCM Hospital, Jianyang Second People's Hospital, Zigong TCM Hospital, Ziyang First People's Hospital, Cangxi County TCM Hospital, Zitong County TCM Hospital, Pengshan District Chinese Medicine Hospital of Meishan City, Sichuan Province, Yanting County Maternal and Child Health Planned Childbirth Service Center, Qu County People's Hospital, Guanghan Orthopaedic Hospital, Sichuan Tianxiang Orthopedic Hospital, Xuanhan County People's Hospital, China Railway Second Bureau Group Central Hospital, Chinese Medicine Hospital, Qingshen County People's Hospital, Deyang People's Hospital, Liangshan Second People's Hospital, Deyang City Chinese and Western Medicine Hospital, Xuanhan County Hospital, Sichuan Provincial Judicial Police General Hospital, Ganluo County People's Hospital, Linshui County People's Hospital.

Funding

This project has received funding from the Health and Family Planning Commission of Sichuan Province (18PJ571).

Authors' contributions

WJY conceived the project. LY, XQ developed study design. WH, WC, CJ assisted with information collection. LY, XQ, CMH co-wrote the manuscript text. ZK, WDQ, ZZH, CJ edited and revised the manuscript. All authors had final approval of the submitted manuscript.

Consent for publication

Not applicable.

Competing interests

The authors declare that they have no competing interests.

References

1. Office of the Sichuan Provincial People's Government. Notice on Printing and Distributing the Implementation Plan for Further Deepening the Reform of Payment Methods for Basic Medical Insurance. Available from: http://www.sc.gov.cn/10462/12771/2018/1/8/10442346.shtml(2018). Accessed 26 July 2018.
2. Di X. The development of specific disease payment and its key issues of management. Chinese Health Resources. 2018;21:27–31.
3. LIU Zhi-jian. Study on the Effect of New Health Payment Scheme on Medical Costs. D. University of Science and Technology of China (2017).
4. Allegranzi B, Bagheri NS, Combescure C, et al. Burden of endemic health-care-associated infection in developing countries: systematic review and meta-analysis. Lancet. 2011;377(9761):228.
5. Guo C, Liu YH, Tian DS. Statistical research on direct economic loss due to nosocomial infections. Chinese Journal of Nosocomiology. 2012;22(8):1651–3.
6. Vrijens F, Hulstaert F, Sande SVD, et al. Hospital-acquired, laboratory-confirmed bloodstream infections: linking national surveillance data to clinical and financial hospital data to estimate increased length of stay and healthcare costs. J Hosp Infect. 2010;75(3):158.
7. Gabriel L, Beriot-Mathiot A. Hospitalization stay and costs attributable to Clostridium difficile infection: a critical review. J Hosp Infect. 2014;88(1):12.

8. Health and Family Planning Commission of Sichuan Province. Statistical communique on the development of health and family planning in Sichuan province in 2016.[EB/OL]. 2017–03-30. Available from: http://www. scwst.gov.cn/xx/tjxx/tjnj/201703/t20170330_13407.html. Accessed 26 July 2018.

9. Sichuan Provincial Healthcare-associated Infections Quality Control Center. Report of 2016 Cross-sectional survey of healthcare-associated infection in Sichuan province. Sichuan Nosocomial Infection Control Network, 2017–06-26. Available from: http://www.scnicn.com:8081/zhuzhan/middlenews/20170626/812.shtml. Accessed 26 July 2018.

10. Liuyi LI. New technique and progress of prevention and control of healthcare-associated infection. West China Medicine. 2018;33(3):240–43.

11. Health and Family Planning Commission of Sichuan Province. Action Plan for Prevention and Control of Healthcare Associated Infection in Sichuan Province (2012–2015). [Z]. 2013–02-01. Available from: http://www.scnicn. com:8081/zcfl/836.jhtml. Accessed 26 July 2018.

12. National Health and Family Planning Commission of the People's Republic of China. Notice on Issuing Diagnostic Criteria for Nosocomial Infection (Trial). [Z].2001–11-07. Available from: http://www.moh.gov.cn/yzygj/s3593/200804/e19e4448378643a09913ccf2a055c79d.shtml. Accessed 26 July 2018.

13. Ministry of Health P.R. China. WS/T 312–2009.Standard for nosocomial infection surveillance. Beijing: People's Medical Publishing House; 2009.

14. Judd WR, Ratliff PD, Hickson RP, et al. Clinical and economic impact of meropenem resistance in Pseudomonas aeruginosa-infected patients. Am J Infect Control. 2016;44(11):1275–9.

15. Marta R, Pietro C, Roser T, et al. Cost Attributable to Nosocomial Bacteremia. Analysis According to Microorganism and Antimicrobial Sensitivity in a University Hospital in Barcelona. Plos One. 2016;11(4):e0153076.

16. Stewardson AJ, Allignol A, Beyersmann J, et al. The health and economic burden of bloodstream infections caused by antimicrobial-susceptible and non-susceptible Enterobacteriaceae and *Staphylococcus aureus* in European hospitals, 2010 and 2011: a multicentre retrospective cohort study. Euro surveillance. 2016;21(33):1–12.

17. Vasudevan A, Memon BI, Mukhopadhyay A, et al. The costs of nosocomial resistant gram negative intensive care unit infections among patients with the systemic inflammatory response syndrome- a propensity matched case control study. Antimicrobial Resistance and Infection Control. 2015;4(1):3.

18. Morales E, Cots F, Sala M, et al. Hospital costs of nosocomial multi-drug resistant Pseudomonas aeruginosa acquisition. BMC Health Serv Res. 2012; 12(1):122.

19. Wu AH. Economicevaluation onthe costs of healthcareassociated infection. Chinese Journal of Infection Control. 2016;5(3):193–7.

20. Stone PW, Glied SA, Mcnair PD, et al. CMS changes in reimbursement for HAIs: setting a research agenda. Med Care. 2010;48(5):433.

21. Zhang XJ, Qiu TF. Application of incentive mechanism in control of nosocomial infections. Chinese Journal of Nosocomiology. 2012;22(5):1001–2.

22. Qiang FU, Guo YH. National strategy for nosocomial infection control in new era. Chinese Journal of Nosocomiology. 2013;23(20):4861–4.

23. Schulgen G, Kropec A, Kappstein I, et al. Estimation of extra hospitalization stay attributable to nosocomial infections: heterogeneity and timing of events. J Clin Epidemiol. 2000;53(4):409–17.

24. Barnett AG, Beyersmann J, Allignol A, et al. The time-dependent bias and its effect on extra length of stay due to nosocomial infection. Value in Health the Journal of the International Society for Pharmacoeconomics & Outcomes Research. 2011;14(2):381.

21

Surface area wiped, product type, and target strain impact bactericidal efficacy of ready-to-use disinfectant Towelettes

Alyssa M West[1], Carine A Nkemngong[1], Maxwell G Voorn[1], Tongyu Wu[1], Xiaobao Li[2], Peter J Teska[2] and Haley F Oliver[1,3*] (iD)

Abstract

Background: Disinfectant products are often used on environmental surfaces (e.g. countertops, patient beds) and patient care equipment in healthcare facilities to help prevent the transmission of healthcare-associated infections. Ready-to-use (RTU) disinfectants in the form of pre-wetted towelettes are increasingly popular among healthcare facilities. Currently, the EPA does not require disinfectant manufacturers to include a recommended maximum surface area per towelette on their product labels. The objective of this study was to investigate the efficacy of disinfectant towelette products on a hard non-porous surface across different coverage areas using a quantitative EPA method. We hypothesized that there would be significant differences in the efficacy of disinfectant towelette products, and that the greater surface area(s) wiped would result in reduced bactericidal efficacy.

Methods: This study tested ten disinfectant towelette products against *Staphylococcus aureus* strain ATCC CRM-6538 and *Pseudomonas aeruginosa* strain ATCC 15442 on Formica surfaces. Defined surface areas were wiped and the towelette weighed before and after wiping to determine the amount of liquid released. Bactericidal efficacy testing was also performed after wiping following standard EPA protocols.

Results: We found that disinfectant product, area of surface wiped, and strain impacted the bactericidal efficacy achieved. Disinfectant product type and area of surface wiped significantly impacted the percent of liquid released per ft^2 from the towelette.

Conclusion: Overall, bactericidal efficacy varied by towelette product, surface area wiped, and strain. This study also found that wiping larger surface areas may lead to decreased bactericidal efficacy. Further research is needed to test its implication.

Keywords: Disinfectant, Towelette, Efficacy

Background

Healthcare-associated infections (HAIs) are reported to occur in one out of 25 patients every day in the United States [1]. It is estimated that in 2011, 721,000 cases of HAIs occurred in United States acute care hospitals [2]. Healthcare-associated pathogens can colonize a vast array of environmental surfaces and patient care equipment in healthcare facilities and transmission from these

surfaces to patients can lead to HAIs [3, 4]. Disinfectant products are often used on environmental surfaces (e.g. countertops, patient beds) and patient care equipment in healthcare facilities to help prevent the transmission of healthcare-associated pathogens. Although disinfectants are generally accepted to be effective against a wide range of pathogens, major factors exist that can cause differences and reductions in bactericidal efficacy. For example, disinfectant concentration can affect the bactericidal efficacy achieved. Concentrations that are lower than the label-use have been shown not to be as effective [5–9]. Reduced contact times (as compared to label instructions) can lower a product's efficacy as well [5–9].

* Correspondence: hfoliver@purdue.edu
[1]Department of Food Science, Purdue University, West Lafayette, IN 47907, USA
[3]Department of Food Science, Purdue University, 745 Agriculture Mall Drive, West Lafayette, IN 47907, USA

Furthermore, a product's overall formulation and active ingredients play a role in bactericidal efficacy. Previous work by our group demonstrated that a sodium hypochlorite-based disinfectant product was significantly more effective against multiple MRSA strains than a quaternary ammonium compounds (quat)- based product [5]. Other published studies have also shown that disinfectants with differing active ingredients have different bactericidal efficacies against the same microorganism [6, 7, 10, 11]. Thus, understanding factors that can reduce bactericidal efficacy are important to help understand how to optimize the performance of a disinfectant.

Ready-to-use (RTU) disinfectants in the form of pre-wetted towelettes are increasingly popular among healthcare facilities. A 2014 study determined that the use of RTU disinfectant towelette products led to a faster disinfection process, higher compliance with disinfection standards, and overall cost savings as compared to traditional disinfection methods [12]. The CDC specifically recommends using an Environmental Protection Agency (EPA)-registered disinfectant product for environmental cleaning in healthcare facilities [6]. The current EPA methodology used to register a disinfectant towelette product is the qualitative AOAC Germicidal Spray Products as Disinfectants Test modified for towelettes [13]. This protocol only requires testing of small carriers (25 mm × 75 mm glass slides) as opposed to larger surfaces areas that are more representative of actual product usage. Currently, the EPA does not require disinfectant manufacturers to include a recommended maximum surface area per towelette on their product labels. Thus, there are a number of important application considerations that are not informed by the current EPA wipe testing method.

To our knowledge, there are no prior peer-reviewed studies that have examined the effectiveness of towelettes over defined coverage areas typical of healthcare facilities. The objective of this study was to investigate the efficacy of disinfectant towelette products on a hard non-porous surface across different coverage areas using a quantitative EPA method. We hypothesized that (i) there would be significant differences in the efficacy of disinfectant towelette products against both S. aureus and P. aeruginosa and (ii) the greater surface area(s) wiped, the less bactericidal efficacy.

Methods
Disinfectants, bacterium, and surface used in study
This study tested ten disinfectant towelette products described below (Table 1). Diversey EasyWipes wetted with phosphate buffered saline (PBS; 4.85 mL per Easy-Wipe towelette) were used as a control. S. aureus strain ATCC CRM-6538 and P. aeruginosa strain ATCC 15442 were used to measure towelette disinfectant efficacy.

These strains were chosen as both are currently required by the EPA to be used in testing base disinfectant efficacy claims for EPA registration [14]. Additionally, S. aureus is the second most common pathogen associated with HAIs [2]. The surfaces used for testing were sheets of Formica cut down to size as detailed below.

Towelette disinfectant load and surface coverage measurements
The initial amount of liquid loaded on the disinfectant wipes was determined based on a modified technique that was used in an EPA efficacy study of sporicidal wipes [15]. The first towelette from each disinfectant container was discarded and the subsequent towelettes were used to ensure towelettes were fully wet. For each of the products, ten wipes were pre-weighed individually using a Mettler-Toledo AG204 analytical balance

Table 1 Active ingredients and contact times for disinfectant towelettes tested in this study

Disinfectant Product "Name" (used throughout manuscript) [a]	Disinfectant Active Ingredient(s)	Label Contact Time [b]
0.5% quat + 55% alcohol	- 0.25% n-alkyl dimethyl ethylbenzyl ammonium chlorides - 0.25% n-alkyl dimethyl benzyl ammonium chlorides - 55% isopropyl alcohol	2 min
0.76% quat + 22.5% alcohol	- 0.76% didecyldimethylammonium chlorides - 7.5% ethanol - 15% isopropyl alcohol	1 min
1.4% hydrogen peroxide	- 1.4% hydrogen peroxide	1 min
1.312% sodium hypochlorite	- 1.312% sodium hypochlorite	1 min
0.5% hydrogen peroxide	- 0.5% hydrogen peroxide	1 min
0.55% sodium hypochlorite	- 0.55% sodium hypochlorite	30 s
0.28% quat	- 0.14% n-alkyl dimethyl ethyl benzyl ammonium chlorides - 0.14% n-akyl dimethyl benzyl ammonium chlorides	3 min
0.21% quat	- 0.105% n-alkyl dimethyl ethyl benzyl ammonium chlorides - 0.105% n-alkyl dimethyl benzyl ammonium chlorides	3 min
0.61% quat + 56% alcohol	- 0.61% dodecyl dimethyl ammonium chloride - 27.3% ethyl alcohol - 28.7% isopropyl alcohol	1 min
0.308% quat + 21% alcohol	- 0.154% n-alkyl dimethyl benzyl ammonium chlorides - 0.154% n-alkyl ethylbenzyl ammonium chlorides - 21.000% isopropyl alcohol	2 min

[a] Abbreviated naming scheme reflects aggregated active ingredients for commercially available EPA registered disinfectants used in this study;
[b] Defined label contact time for S. aureus and P. aeruginosa

(accurate to 0.01 g; Mettler-Toledo LLC, Columbus, OH). After being weighed, the towelettes were rinsed under running tap water for 30 s to remove the liquid disinfectant from the towelette. Once rinsed, the towelettes were placed in a drying oven at 37 C° for 24 h. Each wipe was individually re-weighed to determine the liquid weight loaded on each wipe.

To determine the amount of liquid disinfected deposited on a defined surface area, approximately six by seven inch towelettes were wiped across textured Formica sheet surfaces ranging from one to eight feet. Formica sheets were cut to eight ft. (approx. 243.8 cm^2) in length and marked into one foot square areas (0.5 ft. by two ft.; approx. 929.0 cm^2). To measure the amount of liquid disinfectant deposited on the surface, the first towelette from the disinfectant container was discarded and subsequent towelettes were used to ensure the towelettes were fully wet. Each towelette was pre-weighed on an analytical balance (Mettler-Toledo LLC, Columbus, OH). Each one ft^2 section (approx. 929.03 cm^2) was wiped once in a down and back pattern. The same wiping pattern was used for all products tested and all sections wiped. The towelette was weighed before and after wiping a defined number of sections: one ft^2 (~ 929.0 cm^2), two ft^2 (~ 1858.1 cm^2), three ft^2 (~ 2787.1 cm^2), four ft^2 (~ 3716.1 cm^2), five ft^2 (~ 4645.1 cm^2), six ft^2 (~ 5574.2 cm^2), seven ft^2 (~ 6503.2 cm^2), and eight ft^2 (~ 7432.2 cm^2) to determine liquid weight deposited on the surface. Each of the increasing number of sections was wiped independently using a new towelette each time (e.g. a single towelette was used on an eight square foot surface). The Formica was washed with 75% ethanol and left until dry to touch between each surface area tested. Five replicates of surface coverage testing were conducted independently for the ten disinfectant products and PBS-wetted control towelette.

Towelette bactericidal efficacy
A modified version of the EPA SOP MB-33-00 was used to conduct bactericidal efficacy testing [16]. The surface wiping method described above was used to measured bactericidal efficacy on one, two, four, and eight ft^2 areas. After the designated Formica surface area had been wiped, the same towelette was used to wipe a 97 mm diameter Formica disc that was independently inoculated with either 50 μL of S. aureus culture or 50 μL of P. aeruginosa culture (both approximately 5.5 log CFU following EPA MB-33-00) [16]. The Formica discs were wiped, with consistent pressure, in a circular pattern (as defined in EPA MB-33-00), and the discs were left at room temperature for the disinfectant's label contact time [16]. After the contact time was reached, the discs were swabbed using PUR-Blue Swabs (World

BioProducts, Libertyville, IL) containing 10 mL sterile HiCap neutralizing buffer. The swab samplers were vortexed for 30s to release the bacteria from the sponge and the solution was vacuum-filtered onto a membrane filter (0.2 μm pore size, 47 mm grid, individual sterile pack; Pall Corporation, Port Washington, NY) following EPA MB-33-00 [15]. TSA plates (BD Biosciences, San Jose, CA) containing the plated membrane filter were incubated for 24–48 h at 37 °C, then colonies were counted. Two positive controls were conducted by directly swabbing an inoculated Formica disc with the PUR-Blue swab sampler containing 10 mL sterile HiCap neutralizing buffer. Five biological replicates were conducted for each of the disinfectant products tested and three technical replicates were performed within each biological replicate for every surface area for testing both S. aureus and P. aeruginosa.

Statistical analyses
SAS v. 9.4 (SAS Institute, Cary, NC) was used to perform all statistical analyses. The percent liquid in grams released from the towelette for each surface area was calculated, normalized to the amount of liquid originally loaded onto the towelette (as determined by the drying method mentioned above in grams). All bactericidal efficacy data (bacterial kill) were transformed into log$_{10}$ reduction values for analyses. All analyses had a defined significance level of α = 0.05. Data were fitted into a generalized linear mixed model with Proc Glimmix to determine the significant factors impacting the percent of liquid expended (n = 800). The amount of liquid released was log transformed to maximize data fitness. Least square means comparison with Tukey-Kramer adjustment was used to determine significant differences in the percent of liquid deposited onto a surface across eight areas, ten disinfectant products (with PBS wetted wipes as the control), and combinations of their interaction. To determine the factors significantly impacting bacteria reduction, a separate generalized linear mixed model was developed, with least squares means comparison and Tukey adjustment detecting significant differences in bacteria log$_{10}$ reduction due to area, disinfectant, strain, and their interaction (n = 399).

Results
Disinfectant product, surface area wiped, and strain significantly impacted bactericidal efficacy
Data fitted Proc Glimmix with adequate robustness. Bacteria log$_{10}$ reduction was significantly affected by disinfectant product (p < 0.0001), area (p = 0.0003), and strain (p = 0.0083). Two-level interactions disinfectant*area and disinfectant*strain were also significant (p = 0.0474 and p < 0.0001, respectively). Irrespective of area and strain, 0.55% sodium hypochlorite product (Fig. 1a)

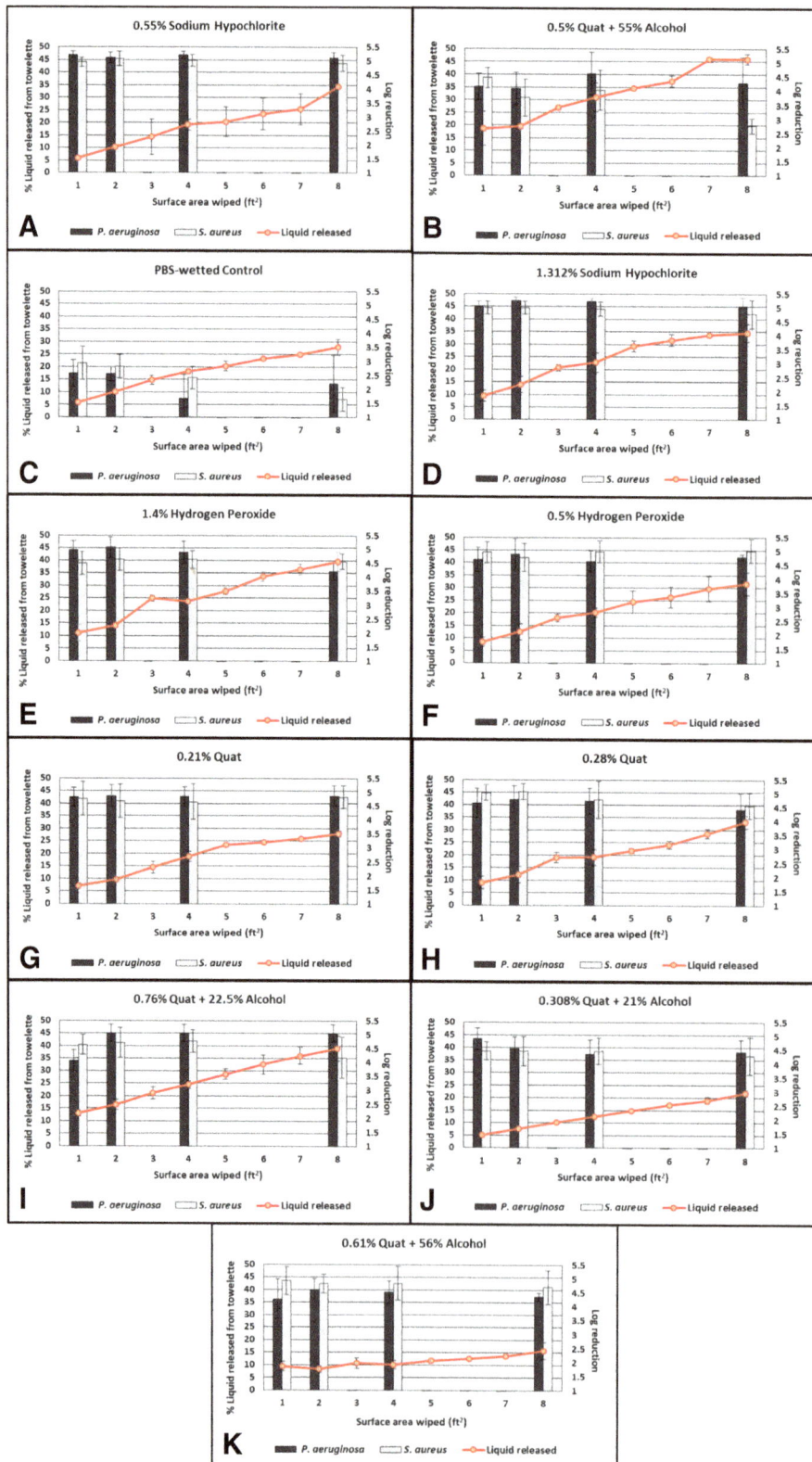

Fig. 1 (See legend on next page.)

(See figure on previous page.)
Fig. 1 Percent of total liquid released from towelette after wiping and bactericidal efficacy against *S. aureus* and *P. aeruginosa* (expressed as $\log_{10}$ reduction values) over varying surface areas wiped for each disinfectant towelette product tested. To determine the factors significantly impacting bacteria reduction, a generalized linear mixed model was developed with least squares means comparison and Tukey adjustment detecting significant differences in bacteria log10 reduction due to area, disinfectant, strain, and their interaction ($n = 399$). Data were fitted into a generalized linear mixed model with Proc Glimmix to determine the significant factors impacting the percent of liquid expended ($n = 800$). Least square means comparison with Tukey-Kramer adjustment was used to determine significant differences in the percent of liquid deposited onto a surface across eight areas, ten disinfectant products (with PBS wetted wipes as the control), and combinations of their interaction. **a** Percent of liquid released and efficacy over varying surface areas for a 0.55% sodium hypochlorite product; **b** Percent of liquid released and efficacy over varying surface areas for a 0.5% quat product + 55% alcohol; **c** Percent of liquid released and efficacy over varying surface areas for PBS-wetted control towelette; **d** Percent of liquid released and efficacy over varying surface areas for a 1.312% sodium hypochlorite product; **e** Percent of liquid released and efficacy over varying surface areas for a 1.4% hydrogen peroxide product; **f** Percent of liquid released and efficacy over varying surface areas for a 0.5% hydrogen peroxide product; **g** Percent of liquid released and efficacy over varying surface areas for a 0.21% quat product; **h** Percent of liquid released and efficacy over varying surface areas for a 0.28% quat product; **i** Percent of liquid released and efficacy over varying surface areas for a 0.76% quat + 22.5% alcohol product; **j** Percent of liquid released and efficacy over varying surface areas for a 0.308% quat + 21% alcohol product; **k** Percent of liquid remaining and efficacy over varying surface areas for 0.61% quat + 56% alcohol product

most effectively reduced bacterial load, while 0.5% quat + 55% alcohol product (Fig. 1b) was the least effective (both $p < 0.0001$). All of the disinfectants were significantly more bactericidal than PBS-wetted control wipe ($p < 0.0001$) (Fig. 1c). Notably, the sodium hypochlorite-based products (Fig. 1a and d), hydrogen peroxide-based (Fig. 1e and f), and quat-based products (Fig 1g and h) achieved a higher bactericidal efficacy than the quat alcohol-based products ($p < 0.05$) (Fig. 1i, j, k). Regardless of disinfectant product and strain, a higher $\log_{10}$ reduction value was reached when wiping one ft^2 and two ft^2 areas ($p = 0.0006$, $p = 0.0015$, respectively) compared to eight ft^2. Aside from the PBS-wetted control wipe, 0.5% quat + 55% alcohol product (Fig. 1b) was the only disinfectant significantly impacted by area wiped. Specifically, the bactericidal efficacy for this product decreased as the area wiped increased. The 0.5% quat + 55% alcohol product was significantly more bactericidal when wiping one ft^2 ($p < 0.0001$), two ft^2 ($p = 0.0166$), and four ft^2 ($p = 0.0017$) areas compared to eight ft^2.

Bactericidal efficacy varied between *P. aeruginosa* and *S. aureus* by disinfectant

Overall, all products were more effective against *P. aeruginosa* than *S. aureus* ($p = 0.0083$). While all disinfectants were more effective than the PBS-wetted control wipe in reducing both *P. aeruginosa* and *S. aureus* ($p < 0.0001$) (Fig. 1c), bactericidal efficacy differed among disinfectants for both strains tested. For *P. aeruginosa*, both sodium hypochlorite products achieved significantly higher $\log_{10}$ reduction values than most quat alcohol products. Specifically, the 1.312% sodium hypochlorite (Fig. 1d) and 0.55% sodium hypochlorite products (Fig. 1a) were significantly more effective than the 0.28% quat (Fig. 1h), 0.308% quat + 21% alcohol (Fig. 1j), 0.61% quat + 56% alcohol (Fig. 1k), and 0.5% quat + 55% alcohol products (Fig. 1b) (all $p < 0.05$). For *S. aureus*, the 0.5% quat + 55% alcohol product (Fig. 1b) was the least

effective compared to all other disinfectants tested (all $p < 0.05$). Sodium hypochlorite, hydrogen peroxide and quat products yielded significantly higher log reduction than 0.308% quat + 21% alcohol and 0.5% quat + 55% alcohol products ($p < 0.05$).

Percent of liquid released per ft^2 from towelettes decreased as area wiped increased and varied among disinfectant products

Data adequately fit in the generalized linear mixed model. Overall, average liquid released per ft^2 was significantly impacted by area wiped ($p < 0.0001$), disinfectant product ($p < 0.0001$), and their interaction ($p < 0.0001$). Greater amounts of liquid were released per ft^2 on smaller areas wiped, compared to larger areas (Table 2). Specifically, greater liquid was released per ft^2 when wiping the one ft^2 area, compared to wiping all other areas respectively ($p < 0.0001$). More liquid was released per ft^2 when wiping the two ft^2 area, compared to wiping four, five, six, seven, and eight ft^2 areas (all $p < 0.0001$). When wiping the three ft^2 area, more liquid was released per ft^2 compared to four, five, six, seven, and eight ft^2 areas (all $p < 0.0001$). Wiping the four ft^2 area released more liquid per ft^2 than wiping the six, seven, and eight ft^2 areas (all $p = 0.001$). Finally, wiping the five ft^2 area released more liquid per ft^2 compared to wiping seven ft^2 ($p = 0.0012$) and eight ft^2 areas ($p < 0.0001$).

There was a greater amount of liquid released per ft^2 from the sodium hypochlorite-based products than quat-, quat-alcohol-, and hydrogen peroxide-based products ($p < 0.05$). Notably, the 1.312% sodium hypochlorite-based product released less liquid per ft^2 compared to the 0.55% sodium hypochlorite product ($p < 0.0001$). Hydrogen peroxide-based products released more liquid per ft^2 than 0.28% quat product, but less compared to 0.5% quat + 55% alcohol product ($p < 0.05$). The 0.308% quat + 21% alcohol product released less liquid per ft^2 compared to the other quat alcohol products, quat-based products, and hydrogen peroxide-based

Table 2 Average liquid released per ft^2

Average liquid released per ft^2 Average liquid released (g/ft^2)[a]								
Towelette Product	1	2	3	4	5	6	7	8
0.55% sodium hypochlorite	0.51 ± 0.09	0.43 ± 0.08	0.40 ± 0.14	0.40 ± 0.07	0.34 ± 0.09	0.32 ± 0.08	0.37 ± 0.06	0.36 ± 0.05
0.5% quat + 55% alcohol	0.72 ± 0.54	0.38 ± 0.52	0.35 ± 0.04	0.29 ± 0.09	0.27 ± 0.02	0.24 ± 0.02	0.25 ± 0.06	0.22 ± 0.04
PBS-wetted towelettes	0.27 ± 0.06	0.22 ± 0.05	0.22 ± 0.08	0.20 ± 0.04	0.18 ± 0.03	0.17 ± 0.03	0.16 ± 0.03	0.16 ± 0.03
1.312% sodium hypochlorite	0.16 ± 0.16	0.33 ± 0.06	0.33 ± 0.03	0.27 ± 0.06	0.28 ± 0.03	0.25 ± 0.02	0.23 ± 0.01	0.21 ± 0.04
1.4% hydrogen peroxide	0.40 ± 0.21	0.26 ± 0.06	0.30 ± 0.01	0.21 ± 0.04	0.20 ± 0.03	0.20 ± 0.02	0.19 ± 0.03	0.18 ± 0.03
0.5% hydrogen peroxide	0.36 ± 0.12	0.26 ± 0.07	0.26 ± 0.05	0.22 ± 0.04	0.21 ± 0.04	0.19 ± 0.04	0.18 ± 0.03	0.17 ± 0.02
0.21% quat	0.32 ± 0.08	0.22 ± 0.05	0.22 ± 0.05	0.21 ± 0.06	0.21 ± 0.04	0.18 ± 0.03	0.17 ± 0.04	0.16 ± 0.05
0.28% quat	0.35 ± 0.12	0.24 ± 0.01	0.25 ± 0.06	0.19 ± 0.06	0.17 ± 0.03	0.16 ± 0.01	0.16 ± 0.02	0.16 ± 0.03
0.76% quat + 22.5% alcohol	0.50 ± 0.12	0.31 ± 0.04	0.27 ± 0.04	0.23 ± 0.03	0.22 ± 0.02	0.21 ± 0.03	0.20 ± 0.02	0.19 ± 0.02
0.308% quat + 21% alcohol	0.25 ± 0.03	0.19 ± 0.02	0.17 ± 0.01	0.16 ± 0.01	0.15 ± 0.01	0.14 ± 0.01	0.13 ± 0.01	0.14 ± 0.01
0.61% quat + 56% alcohol	0.72 ± 0.39	0.32 ± 0.09	0.27 ± 0.09	0.19 ± 0.04	0.18 ± 0.04	0.16 ± 0.01	0.15 ± 0.01	0.15 ± 0.05

[a]Average liquid released per ft^2 was calculated by measuring total liquid released (measured in g) onto a total area wiped divided by the number of ft^2 wiped

products (all $p < 0.0001$). Additionally, 0.76% quat + 22.5% alcohol and 0.5% quat + 55% alcohol products released more liquid per ft^2 than 0.21% quat product ($p < 0.0001$). The 0.76% quat + 22.5% alcohol, 0.61% quat + 56% alcohol, and 0.5% quat + 55% alcohol products released more liquid per ft^2 than the 0.28% quat product ($p < 0.05$). The 0.61% quat + 56% alcohol product released less liquid per ft^2 compared to the 0.5% quat + 55% alcohol product ($p < 0.0001$).

The interaction affect between disinfectant and area was significantly ($p < 0.0001$). The amount of liquid released per ft^2 decreased as the area wiped increased among all of the disinfectant products tested ($p < 0.05$). Across all disinfectant products, there was a significantly greater liquid released per ft^2 when wiping one ft^2 compared to eight ft^2 ($p < 0.05$).

Discussion

In this study we tested ten RTU disinfectant towelette products to determine the impact of surface area wiped on bactericidal efficacy using quantitative methodology. Bactericidal efficacy varied among RTU towelette products tested, the size of surface wiped, and by strain. Further, we found significant differences in the percentage of liquid released per ft^2 among wipes across various surface areas. There is not, to our knowledge, any peer-reviewed literature currently published that has examined the impact of surface area on a disinfectant's bactericidal efficacy. We believe this is the first study to use the EPA disinfectant towelette methodology in scenarios relevant to healthcare facilities.

Bactericidal efficacy varies by towelette product and total surface area wiped

There were statistically significant differences in bactericidal efficacy among the ten disinfectant towelette products tested. Overall, the 0.5% quat+ 55% alcohol product had the lowest bactericidal efficacy compared to all other tested products. The 0.55% sodium hypochlorite product tested achieved the highest bactericidal efficacy. This is consistent with our prior work [5] and other published literature [17, 18]. We elected to test bactericidal efficacy at one, two, four, and eight ft^2 as opposed to all continuous ft^2 based on preliminary data that indicated differences in efficacy was marginal among some surface areas. This was also consistent with the percent liquid released per ft^2 where there was no significant differences in percent released per ft^2 among the six, seven, and eight ft^2 areas.

The 0.5% quat + 55% alcohol product achieved the lowest bactericidal efficacy overall and across all surface areas tested for *S. aureus*, with only an ~ 3 $\log_{10}$ reduction achieved after wiping the eight ft^2 area. However, this product released one of the highest percentages of liquid per ft^2. This inverse relationship may indicate that although liquid is being released from the disinfectant towelette, the liquid may not contain enough active ingredients to achieve the ~ 5–6 $\log_{10}$ reduction performance standard [19] for *S. aureus*. Although previous studies have shown that the addition of other active ingredients with bactericidal properties to quat-based products enhances their bactericidal efficacy [20]), our results indicate the opposite. It is worth noting that quat-based disinfectant products are reported to be among the most commonly used in healthcare facilities for cleaning surfaces [21, 22], although some products such as the 0.5% quat + 55% alcohol product tested in this study may not be achieving a ~ 5–6 $\log_{10}$ reduction for all bacterial species. These results might also be due to the high alcohol content of this product. The alcohol may be evaporating too quickly to achieve the ~ 5–6

$\log_{10}$ kill needed to meet the performance standard guidelines [19, 23–25].

Towelettes were less effective as surface area increased, which may have implications for disinfection of large surfaces

Overall, there was a higher log reduction achieved when wiping the one and two ft^2 surface areas compared to the eight ft^2 surface area. Although the extent to which bactericidal efficacy is impacted is product dependent, it indicates that wiping a larger surface will lead to reduced bactericidal efficacy. The current EPA testing requirements for product registration do not consider varying surface areas. In fact, only a small glass slide is tested in the current protocol, which is not representative of a large surface area (such as a countertop) that would be wiped in a healthcare setting. Additionally, towelette bactericidal efficacy is interpreted based on the EPA's product performance test guidelines (OCSPP 810.2200) for disinfectants used on environmental surfaces [19]. For the AOAC Germicidal Spray Products as Disinfectants test and towelette methods (used for hospital disinfectant validation), "the product should kill all of the test microorganisms on 59 out of each set of 60 carriers", which is repeated three times with starting carrier inoculums of ~ 5–6 log bacteria) [14]. Multiple products tested narrowly made or did not meet a 5–6 log reduction performance standard when tested on larger surface areas. This indicates a need for the performance standards to include larger surface areas in disinfectant towelette validation testing, which is more "real-world applicable" to how the towelettes are used in the healthcare industry.

We noted during our wiping process that certain towelettes became harder to move across the Formica surface as the surface area became larger. This was particularly noticeable when wiping with the 0.55% sodium hypochlorite towelette, which had a lower percentage of liquid released per ft^2 overall yet achieved the highest bactericidal efficacy. Taken together, we hypothesize that the towelette itself, as it becomes dryer, is physically removing bacteria from the surface via friction and contact. Conversely, we suggest the 0.5% quat + 55% alcohol towelette, which released a higher percentage of liquid per ft^2, may have allowed it to "glide" over the surface thus reducing physical removal of microorganisms. The PBS-wetted control towelette achieved an approximate two log reduction overall. The PBS control results are similar to Rutala et al., who investigated the efficacy of a non-germicidal product against *Clostridium difficile* spores on Formica surfaces [26]. They found that physical removal via wiping led to a three log reduction in spores from environmental surfaces [26]. This further substantiates that the towelette

substrate and physical wiping motion are contributing to microbial reduction.

Disinfectant efficacy is bacterial species-dependent

Overall, disinfectant towelettes were more effective against *P. aeruginosa* than *S. aureus*. *P. aeruginosa* was reduced a range of 0.12–0.80 $\log_{10}$ more than *S. aureus*. The CDC's Guidelines for Disinfection and Sterilization in Healthcare Facilities acknowledges that disinfectant efficacy can vary depending on the target microorganism [27]. Our prior work on bactericidal efficacy of products against *P. aeruginosa* versus *S. aureus* [5] and study by Hong [7] are consistent with the findings in this study. This implies the need to investigate more strains and species in future research to determine the full implications of species-dependent differences. We acknowledge that our study was limited to two bacterial species and only one strain of each species underscoring the need for further work. Testing was also done using pure bacterial cultures of each species, per EPA methodology [15]. Therefore, we cannot determine the impact a mixed bacterial culture or more complex matrices such as a biofilm would have on disinfectant products' efficacies.

Conclusions

Overall, a disinfectant towelette bactericidal efficacy varies by product used, size of surface area wiped, and by target bacterial species. The results in this study indicate a clear need for further research to determine the efficacy constraints of these products, particularly as they become more frequently used in health care settings.

Abbreviations
EPA: Environmental Protection Agency; HAI: Healthcare-associated infection; PBS: Phosphate buffered saline; Quat: Quaternary ammonium compounds; RTU: Ready-to-use

Acknowledgements
Dr. Oliver is supported by the USDA National Institute of Food and Agriculture Hatch project 2016-67017-24459.

Funding
This work was supported by Diversey Inc., Charlotte, NC, USA.

Authors' contributions
AW, CN, MV and STW performed the disinfectant efficacy testing, analysed and interpreted the data generated, and wrote the manuscript. XL provided industry experience, designed elements of the experimental protocol, and was a contributor in writing and editing the manuscript. PT provided testing materials, industry experience, and was a contributor in writing and editing the manuscript. HO served as the principle investigator for the study and was a contributor in writing and editing the manuscript. All authors read and approved the final manuscript.

Consent for publication
Not applicable.

Competing interests
HO, CN, STW, MV, and AW all report grants from Diversey, Inc. during the conduct of the study. PT and XL reports grants from Diversey, Inc. during the conduct of the study; personal fees from Diversey, Inc., outside the submitted work.

Author details
[1]Department of Food Science, Purdue University, West Lafayette, IN 47907, USA. [2]Diversey Inc., Charlotte, NC 28273, USA. [3]Department of Food Science, Purdue University, 745 Agriculture Mall Drive, West Lafayette, IN 47907, USA.

References
1. Center for Disease Control. Healthcare associated infection progress report. CDC. 2014. https://www.cdc.gov/hai/surveillance/progress-report/index.html Published 2016. Accessed 20 Apr 2018.
2. Magill SS, Edwards JR, Bamberg W, et al. Multistate point-prevalence survey of healthcare-associated infections. N Engl J Med. 2014;370:1198–208.
3. Monk AB, Kanmukhla V, Trinder K, Borkow G. Potent bactericidal efficacy of copper oxide impregnated non-porous solid surfaces. BMC Microbiol. 2014;14:57.
4. Oliveira ES, Araujo EHV, Garcia JNR, et al. Disinfectant use in the hospital environment for microorganisms control. J Bacteriol Parasitol. 2017;8:5.
5. West AM, Teska PJ, Lineback CB, Oliver HF. Strain, disinfectant, concentration, and contact time quantitatively impact disinfectant efficacy. Antimicrob Resist Infect Control. 2018;7:49.
6. Rutala WA, Weber DJ, and the HICPAC. Guideline for disinfection and sterilization in healthcare facilities. CDC. 2008. https://www.cdc.gov/infectioncontrol/pdf/guidelines/disinfection-guidelines.pdf. Accessed 4 May 2018.
7. Hong Y, Teska PJ, Oliver HF. Effects of contact time and concentration on bactericidal efficacy of 3 disinfectants on hard nonporous surfaces. Am J Infect Control. 2017;45:1284–5.
8. Havill NL. Best practices in disinfection of noncritical surfaces in the health care setting: creating a bundle for success. Am J Infect Control. 2013;41:S26–30.
9. Dvorak G. Disinfection 101. In: Iowa State University: Center for Food Security and Public Health website; 2008. http://www.cfsph.iastate.edu/Disinfection/Assets/Disinfection101.pdf. Accessed 2 Feb 2018.
10. Bocian E, Grzybowska W, Tyski S. Evaluation of mycobactericidal activity of selected chemical disinfectants and antiseptics according to European standards. Med Sci Monit. 2014;20:666–73.
11. Gonzalez EA, Nandy P, Lucas AD, Hitchins VM. Ability of cleaning-disinfecting wipes to remove bacteria from medical device surfaces. Am J Infect Control. 2015;43:1331–5.
12. Wiemken TL, Curran DR, Pacholski EB, et al. The value of ready-to-use disinfectant wipes: compliance, employee time, and costs. Am J Infect Control. 2014;42:329–30.
13. Environmental Protection Agency. Standard operating procedure for AOAC use dilution method for testing disinfectants: MB-05-14. EPA. 2016. https://www.epa.gov/sites/production/files/2016-08/documents/mb-05-14.pdf. Accessed 7 May 2018.
14. Environmental Protection Agency. Product performance test guidelines-OCSPP 810.2100: Sterilants-efficacy data recommendations. EPA 2018. https://www.regulations.gov/document?D=EPA-HQ-OPPT-2009-0150-0020. Accessed 28 Feb 2018.
15. Environmental Protection Agency. Operational testing of sporicidal wipes for decontamination of surfaces contaminated with Bacillus anthracis surrogate spores. 2015. https://cfpub.epa.gov/si/si_public_record_report.cfm?dirEntryId=309230&address=nhsrc/si/&view=desc&sortBy=pubDateYear&showCriteria=1&count=25&searchall=%27Biological%20inactivation%27&. Accessed 17 Sept 2018.
16. Environmental Protection Agency. Standard operating procedure for quantitative petri plate method for determining the effectiveness of antimicrobial towelettes against vegetative bacteria on inanimate, hard, non-porous surfaces: MB-33-00. EPA. 2014. https://www.epa.gov/sites/production/files/2014-12/documents/mb-33-00.pdf. Accessed 15 Jan 2018.
17. World Health Organization. Infection prevention and control of epidemic- and pandemic- prone acute respiratory infections in health care. 2014. https://www.ncbi.nlm.nih.gov/books/NBK214359/. Accessed 7 May 2018.
18. Hacek DM, Ogle AM, Fisher A, Robicsek A, Peterson LR. Significant impact of terminal room cleaning with bleach on reducing nosocomial Clostridium difficile. Am J Infect Control. 2010;38:350–3.
19. Environmental Protection Agency. Product performance test guidelines-OCSPP 810.2200: Disinfectants for use on environmental surfaces, guidelines for efficacy testing. EPA. 2018. https://www.regulations.gov/document?D=EPA-HQ-OPPT-2009-0150-0036. Accessed 28 Feb 2018.
20. Environmental Protection Agency. Product performance test guidelines-OCSPP 810.2200: Disinfectants for use on environmental surfaces, guidance for efficacy testing. EPA. 2018. https://www.regulations.gov/document?D=EPA-HQ-OPPT-2009-0150-0036. Accessed 28 Feb 2018.
21. Moore LE, Ledder RG, Gilbert P, McBain AJ. In vitro study of the effect of cationic biocides on bacterial population dynamics and susceptibility. Appl Environ Microbiol. 2008;74(1):4825–34.
22. McBain AJ, Ledder RG, Moore LE, Catrenich CE, Gilbert P. Effects of quaternary-ammonium-based formulations on bacterial community dynamics and antimicrobial susceptibility. Appl Environ Microbiol. 2004;70(6):3449–56.
23. Gerba CP. Quaternary ammonium biocides: efficacy in application. Appl Environ Microbiol. 2015;81:464–9.
24. Boyce JM. Alcohols as surface disinfectants in healthcare settings. Infect Control Hosp Epidemiol. 2018;39:323–8.
25. Rutala WA, Weber DJ. Selection of the ideal disinfectant. Infect Control Hosp Epidemiol. 2014;35:855–65.
26. Rutala WA, Gergen MF, Weber DJ. Efficacy of different cleaning and disinfection methods against Clostridium difficile spores: importance of physical removal versus sporicidal inactivation. Infect Control Hosp Epidemiol. 2012;33:1255–8.
27. Center for Disease Control. Guideline for disinfection and sterilization in healthcare facilities. CDC. 2008. https://www.cdc.gov/infectioncontrol/guidelines/disinfection/efficacy.html. Accessed 16 Sept 2018.

22

Alcohol-based surgical hand preparation: translating scientific evidence into clinical practice

Gilberto G. Gaspar[1,6*], Mayra G. Menegueti[1], Ana Elisa R. Lopes[1], Roberto O. C. Santos[2], Thamiris R. de Araújo[3], Aline Nassiff[3], Lécio R. Ferreira[1], Maria Eulalia L. V. Dallora[4], Silvia R. M. S. Canini[3] and Fernando Bellissimo-Rodrigues[5]

Abstract

Background: Although alcohol-based surgical hand preparation offers potential advantages over the traditional surgical scrubbing technique, implementing it may be challenging due to resistance of surgeons in changing their practice. We aimed to implement alcohol-based surgical hand preparation in the hospital setting evaluating the impact of that on the quality and duration of the procedure, as well as on the prevention of surgical site infections.

Methods: A quasi-experimental study conducted at a tertiary-care university hospital from April 01 to November 01, 2017. Participants were cardiac and orthopedic surgical teams ($n = 56$) and patients operated by them ($n = 231$). Intervention consisted of making alcohol-based handrub available in the operating room, convincing and training surgical teams for using it, promoting direct observation of surgical hand preparation, and providing aggregated feedback on the quality of the preparation. The primary study outcome was the quality of the surgical hand preparation, inferred by the compliance with each one of the steps predicted in the World Health Organization (WHO) technique, evaluated through direct observation. Secondary study outcome was the patient's individual probability of developing surgical site infection in both study periods. We used the Wilcoxon for paired samples and McNemar's test to assess the primary study outcome and we build a logistic regression model to assess the secondary outcome.

Results: We observed 534 surgical hand preparation events. Among 33 participants with full data available for both study periods, we observed full compliance with all the steps predicted in the WHO technique in 0.03% (1/33) of them in the pre-intervention period and in 36.36% (12/33) of them in the intervention period (OR:12.0, 95% CI: 2. 4-59.2, $p = 0.002$). Compared to the pre-intervention period, the intervention reduced the duration of the preparation (4.8 min vs 2.7 min, respectively; $p < 0.001$). The individual risk of developing a surgical site infection did not significantly change between the pre-intervention and the intervention phase (Adjusted RR = 0.66; 95% CI 0. 16-2.70, $p = 0.563$).

Conclusion: Our results demonstrate that, when compared to the traditional surgical scrub, alcohol-based surgical hand preparation improves the quality and reduces the duration of the preparation, being at least equally effective for the prevention of surgical site infections.

* Correspondence: ggaspar@hcrp.usp.br
[1]Infection Control Service, University Hospital of the Ribeirão Preto Medical School, University of São Paulo, Ribeirão Preto, SP, Brazil
[6]University Hospital of Ribeirão Preto Medical School, Avenida Bandeirantes, 3900 – Vila Monte Alegre, Ribeirão Preto, SP 14048-900, Brazil

Background

Surgical site infection (SSI) is a worldwide concern. A study conducted in 16 European countries identified that 20% of all notified healthcare-associated infections were related to surgical procedures [1]. In Florida, SSI represented one-third of all cases of healthcare-associated infections [2].

Surgical hand preparation is recommended by both the Centers for Disease Control and Prevention (CDC) and the World Health Organization (WHO) for preventing SSI in all kinds of surgical procedures [3]. There are two well-recognized methods for performing surgical hand preparation. The most traditional one is scrubbing hands and forearms with antimicrobial soap, usually 2% chlorhexidine or 10% povidone-iodine (PVPI). More recently, alcohol-based surgical hand preparation has been proposed as an alternative to surgical scrub [3–8]. Among potential advantages of the alcohol-based procedure are: less skin irritation, less time-consuming, economy of tap water, and more potent antimicrobial effect [9].

However, surgeons may be skeptical about adopting alcohol-based surgical hand preparation, and this may represent a challenge for implementing such a strategy in the operating room. A study carried out among 156 healthcare professionals in a medical center in Taiwan identified that a higher number of nurses employed alcohol-based handrub (ABHR) for surgical hand preparation as compared to surgeons. The authors attributed this finding to the greater familiarity of surgeons with the traditional surgical hand preparation technique and to their higher reliability on the antiseptic effect thereof [10].

Therefore, studies performed in the real world scenario are necessary to confirm the benefits of using ABHR for surgical hand preparation, predicted mostly by lab studies. Implementation research studies entail: (i) testing strategies to face obstacles and (ii) determining the best strategy to introduce innovations or to promote sustainable changes [11].

The present study aimed to implement the exchange of using antimicrobial soap for using ABHR in the context of surgical hand preparation and to evaluate the impact of that on the quality and duration of the procedure, as well as on the prevention of surgical site infections.

Methods

This quasi-experimental study was conducted from April 01 to November 01, 2017 in a tertiary-care public-affiliated university hospital in Brazil. The Research Ethics Committee of the study institution approved its protocol before the study implementation (n° 64,964,217.9.0000.5440).

The study population consisted of all members of the cardiac and orthopedic surgical teams of the study facility and all patients operated by them during the study period. Each patient was included just one time in the study, so re-operations during the study period were not considered in the data analysis.

In the pre-intervention period, which lasted 3 months, traditional surgical scrub was performed with antimicrobial soap (either 2% chlorhexidine or 10% PVPI) before every surgery and ABHR was not available for surgical hand preparation. Direct observation of the procedures was implemented as a part of the data collection.

Just after the pre-intervention period, we started the implementation period, which lasted 1 month, and during it no data was collected. The intervention consisted of making ABHR available in the operating room, convincing and training the selected surgical teams for using it, promoting direct observation of surgical hand preparation, and providing them aggregated feedback on the quality of the preparation. The training consisted of a 4 h workshop, repeated five times, when the scientific literature about surgical hand preparation was reviewed and the participants were instructed about how to apply ABHR for this purpose, according to the WHO technique. To ensure the covering of all hand and forearms surface, we asked all participants to apply a fluorescent ABHR simulating the surgical hand preparation, which was afterwards revealed by a fluorescence apparatus.

Just after the implementation period, the intervention period began, and the data collection re-started. The intervention period also lasted 3 months.

The primary study outcome was the quality of the surgical hand preparation, inferred by the compliance with each one of the steps predicted in the WHO technique, evaluated through direct observation in the operating room. Secondary study outcome was the patient's individual probability of developing SSI in both study periods.

The following instruments were employed for data collection:

1) Surgical site infection (SSI) – we followed up operated patients for 1 month to verify whether they had developed SSI or not, according to the CDC criteria, including post-discharge surveillance. Patients were screened by an infection control nurse, and SSI episodes were confirmed by an infectious disease specialist of the Infection Control Service.

2) Risk factors for SSI – an instrument containing the following items was designed: study phase, surgical procedure, extracorporeal circulation time (min), surgical time (min), American Society of Anesthesiologists physical status classification system (ASA), comorbidities, use of immunosuppressive

drugs, Body Mass Index (BMI), preoperative hospital stay (in days), presence of infection before the surgery, antibiotic prophylaxis, surgical complications and SSI by a multidrugresistant microorganism (carbapenem-resistant Enterobacteria, *Pseudomonas* spp., or *Acinetobacter baumannii*; methicillin-resistant *Staphylococcus aureus*; or vancomycin-resistant *Enterococcus* spp.). Two investigators from the Infection Control Service collected these data.

3) Surgical hand-preparation quality assessment – an instrument based on the WHO technique and framing the following items was designed: time spent on surgical hand preparation, use of jewelry (e.g., rings, wristwatch, and bracelets), short nails, and compliance with all the antisepsis steps (palm to palm; right palm over back of left hand and vice-versa; interdigital spaces, thumb, nails, fingertips, wrist, and forearm). Two investigators with extensive training in hand hygiene and surgical hand preparation performed these observations in both study periods.

Taking into account the previously unknown baseline status of the quality of the surgical hand preparation (primary study outcome) in the study facility, we could not estimate a sample size for the study. The period of 3 months for the pre-intervention and 3 months for the intervention was chosen for convenience. Data were analyzed with the STATA SE® software version 14. First, a descriptive analysis was accomplished. Then, we calculated the weighted average for each surgical team member of the compliance with each one of the steps of the WHO technique for surgical hand preparation (primary study outcome) and we used the Wilcoxon test for paired samples to compare it between the two study periods. We also used McNemar's test to compare full compliance with the WHO technique observed before and after the intervention. Finally, we build a logistic regression model to assess the secondary study outcome (SSI risk) on the patient level, adjusting it for surrogate markers of baseline severity status, such as pre-operative length of stay, ASA score, and other potential risk factors for SSI implicated in univariate analysis ($p < 0.10$).

Results

All cardiac and orthopedic surgery staff members agreed to participate in the study and were included in the pre-intervention and intervention phases, totaling 56 participants. All the 231 patients who had undergone cardiac (85 patients) or orthopedic (146 patients) surgeries during the study period were also included.

Table 1 contains a descriptive analysis of selected demographical and clinical characteristics of the patients operated in pre-intervention (132 patients) and intervention (99 patients) phases. Although a reasonable balance was observed for most of these variables between the two study periods, we have detected some important differences. Median age was higher in the pre-intervention (53.7 years old) than in the intervention phase (46.9 years old). Orthopedic surgery was less frequent in the pre-intervention (57.6%) than in the intervention phase (70.7%). The average duration of the procedures was shorter in the pre-intervention (median time: 175 min) compared to the intervention phase (median time: 240 min). Technical complications during procedure were more frequent in the pre-intervention phase (3.8% vs 1%) than in the intervention phase. In addition, finally, post-discharge follow-up reached more patients in the pre-intervention (86.4%) than in the intervention phase (73.7%).

Surgical hand preparation quality assessment

We directly observed 534 surgical hand preparation events. In the pre-intervention phase, 303 events were observed, and in most of them 2% chlorhexidine ($n = 180$) was employed for surgical scrub and, in the remaining events, 10% PVPI ($n = 123$) was used. In the intervention phase, we observed 231 events of alcohol-based surgical hand preparation (Table 2). Compliance with most of the steps predicted by the WHO technique did not significantly varied between the two study periods. However, average compliance with the scrubbing of the thumb in the pre-intervention period (86.2%) was lower than the rubbing of the thumb in the intervention period (96.9%), and that difference was borderline statistically significant ($p = 0.052$). Nail scrubbing was observed in only 33.7% of events when chlorhexidine was employed and in only 41.5% of the events when PVPI was used. Interestingly, hands rinsing at the end of surgical hand preparation was performed only in 72.3% of the events in which PVPI was used. Another problem detected in the scrubbing period was that only 13.5 and 18.0% of the participants did not get back to hands after scrubbing the forearms, while using chlorhexidine and PVPI, respectively.

Considering a subset of 33 participants with full data available for both study periods, we observed a full compliance with all the steps predicted in the WHO technique for surgical hand preparation in 0.03% (1/33) of them in the pre-intervention period and in 36.36% (12/33) of them in the intervention period (OR:12.0; 95% CI: 2. 4-59.2; $p = 0.002$).

The median scrubbing time was 4.8 min when the surgical team used chlorhexidine, and 4.9 min when they used PVPI. This was significantly longer than the median 2.7 min spent on rubbing hands and forearms, in the intervention period ($p = 0.001$).

Table 1 Demographical and clinical aspects of the patients operated in the pre-intervention and intervention phases of the study

Patients characteristics	Pre-intervention phase Surgical scrub (n = 132)		Intervention phase Alcohol-based surgical hand preparation (n = 99)	
	Number	Percent	Number	Percent
Sex				
Male	74	56.0	62	62.6
Female	58	44.0	37	37.4
Age (years)[a]	53.7 (25.0–65.9)		46.9 (20. 4-63.5)	
Surgical specialty				
Orthopedics	76	57.6	70	70.7
Cardiac	56	42.4	29	29.3
Post-discharge follow-up	114	86.4	73	73.7
Duration of surgery (min)[a]	180 (122–263)		200 (130–255)	
Duration of extracorporeal circulation (min)[a] (n = 41)	115 (80–140.5)		125 (95–155)	
Preoperative length of stay (days)[a]	2 (1-8)		2 (1-4)	
Body Mass Index – BMI	26.7 (23. 8-31.7)		27.2 (23. 2-30.5)	
Technical complication during procedure	5	3.8	1	1
Urgent procedure	8	6	8	8.1
Chronic hepatopathy	2	1.5	5	5
Malignancy	10	7.6	5	5
Diabetes Mellitus	32	24.2	27	27.3
Use of immunosuppressive drug	5	3.8	2	2
Smoking	31	23.5	20	20.2

[a]Median (interquartile range)

Table 2 Percentage of weighted average compliance with each one of the steps of the WHO technique for surgical hand preparation according to the study phase and product employed

Compliance with each one of the steps of the WHO technique for surgical hand preparation	Pre-intervention phase (n = 303)		Intervention phase (n = 231)	P-Value[c]
	Surgical scrub with 2% chlorhexidine (%) (n = 180)[a]	Surgical scrub with 10% PVPI (%) (n = 123)[b]	Alcohol-based surgical hand preparation (%) (n = 231)[b]	
Removed jewelry	99.4	100	100	1.000
Short nails	95	100	97.8	0.341
Finger	96.6	95.9	98.2	0.762
Palm	100	100	99	0.157
Back of hand	96.6	97.4	98.2	0.946
Interdigital space	82.1	85.5	93	0.948
Thumb	85.7	87.2	96.9	0.052
Wrist	95.5	98.3	99.1	0.247
Did not get back to hands after donning forearms	13.5	18	NA	NA
Nail scrubbing	33.7	41.5	NA	NA
Hands rinsing	98.8	72.3	NA	NA
Time (min)	4.8	4.9	2.7	0.001

NA not applicable
[a]The number of surgical hand preparation events observed per participant ranged from 1 to 24
[b]The number of surgical hand preparation events observed per participant ranged from 1 to 16
[c]Comparison between the pre-intervention and intervention phases by the Wilcoxon for paired samples test

Analysis of potential risk factors for surgical site infection

We analyzed all 231 patients operated during the study period. Among patients operated in the pre-intervention period, 8.3% (11/132) developed SSI, while during the intervention period, SSI rate was reduced to 4.0% (4/99), although those differences did not reach statistical significance (RR = 0.48, 95% CI 0. 16-1.48).

Table 3 exhibits the univariate analysis of the potential risk factors for SSI observed during the study implementation. According to that analysis, no variable was implicated as a predictor of SSI and the alcohol-based surgical hand preparation, implemented in the intervention period, was not considered to impact on the individual probability of developing SSI (RR = 0.48, 95% CI 0. 16-1.48, $p = 0.281$).

Table 4 presents the multivariate analysis of the impact that alcohol-based surgical hand preparation could have over the individual probability of developing SSI, adjusted for pre-operative length of stay and ASA score. This analysis was performed for a subset of 150 patients, for whom all the data, including ASA score, was available. According to that, alcohol-based surgical hand preparation was not predictor nor protective against the individual risk of developing SSI (adjusted RR = 0.66, 95% CI 0. 16-2.70, $p = 0.563$).

The incidence of SSI caused by multidrug-resistant microorganisms was 6.06% (8/132) in the pre-intervention period, dropping to 1.01% (1/99) in the intervention period (RR = 0.17, 95% CI 0. 21-1.31, $p = 0.082$).

Difficulties faced during implementation of an ABHR for surgical hand preparation

Two surgeons, one of the orthopedic surgery staff and another of the cardiac surgery staff, at first, reported that they did not rely on the ABHR effectiveness. Therefore, we scheduled meetings to show them that ABHR was actually efficient for surgical hand preparation. The professionals received all the information via email or printed articles. After this approach, these two surgeons complied with the use of ABHR during the intervention phase.

Discussion

Many advantages of using ABHR for surgical hand preparation have been proposed by scientific literature, mostly based on laboratory-based studies [12–16].

Table 3 Univariate statistical analysis of risk factors for surgical site infection (SSI) among 231 patients operated during the study period

Variable	Patients characteristics		With SSI ($n = 15$)	Without SSI ($n = 216$)	Relative risk (95% CI) or p-value
	Situation	Total n (%)			
Chronic Hepatopathy	Present	4 (1.7%)	1 (6.6%)	3 (1.3%)	4.05 (0.68–23.80)
	Absent	227 (98.3%)			
Malignance	Present	15 (6.5%)	1 (6.6%)	14 (6.4%)	1.02 (0.14–7.30)
	Absent	216 (93.5%)			
Diabetes Mellitus	Present	59 (25.5%)	2 (13.3%)	57 (26.3%)	0.44 (0.10–1.92)
	Absent	172 (74.4%)			
Use of immunosuppressive drugs	Present	7 (3%)	1 (6.6%)	6 (2.7%)	2.28 (0.34–15.04)
	Absent	224 (97%)			
Smoking	Present	53 (22.9%)	5 (33.3%)	48 (22.2%	1.67 (0.60–4.69)
	Absent	178 (77.1%)			
Urgent surgery	Present	16 (6.9%)	1 (6.6%)	15 (6.9%)	0.95 (0.13–6.84)
	Absent	215 (93,1%)			
Technical complications during surgery	Present	8 (3.4%)	1 (6.6%)	7 (3.3%)	1.99 (0.29–13.34)
	Absent	223 (96.6%)			
Alcohol-based surgical hand preparation	Present	99 (42.8%)	4 (26.6%)	95 (43.9%)	0.48 (0.16–1.48)
	Absent	132 (57.2%)			
Extracorporeal circulation time (min)[a]			130 (65–210)	117 (80–145)	$p = 0.688$
ASA score[a]			2 (2-2)	2 (2-2)	$P = 0.932$
Pre-operative length of stay (days)[a]			3 (1–7)	2 (1–6)	$p = 0.356$
Duration of surgery (min)[a]			195 (129–285)	190 (125–261)	$p = 0.778$
Body Mass Index – BMI[a]			28.5 (25.3–30.1)	26.6 (23.6–31.2)	$p = 0.802$

[a]Median (interquartile range)

Table 4 Multivariate statistical analysis (logistic regression) of risk factors for surgical site infections (SSI) among 150 patients operated in the study period

Variable	Odds ratio (95% CI)	P-value
Alcohol-based surgical hand preparation	0.66 (0.16–2.70)	0.563
ASA score	1.09 (0.41–2.90)	0.862
Pre-operative length of stay (days)	0.92 (0.75–1.15)	0.493

Among those advantages, we can highlight less skin irritation, less time-consuming, economy of tap water, and more potent antimicrobial effect. However, only a few studies have attempted to implement and evaluate alcohol-based surgical hand preparation in a real world scenario [17, 18]. The present study adds evidence on this topic, confirming some of the predicted benefits. The studied intervention consisted of making ABHR available in the operating room, training surgical teams for using it, promoting direct observation of the preparation, and providing them aggregated feedback on the quality of the preparation. That intervention was demonstrated effective for enhancing the quality of the preparation, and for shortening the time spent on the preparation. Regarding SSI prevention, the intervention was proven at least equivalent to the previous protocol, focused on the surgical scrub with antimicrobial soap.

An observational study of traditional surgical hand preparation by scrubbing with chlorhexidine solution detected unsatisfactory preparation, especially with respect to the mean scrubbing time, which was lower than the time advocated in the literature [13]. In another study. Nail scrubbing was observed in 33.7 and 41.5% for 2% chlorhexidine and 10% PVPI solutions, respectively. Most healthcare professionals followed all the scrub steps during surgical hand preparation, which promoted an abrasive effect of scrub brush on their skin. This is the reason why the WHO does not recommend the use of scrub brushes [19, 20].

A study involving 156 healthcare professionals in southern Taiwan evaluated the microbial load reduction after surgical hand preparation and found that ABHR had a highly persistent effect ($P = 0.001$) [12]. Another study verified an improved microbial load reduction when an ABHR was employed (1.91–1.52 log10), as compared to chlorhexidine (0.82–1.16 log10) and PVPI (0.52–0.92) solutions [21].

A systematic review of 14 randomized clinical trials compared the efficacy of chlorhexidine, PVPI, and ABHRs. ABHR was as effective as or more effective than antiseptic agent solutions. Nail scrubbing was the surgical hand asepsis step with the lowest evidence level. Moreover, the SSI rates were similar in all cases [17].

In a randomized clinical trial conducted in France between January 01 of 2000 and March 01 of 2001 with 4387 surgical patients, the SSI rates were similar for antiseptic agent solution and ABHR [55 cases (2.4%) vs 53 cases (2.48%)], respectively [18].

Our study presents some important limitations. First, a small imbalance was observed in some of the clinical and demographical features of the patients included in the pre- and in the intervention phases. However, none of those characteristics could affect the primary study outcome, and none of them was actually demonstrated to interfere with the secondary study outcome, in multivariate analysis. Second, compliance with post-discharge follow-up was greater in the pre-intervention than in the intervention period, which could lead to an underestimation of the SSI rate in the intervention period. Third, as the intervention was multifaceted, we are not able to infer the individual impact of each one of its components over the study outcomes.

Conclusion
The present study provides support for the routine use of ABHR for surgical hand preparation. Our results demonstrate that, when compared to the traditional surgical scrubbing with antimicrobial soap, alcohol-based surgical preparation, along with proper training, may improve the quality of the preparation, reduce the time spent on the preparation, and it is at least equally effective for the prevention of surgical site infections.

Abbreviations
95% CI: 95% Confidence Interval; ABHR: Alcohol-Based Handrub; Adjusted RR: Adjusted Relative Risk; ASA: American Society of Anesthesiologists physical status classification system; BMI: Body Mass Index; PVPI: Povidone-Iodine; SSI: Surgical Site Infection; WHO: World Health Organization

Acknowledgements
The authors thank the Infection Control Service team of the study facility for their assistance on the study implementation.

Funding
The University Hospital of the Ribeirão Preto Medical School provided the ABHR for the study. Other study costs were covered by a research grant issued by the World Health Organization Implementation Research Regional Training Centre for the Americas' Region.

Authors' contributions
Study concept and design: FBR; GGG. Acquisition of data: AN; TRA. Drafting of the manuscript: GGG; MGM; AERL. Statistical analysis: FBR;. Critical revision of the manuscript for important intellectual content: GGG; MGM; AERL; ROCS; TRA; AN; LRF; MED; FBR; SRMSC. All authors read and approved the final manuscript.

Consent for publication
Not applicable.

Competing interests
The authors declare that they have no competing interest. None of the authors have any conflicts of interest to disclose.

Author details

[1]Infection Control Service, University Hospital of the Ribeirão Preto Medical School, University of São Paulo, Ribeirão Preto, SP, Brazil. [2]Department of Surgery and Anatomy, Ribeirão Preto Medical School, University of São Paulo, Ribeirão Preto, SP, Brazil. [3]Department of Fundamental Nursing, Ribeirão Preto College of Nursing, University of São Paulo, Ribeirão Preto, SP, Brazil. [4]Hospital Administration, University Hospital of the Ribeirão Preto Medical School, University of São Paulo, Ribeirão Preto, SP, Brazil. [5]Social Medicine Department, Ribeirão Preto Medical School, University of São Paulo, Ribeirão Preto, SP, Brazil. [6]University Hospital of Ribeirão Preto Medical School, Avenida Bandeirantes, 3900 – Vila Monte Alegre, Ribeirão Preto, SP 14048-900, Brazil.

References

1. European Centre for Disease Prevention and Control. Point prevalence survey of healthcare-associated infections and antimicrobial use in European acute care hospitals. Stockholm: ECDC; 2013. Available from: https://ecdc.europa.eu/sites/portal/files/media/en/publications/Publications/healthcare-associated-infections-antimicrobial-use-PPS.pdf

2. Magill SS, Hellinger W, Cohen J, et al. Prevalence of healthcare-associated infections in acute care hospitals in Jacksonville, Florida. Infect Control Hosp Epidemiol. 2012;33(3):283–91. https://doi.org/10.1086/664048.

3. WHO guidelines on hand hygiene in healthcare. Geneva: World Health Organization; 2009 (http://apps.who.int/iris/bitstream/handle/10665/44102/9789241597906_eng.pdf;jsessionid=8DFE9483D36DB1E696E2FD777FEFEC56?sequence=1. Accessed 20 Dec 2017).

4. Rotter ML. Arguments for alcoholic hand disinfection. J Hosp Infect. 2001;48(Suppl A):S4–8.

5. Widmer AF. Surgical hand hygiene: scrub or rub? J Hosp Infect. 2013; 83(Suppl 1):S35–9.

6. Hsieh HF, Chiu HH, Lee FP. Surgical hand scrubs in relation to microbial counts: systematic literature review. J Adv Nurs. 2006;55(1):68–78. 9.

7. Graf ME, Machado A, Mensor LL, Zampieri D, Campos R, Faham L. Surgical hands antisepsis with alcohol-based preparations: cost-effectiveness, compliance of professionals and ecological benefits in the Brazilian healthcare scenario (in Portuguese). J Bras Econ Saúde. 2014;6(2):71–80.

8. Hennign TJ, Werner S, Naujox K, Arndt A. Chlorhexidine is not an essential component in alcohol-based surgical hand preparation: a comparative study of two handrubs based on a modified EN 12791 test protocol. Antimicrob Resist Infect Control. 2017;6:96.

9. Suchomel M, Gnant G, Weinlich M, Rotter M. Surgical hand disinfection using alcohol: the effects of alcohol type, mode, and duration of application. J Hosp Infect. 2009;71(3):228–33. https://doi.org/10.1016/j.jhin.2008.11.006. Epub 2009 Jan 13

10. Chen SH, Chou CY, Huang JC, Tang YF, Kuo YR, Chien LY. Antibacterial effects on dry-fast and traditional water-based surgical scrubbing methods: a two-time points experimental study. Nurs Health Sci. 2014;16:179–85.

11. Peters DH, Tran NT, Adam T. Implementation research in health: a practical guide Alliance for Health Policy and Systems Research. Geneve: World Health Organization; 2013.

12. Barbadoro P, Martin E, Savini S, Marigliano A, Ponzio E, Prospero E, D'Errico MM. In vivo comparative efficacy of three surgical hand preparation agents in reducing bacterial count. J Hosp Infect. 2014;86:64–7.

13. Pietsch HJ. Hand antiseptics: rubs versus scrubs, alcoholic solutions versus alcoholic gels. Hosp Infect. 2001;48(Suppl A):S33–6.

14. Marchetti MG, Kampf G, Finzi G, Salvatorelli GJ. Evaluation of the bactericidal effect of five products for surgical hand disinfection according to prEN 12054 and prEN 12791. Hosp Infect. 2003;54(1):63–7.

15. Lai KW, Foo TL, Low W, Naidu G. Surgical hand antisepsis–a pilot study comparing povidone iodine hand scrub and alcohol-based chlorhexidine gluconate hand rub. Ann Acad Med Singap. 2012;41(1):12–6.

16. Suchomel M, Kundi M, Allegranzi B, Pittet D, Rotter ML. Testing of the World Health Organization-recommended formulations for surgical handpreparation and proposals for increased efficacy. J Hosp Infect. 2011;79(2):115–8. https://doi.org/10.1016/j.jhin.2011.05.005. Epub 2011 Jul 7

17. Gonçalves KJ; Graziano KU; Kawagoe JK. Revisão sistemática sobre antissepsia cirúrgica das mãos com preparação alcoólica em comparação aos produtos tradicionais. Rev. esc. enferm. USP vol.46 no.6 São Paulo Dec. 2012.

18. Parienti JJ, Thibon P, Heller R, et al. Hand-rubbing with an aqueous alcoholic solution vs traditional surgical hand-scrubbing and 30-day surgical site infection rates: a randomized equivalence study. JAMA. 2002;288:722.

19. World Health Organization (WHO). WHO guidelines on hand hygiene in health care. First global patient safety challenge. Clean care is safe care, Geneva: World Health Organization (WHO); 2009.

20. Boyce JM, Pittet D. Guideline for Hand Hygiene in Health- Care Settings. Recommendations of the Healthcare Infection Control Practices Advisory Committee and the HICPAC/SHEA/ APIC/IDSA Hand Hygiene Task Force. Society for Healthcare Epidemiology of America/Association for Professionals in Infection Control/Infectious Diseases Society of America. MMWR Recomm Rep. 2002;51(RR-16):1–45. quiz CE1–4. https://www.cdc.gov/mmwr/PDF/rr/rr5116.pdf pubmed/12418624

21. Tanner J, Dumville JC, Norman G, Fortnam M. Surgical hand preparation to reduce surgical site infection. Cochrane Database Syst Rev. 2016;(1)Art. No.: CD004288.

23

Large variations in the practice patterns of surgical antiseptic preparation solutions in patients with open and closed extremity fractures

Maria Jurado-Ruiz[1], Gerard P. Slobogean[2], Sofia Bzovsky[3], Alisha Garibaldi[3], Nathan N. O'Hara[2], Andrea Howe[2], Brad Petrisor[3] and Sheila Sprague[3,4,5*]

Abstract

Background: Surgically-managed fractures, particularly open fractures, are associated with high rates of surgical site infections (SSIs). To reduce the risk of an SSI, orthopaedic surgeons routinely clean open fracture wounds in the emergency department (ED) and then apply a bandage to the open wound. Prior to the surgical incision, it is standard practice to prepare the fracture region with an antiseptic skin solution as an additional SSI prevention strategy. Multiple antiseptic solutions are available.

Objectives: To explore the variation in practice patterns among orthopaedic surgeons regarding antiseptic solution use in the ED and antiseptic preparatory techniques for fracture surgery.

Methods: We developed a 27-item survey and surveyed members of several orthopaedic associations.

Results: Two hundred and-ten surveys were completed. 71.0% of respondents irrigate the open wound and skin in the ED, primarily with saline alone (59.7%) or iodine-based solutions (32.9%). 90.5% of responders indicated that they dress the open wound in the ED, with 41.0% applying a saline-soaked bandage and 33.7% applying an iodine-soaked dressing (33.7%). In their surgical preparation of open fractures, 41.0% of respondents used an iodine-based solution, 26.7% used a chlorhexidine gluconate (CHG)-based solution, and 31.4% used a combination of the two. In closed fractures, 43.8% of respondents used a CHG-based solution, 28.1% used an iodine-based solution, and 27.1% used a combination. Despite theoretical concerns about the use of alcohol in open wounds, 51.4% used alcohol-based solutions or alcohol alone during skin preparation of open fractures.

Conclusions: A lack of consensus exists regarding use of antiseptic surgical preparation solutions for fractures. High-quality clinical research is needed to assess the effectiveness of different surgical antiseptic preparation solutions on patient outcomes in fracture populations.

Keywords: Survey, Open fracture, Closed fracture, Antiseptic preparation, Surgical site infection, Surgical preparation, Antiseptic solution

* Correspondence: sprags@mcmaster.ca
[3]Division of Orthopaedic Surgery, Department of Surgery, McMaster University, Hamilton, ON, Canada
[4]Department of Health Research Methods, Evidence, and Impact, McMaster University, Hamilton, ON, Canada

Introduction

Surgically managed fractures have a high incidence of surgical site infections (SSIs) as compared to other surgical specialties [1]. SSIs can be devastating to patients and to their families, as they may lead to use of additional antibiotic use, additional surgical interventions, prolonged morbidity, loss of function, potential limb loss, and even death [2]. Given the negative consequences of an SSI, the prevention of infection is an important focus of perioperative fracture management.

To reduce the risk of an SSI in open fracture management, orthopaedic surgeons often irrigate the open fracture wound in the emergency department and then apply a bandage, either dry or soaked with saline or an antiseptic solution. Additionally, prior to a surgical incision for operative management of either open or closed fractures, it is standard practice to prepare the injured region with an antiseptic solution to reduce the risk of an SSI.

In general, the application of an antiseptic solution prior to surgical incision is known to be effective in preventing SSIs [3]. However, given the many types of antiseptic solutions with different active agents available to surgeons, there is no clear evidence on the best antiseptic solution for fracture patients [3]. Two common preoperative skin antiseptics used are chlorhexidine gluconate (CHG) and iodine-based solutions, both of which have a strong biological rationale [4] and are available in either an aqueous-based or alcohol-based solution.

There is a paucity of compelling clinical evidence regarding which of these surgical antiseptic preparation solutions is more effective at preventing SSIs [3] and the evidence guiding preoperative antiseptic skin solution choice in fracture surgery (either open or closed) is largely extrapolated from other surgical disciplines [3]. Data from the FLOW trial (Fluid Lavage of Open Wounds) of approximately 2500 open fracture patients found great variation in the early management of open fractures and the type of preoperative skin preparations used by surgeons [5].

To quantify this further, we conducted a survey of orthopaedic surgeons to understand the practice patterns regarding use of antiseptic solutions in the emergency department and surgical antiseptic preparatory processes for open and closed extremity fractures.

Materials and methods

Questionnaire development - item generation

We developed a questionnaire using the previous literature and key informants to examine preferences and practices of orthopaedic surgeons for early management of open fracture wounds, and the preoperative antiseptic skin preparation practices for open and closed extremity fractures. The survey was reviewed by five experts, including three orthopaedic surgeons and two epidemiologists, to ensure that nothing vital was missed and to ensure that the wording of the questions was clear and precise.

Pretesting and validity assessments of the questionnaire

We pretested the questionnaire in an independent group of five orthopaedic surgeons with experience in clinical research and the treatment of open and closed fractures to evaluate whether the questionnaire adequately encompassed current management practices (face validity), and whether the individual questions adequately addressed the objectives of the current study (content validity). This group of surgeons also commented on the clarity and comprehensiveness of the questionnaire. The survey was revised based upon the recommendations of this independent group and retested in the same group until no additional issues or concerns were identified.

Survey description

The final survey was comprised of 27 questions using check-boxes and brief open-ended questions. All of the questions used clear and widely recognized terminology to enhance the validity of results. The survey length was kept to a minimum to maximize response rate and to limit respondent fatigue. The survey included questions about the participants' demographics, location of practice, type of practice (community or academic), and their number of years of experience treating fracture patients. It also included questions about early open fracture wound management, the use of single or multiple surgical antiseptics for both open and closed fractures, type(s) of antiseptics used, irrigation procedures, the use of dressings on open wounds, and what typically guides surgeons' clinical decision making, as well as their perceptions on the importance of antiseptic selection in the prevention of an SSI. Finally, respondents were asked several questions about their personal interest in participating in future clinical trials comparing different surgical antiseptic preparation solutions. All questions were in the context of the preoperative surgical care of fracture patients with the focus being on how to prevent SSI of the current fracture rather than the prevention of secondary infections. The questions were not randomized and we used adaptive questioning for certain items. All questions fit an average screen, with 1 question per page. All questions had to be completed, and respondents were able to go back and review their previous answers. Please refer to Additional file 1 for a copy of the survey.

Survey administration

The survey was made available to 2149 active members of the Canadian Orthopaedic Association (COA), Canadian Orthopaedic Trauma Society (COTS), and the Orthopaedic

Trauma Association (OTA) through email messages from the corresponding association. The e-mail included a link to the online survey and information about the survey's purpose, how their data would be stored and used, the length of time required to complete the survey, and the investigators' contact information. Follow-up emails at 2 weeks and at 4 weeks following the initial request were sent to aid in increasing the response rate among survey participants. Participants were assigned a unique ID when opening the link to our survey which they would only be able to answer once; the IP address of each client computer was also used to identify any potential duplicate entries from the same user. Completion of the survey was considered as implicit consent. All surveys were completed using Survey-Monkey, an online survey development cloud-based software that includes data analysis, sample selection, bias elimination, and data representation tools. No monetary incentives or pre-notification telephone calls were used for this survey. Questionnaire completion was voluntary and individual responses were kept confidential, only being accessible through a password protected account. The data was collected from November 2016 to May 2017.

Sample size

To determine the number of respondents needed to sufficiently power our analysis, we assumed that approximately 50% of surgeons surveyed would use a surgical antiseptic preparation solution with chlorhexidine gluconate and 50% of surgeons would use a surgical antiseptic preparation solution with iodine as their preferred choice. The calculation for appropriate sample size was performed according to the following formula, assuming a 95% confidence interval for the estimate: $N = (Z_\alpha/w)^2$ $p(1 - p)$, [Where: $Z = z$ value (1.96 for 95% confidence interval); w = width of the confidence interval, expressed as decimal (0.07 to give ±7); p = hypothesized proportion of who would use a surgical antiseptic preparation solution with chlorhexidine gluconate, expressed in decimal (70% = 0.70)]. According to our calculation, approximately 164 completed questionnaires would facilitate a meaningful analysis.

Statistical analysis

We summarized all categorical and dichotomous variables with frequencies and percentages. Only completed questionnaires were analyzed. Continuous data were described with means and standard deviations (SDs). All analyses were conducted in SPSS Version 25.0 (IBM Corporation, Armonk, NY).

Results

Characteristics of the respondents

A total of 210 surveys were completed. Most of the respondents were from North America (45.2%), Europe (25.7%), or Asia (18.1%) (Table 1). Nearly 93% of the respondents were men and the mean age was 47.7 ± 8.2 years. Approximately three-quarters of the respondents practiced in an academic teaching hospital and most respondents (82.4%) had 10 or more years' experience treating fracture patients.

Solutions used in the emergency room to treat open fracture wounds

More than two-thirds (149/210 = 71.0%) of the responders indicated that they irrigate the open wound and skin in the emergency department. Among these 149 surgeons, almost two-thirds, indicated that the irrigation is conducted following orthopaedic surgeon consultation (95/149 = 63.8%), whereas a third indicated that the irrigation is performed immediately upon arrival to emergency department (52/149 = 34.9%). Among those who irrigated the open wound in the emergency room, more than half (89/149 = 59.7%) used saline alone, 32.9% used an aqueous-iodophor solution (e.g. Betadine®), and 7.4% used either CHG or iodine in an alcohol-based solution (Table 2).

Most surgeons indicated that they always dress the open wound in the emergency department (90.5%) and approximately one-third used a sterile dry-dressing (75/205 = 36.6%). 41.0% (84/205) used a saline-soaked dressing and a third indicated that they use an iodine-soaked dressing (69/205 = 33.7%). Please note that surgeons were able to select more than one response when indicating the type of dressing used.

Table 1 Characteristics of survey respondents

Characteristic	Number of respondents (N = 210), n (%)
Location	
North America	95 (45.2)
Europe	54 (25.7)
Asia	38 (18.1)
Australasia	7 (3.3)
Africa	8 (3.8)
Central and South America	8 (3.8)
Sex	
Male	195 (92.9)
Female	15 (7.1)
Mean age ± SD (years)	47.7 ± 8.2
Location of practice	
Academic	153 (72.9)
Community	57 (27.1)
Number of years treating fracture patients	
< 10 years	37 (17.6)
≥ 10 years	173 (82.4)

Table 2 Agents used among surgeons who irrigate the open fracture wound and skin in the emergency department

Agent	Number of Respondents (N = 149*), n (%)
Saline	89 (59.7)
Iodine Aqueous-Based Solution	37 (24.8)
CHG Alcohol-Based Solution	7 (4.7)
Hydrogen Peroxide	6 (4.0)
Aqueous-Based CHG Solution	5 (3.4)
Iodine Alcohol-Based Solutions	4 (2.7)
Soap	1 (0.7)

*149/210 surgeons irrigate in the emergency department

Open fractures – Surgical preparation practices

Surgeons were asked if it was in their routine practice to use only a single antiseptic surgical preparation solution or multiple antiseptic surgical preparation solutions when preparing an open fracture for surgery. 53.8% (113/210) of the respondents indicated that they routinely use multiple antiseptic surgical preparation solutions when preparing an open fracture for surgery (Table 3). Surgeons were then asked to indicate from the following, 1) CHG in an alcohol-based solution, 2) CHG in an aqueous-based solution, 3) aqueous-iodophor solution, 4) alcohol-iodophor solution, and 5) alcohol, what type of antiseptic surgical preparation solution(s) they used when preparing an open fracture for surgery. For this question, surgeons were able to select more than one antiseptic surgical preparation solution as a response. 41.0% of the respondents indicated that they use only iodine-based solution(s) (either aqueous- or alcohol-based) in their preparation practices for open fractures, 26.7% indicated the use of only CHG-based solution(s) (either aqueous- or alcohol-based), and 31.4% indicated that they use a combination of both CHG-based and iodine-based solutions (either aqueous- or alcohol-based) (Table 4). 51.4% of the respondents indicated that they used an alcohol-based solution or added alcohol alone in

their preparation practices for open fractures. Specifically, 35.7% used an alcohol-CHG preparation solution (Chloraprep®, Soluprep® or equivalents), 7.6% (16/210) used an alcohol-iodophor preparation solution (Duraprep™ and equivalents), and 20.0% added alcohol alone as part of the surgical preparation routine. While the results of this survey suggest that many orthopaedic surgeons use alcohol-containing antiseptics or add alcohol alone for surgical skin preparation of open fractures, the orthopaedic community also indicated in the open-ended questions of the survey that it follows standard precautions regarding the use of alcohol antiseptic solutions in order to prevent pooling of the solutions and ensure that adequate drying (evaporation) takes place to avoid the flammability risks from electrocautery. Of total, we found 20 different preoperative antiseptic regimens in open fractures for preventing SSI in open fractures.

Closed fractures – Surgical preparation practices

Surgeons were asked if it was in their routine practice to use only a single antiseptic surgical preparation solution or multiple antiseptic surgical preparation solutions when preparing a closed fracture for surgery. 65.7% (138/210) of the respondents indicated that they routinely use multiple antiseptic surgical preparation solutions when preparing a closed fracture for surgery (Table 3). Surgeons were then asked to indicate from the following, 1) CHG in an alcohol-based solution, 2) CHG in an aqueous-based solution, 3) aqueous-iodophor solution, 4) alcohol-iodophor solution, and 5) alcohol, what type of antiseptic surgical preparation solution(s) they used when preparing a closed fracture for surgery. For this question, surgeons were able to select more than one antiseptic surgical preparation solution as a response. 43.8% of the respondents indicated that they use only CHG-based solution(s) (either aqueous- or alcohol-based) in their preparation practices for closed fractures, 28.1% indicated the use of only iodine-based

Table 3 Use of single or multiple surgical antiseptics in open and closed fractures

Type of Solution	Single Solution		Multiple Solutions[a]		Total[a]	
	Open Fractures (N = 97) n (%)	Closed Fractures (N = 72) n (%)	Open Fractures (N = 113) n (%)	Closed Fractures (N = 138) n (%)	Open Fractures (N = 210) n (%)	Closed Fractures (N = 210) n (%)
Aqueous-Iodophor Solution (Betadine®, ScrubCare® and equivalents)	66 (68.0)	29 (40.3)	79 (69.9)	73 (52.9)	145 (69.0)	102 (48.6)
Aqueous-CHG Solution (Betasept®, Hibiclens® or equivalents)	11 (11.3)	2 (2.8)	69 (61.1)	89 (64.5)	80 (38.1)	91 (43.3)
Alcohol-Iodophor Solution (Duraprep™ and equivalents)	2 (1.0)	8 (11.1)	14 (12.4)	21 (10.0)	16 (7.6)	29 (13.8)
Alcohol-CHG Solution (Chloraprep®, Soluprep® or equivalents)	16 (7.6)	31 (43.1)	59 (52.2)	90 (42.9)	75 (35.7)	121 (57.6)
Alcohol	2 (1.0)	2 (2.8)	40 (35.4)	51 (24.3)	42 (20.0)	53 (25.2)

[a]Numbers may not add up to N value due to ability to select multiple responses

Table 4 Breakdown of types of surgical antiseptics used in open and closed fractures

Antiseptic surgical preparation solution	Open Fractures N = 210 n (%)	Closed Fractures N = 210 n (%)	Total N = 420 n (%)
Use of CHG-Based Solutions Only	56 (26.7)	92 (43.8)	148 (35.2)
CHG in an Aqueous-Based Solution + CHG in an Alcohol-Based Solution	20 (9.5)	40 (19.0)	60 (14.3)
CHG in an Alcohol-Based Solution	16 (7.6)	31 (14.8)	47 (11.2)
CHG in an Aqueous-Based Solution	11 (5.2)	2 (1.0)	13 (3.1)
CHG in an Aqueous-Based Solution + CHG in an Alcohol-Based Solution + Alcohol	6 (2.9)	10 (4.8)	16 (3.8)
CHG in an Alcohol-Based Solution + Alcohol	3 (1.4)	6 (2.9)	9 (2.1)
CHG in an Aqueous-Based Solution + Alcohol	0 (0.0)	3 (1.4)	3 (0.7)
Use of Iodine-Based Solutions Only	86 (41.0)	59 (28.1)	145 (34.5)
Only Aqueous-Iodophor Solution	66 (31.4)	29 (13.8)	95 (22.6)
Aqueous-Iodophor Solution + Alcohol	11 (5.2)	14 (6.7)	25 (6.0)
Aqueous-Iodophor Solution + Alcohol-Iodophor Solution	4 (1.9)	5 (2.4)	9 (2.1)
Aqueous-Iodophor Solution + Alcohol-Iodophor Solution + Alcohol	3 (1.4)	3 (1.4)	6 (1.4)
Only Alcohol-Iodophor Solution	2 (1.0)	8 (3.8)	10 (2.4)
Combined Use of CHG-Based and Iodine-Based Solutions	66 (31.4)	57 (27.1)	123 (29.3)
CHG in an Aqueous-Based Solution + Aqueous-Iodophor Solution	25 (11.9)	10 (4.8)	35 (8.3)
CHG in an Alcohol-Based Solution + Aqueous-Iodophor Solution	14 (6.7)	13 (6.2)	27 (6.4)
CHG in an Aqueous-Based Solution + Aqueous-Iodophor Solution + Alcohol	9 (4.3)	8 (3.8)	17 (4.0)
CHG in an Alcohol-Based Solution + Aqueous-Iodophor Solution + Alcohol	4 (1.9)	2 (1.0)	6 (1.4)
CHG in an Aqueous-Based Solution + CHG in an Alcohol-Based Solution + Aqueous-Iodophor Solution	3 (1.4)	9 (4.3)	12 (2.9)
CHG in an Alcohol-Based Solution + Alcohol-Iodophor Solution	3 (1.4)	2 (1.0)	5 (1.2)
CHG in an Alcohol-Based Solution + Aqueous-Iodophor Solution + Alcohol-Iodophor Solution	2 (1.0)	3 (1.4)	5 (1.2)
CHG in an Aqueous-Based Solution + Alcohol-Iodophor Solution	2 (1.0)	3 (1.4)	5 (1.2)
CHG in an Alcohol-Based Solution + Alcohol-Iodophor Solution + Alcohol	0 (0.0)	1 (0.5)	1 (0.2)
CHG in an Aqueous-Based Solution + CHG in an Alcohol-Based Solution + Aqueous-Iodophor Solution + Alcohol	4 (1.9)	2 (1.0)	6 (1.4)
CHG in an Aqueous-Based Solution + CHG in an Alcohol-Based Solution + Aqueous-Iodophor Solution + Alcohol-Iodophor Solution	0 (0.0)	1 (0.5)	1 (0.2)
CHG in an Aqueous-Based Solution + Aqueous-Iodophor Solution + Alcohol-Iodophor Solution	0 (0.0)	1 (0.5)	1 (0.2)
CHG Aqueous-Based Solution + Aqueous-Iodophor Solution + Alcohol-Iodophor Solution + Alcohol	0 (0.0)	1 (0.5)	1 (0.2)
CHG in an Aqueous-Based Solution + CHG in an Alcohol-Based Solution + Aqueous-Iodophor Solution + Alcohol-Iodophor Solution + Alcohol	0 (0.0)	1 (0.5)	1 (0.2)
Use of Alcohol Only as a Single Solution	2 (1.0)	2 (1.0)	4 (1.0)

solution(s) (either aqueous- or alcohol-based), and 27.1% of respondents indicated that they use a combination of both CHG-based and iodine-based solutions (either aqueous- or alcohol-based) (Table 4). Most of the respondents used an alcohol-based solution or alcohol alone (169/210 = 80.5%) in their preparation practices for closed fractures. Specifically, 57.6% (121/210) used an alcohol-CHG preparation (Chloraprep®, Soluprep® or equivalents), 25.2% (53/210) added alcohol alone, and 13.8% (29/210) used an alcohol-iodophor preparation (Duraprep™ and equivalents) solution as part of the preparation practices. Of total, we found 26 different preoperative antiseptic regimens in closed fractures for preventing SSI in closed fractures.

Factors influencing surgeons' decision to use surgical antiseptic solution(s)

Surgeons were able to select more than one response when indicating what factors influence their decision to use surgical antiseptic preparation solution(s) when preparing a fracture for surgery. Surgeons indicated that their decision to use antiseptic surgical preparation solution(s) in open fractures was influenced by hospital and/or operating room policy (46.7%), personal experience (43.3%), and experience during training (38.1%). Choice of antiseptic surgical preparation solution(s) in closed fractures was influenced by hospital and/or operating room policy (57.6%), literature (41.9%), and personal experience (39.0%) (Table 5).

The need for future research

More than half of the respondents (54.3%) supported the idea of participating in a randomized controlled trial comparing different surgical antiseptic preparation solutions for both open and closed fractures. Almost half of the surgeons who completed the survey (45.2%) indicated that they would participate in a randomized controlled trial comparing different antiseptic preparation solutions in the emergency room setting.

Table 5 Factors influencing surgeons' decisions to use surgical antiseptic solution(s), consideration in the election of the proper antiseptic, and importance to reduce risk of infection

	Open Fractures (N = 210) n (%)	Closed Fractures (N = 210) n (%)
Factors influencing surgeons' decision[a]		
Hospital policy	98 (46.7)	121 (57.6)
Literature	77 (36.7)	88 (41.9)
Clinical experience	91 (43.3)	82 (39.0)
Practice guidelines	75 (35.7)	67 (31.9)
Experience during training	80 (38.1)	59 (28.1)
Colleague's recommendation	31 (14.8)	20 (9.5)
Suppliers agreement	4 (1.9)	5 (2.4)
How often surgeons consider what type of antiseptic solution to use for open fracture cases		
Never (0%)	31 (14.8)	43 (20.5)
Infrequently (1–25%)	16 (7.6)	20 (9.5)
Sometimes (25–75%)	14 (6.7)	7 (3.3)
Usually (75–99%)	17 (8.1)	19 (9.0)
Always (100%)	132 (62.9)	121 (57.6)
Importance of type of antiseptic used in reducing risk of infection		
Not important	4 (1.9)	8 (3.8)
Slightly important	23 (11.0)	25 (11.9)
Moderately important	49 (23.3)	56 (26.7)
Very important	71 (33.8)	64 (30.5)
Extremely important	63 (30.0)	57 (27.1)

[a]Numbers may not add up to N value due to ability to select multiple responses

Discussion

The results of this survey demonstrate that, 1) there is no established consensus among surgeons regarding the use of antiseptic preparation agents for early open fracture wound management in the emergency room and 2) there is no consensus regarding the use of preoperative skin antiseptics for the prevention of SSIs in the operative treatment of both open and closed fractures. The majority of surveyed surgeons indicated that they routinely perform an irrigation of the open fracture wound in the emergency department; however, there is a lack of consensus on the type of solution used. While most surgeons concur that a dressing should be used; there is a clear divide in the type of dressing they use, as approximately one-third use a sterile dry dressing, one-third use a saline soaked dressing, and the final third use a dressing soaked in an iodophor aqueous-based solution.

Furthermore, we found 20 different preoperative antiseptic regimens in the operative management of open fractures and 26 different preoperative antiseptic routines for preventing SSIs in the operative management of closed fractures. In both open and closed fractures, there was a lack of consensus on the use of iodine-based solutions and CHG-based solutions. In closed fractures, the majority of respondents used an alcohol-based solution. In open fractures, many surgeons are using alcohol-based solutions in this setting (51.4%), with alcohol-based CHG solutions being the most commonly used alcohol-based solutions (35.7%).

Our survey results indicate that when deciding what particular surgical antiseptic solution to use surgeons are less influenced by evidence from the literature for open fractures than for closed fractures; this finding suggests that there is a lack of available clinical evidence on this matter. If present, this evidence could help guide orthopedic surgeons in making decisions regarding what the best antiseptic solutions are for open fractures.

Overall, the results of this study must be interpreted in the context of the study design. Few surgeons outside of North America and Europe completed our survey, limiting the generalizability of our results in other regions. Additionally, orthopaedic organizations distributed the survey to their membership as part of their mailers or posted the survey on their website. This passive approach likely contributed to a low response rate and possible respondent bias. Previous surveys, where the researchers were able to contact potential survey participants directly, have achieved higher response rates [6, 7], which increases generalizability and decreases the risk of bias. This study is strengthened by the use of a rigorous process for the development of the questionnaire and extensive piloting of the survey. Moreover, our survey used open-ended questions about the surgical antiseptic preparation process to allow the participants to describe their practice pattern in detail without being restricted to categorical responses.

Conclusion

In conclusion, there is a paucity of compelling clinical evidence examining which of these surgical antiseptic preparation solutions is more effective at preventing SSIs; we believe this has led to considerable controversy and practice variation among surgeons. High-quality clinical research is needed to resolve this debate and determine the effectiveness of different surgical antiseptic preparation solutions on patient important outcomes in open and closed fracture patients. Approximately half of the respondents endorsed the idea of participating in a randomized controlled trial comparing different surgical antiseptic preparation solutions indicating that the orthopaedic surgery community is interested in definitively resolving this question.

Abbreviations
CHG: Chlorhexidine Gluconate; COA: Canadian Orthopaedic Association; COTS: Canadian Orthopaedic Trauma Society; ED: Emergency Department; FLOW: Fluid lavage of open wounds; OTA: Orthopaedic Trauma Association; SDs: Standard deviations; SSI: Surgical site infection

Acknowledgements
Not applicable.

Funding
No funding is reported for this study.

Authors' contributions
SS, MJ-R, GPS, SB, and AG were responsible for the inception of this study and together led the design of the study, interpreted the results, and drafted the manuscript. BP provided clinical expertise regarding design of the study and interpretation and significance of the results. NNO, AH and the remaining co-authors reviewed the manuscript and provided critical input regarding its intellectual content. All authors read and approved the final manuscript.

Ethics approval and consent to participate
This study was approved by the Hamilton Integrated Research Ethics Board (HiREB #2016–2326). Utilizing SurveyMonkey, the survey was distributed through email which included a link to the online survey and presented information on the survey's purpose, how their data would be stored and used, and the investigator's contact information. Completion of the survey was considered as implicit consent, and no monetary incentives or pre-notification emails were used for this survey. Questionnaire completion was voluntary and individual responses were kept confidential, only being accessible through a password protected account.

Consent for publication
Not Applicable.

Competing interests
The authors declare that they have no competing interests.

Author details
[1]Department of Trauma and Orthopaedic Surgery, Hospital Universitari Vall d'Hebron, Universitat Autonoma de Barcelona, Barcelona, Spain. [2]R Adams Cowley Shock Trauma Center, Department of Orthopaedics, University of Maryland School of Medicine, Baltimore, MD, USA. [3]Division of Orthopaedic Surgery, Department of Surgery, McMaster University, Hamilton, ON, Canada. [4]Department of Health Research Methods, Evidence, and Impact, McMaster University, Hamilton, ON, Canada. [5]McMaster University, 293 Wellington Street North, Suite 110, Ontario, Hamilton L8L 8E7, Canada.

References
1. Uçkay I, Hoffmeyer P, Lew D, Pittet D. Prevention of surgical site infections in orthopaedic surgery and bone trauma: state-of-the-art update. J Hosp Infect. 2013;84:5–12.
2. Whitehouse JD, Friedman ND, Kirkland KB, Richardson WJ, Sexton DJ. The impact of surgical-site infections following orthopedic surgery at a community hospital and a university hospital adverse quality of life, excess length of stay, and extra cost. Infect Control Hosp Epidemiol. 2002;23:183–9.
3. Dumville JC, McFarlane E, Edwards P, Lipp A, Holmes A, Liu Z. Preoperative skin antiseptics for preventing surgical wound infections after clean surgery. Cochrane Database Syst Rev. 2015:CD003949.
4. Hemani ML, Lepor H. Skin preparation for the prevention of surgical site infection: which agent is best? Rev Urol. 2009;11:190–5.
5. FLOW Investigators. A trial of wound irrigation in the initial Management of Open Fracture Wounds. N Engl J Med. 2015;373:2629–41.
6. Petrisor B, Jeray K, Schemitsch E, Hanson B, Sprague S, Sanders D, Bhandari M, FLOW Investigators. Fluid lavage in patients with open fracture wounds (FLOW): an international survey of 984 surgeons. BMC Musculoskelet Disord. 2008;9:7.
7. Busse J, Morton E, Lacchetti C, Guyatt G, Bhandari M. Current management of tibial shaft fractures: a survey of 450 Canadian Orthopaedic trauma surgeons. Acta Orthop. 2008;79:689–94.

24

Non-prescribed sale of antibiotics for acute childhood diarrhea and upper respiratory tract infection in community pharmacies

Daniel Asfaw Erku[1*†] [iD] and Sisay Yifru Aberra[2†]

Abstract

Background: Although prohibited by law and legal regulatory frameworks, non-prescribed sale of antibiotics in community medicine retail outlets (CMROs) remains a serious problem in Ethiopia. The aim of this study was to document the extent of and motivations behind non-prescribed sale of antibiotics among CMROs in Gondar town, Ethiopia.

Methods: A 2 phase mixed-methods study (a simulated patient visit followed by an in-depth interview) was conducted among CMROs in Gondar town, Ethiopia. Two clinical case scenarios (acute childhood diarrhea and upper respiratory tract infection) were presented and the practice of non-prescribed sale were measured and results were reported as percentages. Pharmacy staff (pharmacists and pharmacy assistants) were interviewed to examine factors/motivations behind dispensing antibiotics without a valid prescription.

Results: Out of 100 simulated visits (50 each scenarios) presented to drug retail outlets, 86 cases (86%) were provided with one or more medications. Of these, 18 (20.9%) asked about past medical and medication history and only 7 (8.1%) enquired about the patient's history of drug allergy. The most frequently dispensed medication for acute childhood diarrhoea simulation were oral rehydration fluid (ORS) with zinc ($n = 16$) and Metronidazole ($n = 15$). Among the dispensed antibiotics for upper respiratory infection simulation, the most common was Amoxicillin ($n = 23$) followed by Amoxicillin-clavulanic acid capsule ($n = 19$) and Azithromycin ($n = 15$). Perceived financial benefit, high expectation and/or demand of customers and competition among pharmacies were cited as the main drivers behind selling antibiotics without a prescription.

Conclusions: A stringent law and policy enforcement regarding the sale of antibiotics without a valid prescription should be in place. This will ultimately help to shift the current pharmacy practices from commercial and business-based interests/practices to the provision of primary healthcare services to the community.

Keywords: Community pharmacy, Simulated patient, Antimicrobial, Dispensing Ethiopia

* Correspondence: staymotivated015@gmail.com
†Daniel Asfaw Erku and Sisay Yifru Aberra contributed equally to this work.
[1]School of Pharmacy, University of Gondar, Lideta kebele 16, P.O.Box: 196, Gondar, Ethiopia

Background

The development of antimicrobial agents represents one of the most significant achievements of modern medicine in the past century. Yet, the emergence of antimicrobial resistance (AMR) combined with the downturn in the introduction of new antibiotics to the market poses an unanticipated threat in the treatment of infectious diseases [1]. The emergence and spread of antimicrobial resistance is largely attributed to the use, over use or misuse of antimicrobials [2]. Community medicine retail outlets (CMROs) represent one of the main sources of antimicrobials globally [3]. According to the recent multi-country public awareness survey conducted by the World Health Organization (WHO), 93% of people got their most recently taken antimicrobial from a pharmacy and drug store [4]. In Ethiopia, the widespread access and availability of antibiotics without a valid prescription, coupled with the general public's poor knowledge about antimicrobials, has increased self-medication with these drugs and augmented the risk of the inappropriate antibiotics use in the community [5–7]. Non-prescribed sale and dispensing of antibiotics will not only promote antimicrobial resistance but can also be linked with adverse drug events, significantly increased cost burden and poor health outcome. Thus, by acting as antimicrobial stewardship proponents, community pharmacists can play a significant role in the containment of cost and antimicrobial resistance.

Antimicrobial stewardship (AMS) is the term collectively used for a variety of quality improvement activities aimed at improving and sustaining the appropriate use of antibiotics for the treatment and/or prevention of infectious diseases [8]. One approach to achieving this is through the development of formal institutional AMS programs. The regular correspondence that community pharmacy professionals have with patients, their responsibility for dispensing these agents as well as the training and knowledge they possess, provides a great deal of opportunity to implement interventions for patients in order to slow antimicrobial resistance, verify appropriate usage, recommend alternative over-the-counter (OTC) medications, and educate patients. The majority of AMS programs in Ethiopia have been introduced in institutional settings such as hospitals and health management organizations. In contrast, there are no established antibiotic stewardship programs that formally exist in CMROs. Moreover, a recent national survey conducted in Ethiopian community pharmacies identified a need for incorporation of AMS program in CMROs and implement educational intervention to improve over the counter sale of antimicrobials and reduce the occurrence of antimicrobial resistance in the community [9].

This study is part of a larger investigation focusing on implementing a community pharmacy-based antimicrobial stewardship program in Ethiopia. In this mixed-methods study, we employed a simulated client method to document the extent of non-prescribed sale of antibiotics for the two most common minor ailments encountered in pharmacies (acute childhood diarrhea and uncomplicated upper respiratory infection) [10]. We then employed a qualitative study, using the theory of planned behaviour, to examine factors/motivations behind dispensing antibiotics without a valid prescription. The overarching aim of this study was, therefore, to document the extent and drivers of non-prescribed sale of antibiotics among CMROs in Gondar town, Ethiopia.

Methods

Study design and setting

A 2 phase mixed-methods research design, including a simulated client method (August 2017) and an in-depth interview with community pharmacists (October 2017) was used to comprehensively assess pharmacists' overall practice regarding over the counter sale (OTC) of antibiotics in community pharmacies. The study was conducted in Gondar town, Northwest Ethiopia. The town has a population of approximately 206,987 [11] and the town has 57 CMROs (20 community pharmacies, 35 drug stores and 2 rural drug vendors). Ethical approval to conduct this study was granted by the ethical review committee of School of Pharmacy, University of Gondar. Informed consent was obtained from all participants for the qualitative study. The obtained participant's information were kept confidential.

The simulated patient study

Drug retail outlets in Ethiopia are classified based on the type of medications they are supposed to stock/dispense and qualification of pharmacy staff. Pharmacies were defined as drug retail outlets having at least one licensed pharmacist with a minimum qualification of a bachelor of pharmacy as a pharmacy staff, whereas drug stores are drug retail outlets having at least one licensed pharmacy technician/druggist with a minimum qualification of a diploma in pharmacy as a pharmacy staff. All pharmacies and drug stores located in Gondar town (a total of 50 CMROs) were visited. As each CMROs were visited twice by each simulated patient (SP), a total of 100 simulated visits were conducted over a 2-weeks period.

Two different clinical case scenarios, which are considered to be common (acute childhood diarrhea and uncomplicated upper respiratory infection) were developed and enacted by the simulated patients. In the acute diarrhea scenario, a female simulated patient (31-year-old) asked the pharmacy staff to give her a medication to relieve the acute diarrhea suffered by her 3-year-old son. The scenario was designed to exclude acute bloody, persistent diarrhea and diarrhea due to malnourishment. In the uncomplicated upper respiratory tract infection (URTI) scenario, a male simulated patient (27-year-old) asked for a medication after presenting with a symptom of upper respiratory tract infection. Details of the scenarios, along with the data collection tool used by the SPs are presented in Additional file 1. In both scenarios, the SP noted the queries and recommendations provided by the pharmacist including drug allergies, non-pharmacological advices given and medications dispensed.

Four clinical pharmacists acted as simulated patients. A half-day long discussion and training was given to SPs so that they will be familiar and be able to perform the clinical scenarios given. They were instructed not to give and/ or ask further information unless asked by the pharmacy staff so as to make sure that the information provided by each SPs is uniform across all the visits. In order to avoid depending on the human cognitive processes, which has been mentioned as a potential limitation of the simulated patient method [12], all the visits were audio recorded. Immediately after each visit, the SPs filled the data gathered in a form containing a check list of items (such as queries/patient history requested, medications and/or counselling delivered and duration of the visit) that were intended to assess the practice of pharmacy personnel toward the dispensing of antibiotics for the specified minor ailments. The principal investigator (DAE) compared and validated the data from the check list against audio recordings for the purpose of quality assurance. Data were entered into and analyzed using Statistical Package for Social Studies (SPSS) version 20 for Windows and results are presented as frequencies and percentages.

The qualitative study

In the second phase of the study, we employed a qualitative study using in-depth interviews to examine factors/motivations behind dispensing antibiotics without a valid prescription The interviews were constructed based on the theory of planned behaviour (TPB). TPB is a theory in psychology that links people's belief and their behaviour. It assumes that individuals' attitudes, subjective norms, perceived behavioural control and moral obligation ultimately determines their behavioural intention and/or how they display the behavior [13]. TPB has been employed extensively in pharmacy practice research [14, 15]. To allow for a maximum variation and come up with a richer data [16], we recruited pharmacy staff from different types of drug retail outlets (considering the socioeconomic status of customers served in these CDROs), geographical location (urban/ rural), and varied demographics (such as age, gender, educational level and experience in community pharmacy). From a total of 17 pharmacy staff invited, 15 pharmacy staff (9 pharmacists and 6 pharmacy assistants) agreed to participate. Based on the preliminary data analysis, the

data was saturated after 13th participant was interviewed, after which no new content was identified [17]. All interviews were conducted by the principal author (DAE) in person at either the participant's work place or other convenient locations such as coffee shops. Interviews were recorded and transcribed verbatim immediately following after each interview.

Each interview took approximately 30–45 min. Thematic analysis were performed using individual narratives of interviewed pharmacy staff as the main unit/case of analysis. The content of the interviews were carefully identified and coded in light of the TPB theory constructs, which then yielded the main themes of the analysis. NVivo 11 Software was used to assist the coding process.

Results
Finding of simulated visits

Out of 100 simulated visits (50 scenarios each) presented to drug retail outlets, 86 cases (86%) were provided with one or more antimicrobials. Of the 86 drug retail outlets selling an antibiotic when childhood diarrhea and upper respiratory tract infection was simulated, only 7 (8.1%) enquired about the patient's history of drug allergy, 18 (20.9%) asked about past medical and medication history. Only 9 (10.6%) of the community pharmacy professionals advice simulated patients to visit a physician and only 12 (14%) of them provided advise on non-pharmacological management. The average time taken for pharmacy staff to counsel and dispense were 4 min. The detailed actions and advises provided by the pharmacy staff is presented in Table 1.

A variety of medications were dispensed for acute diarrhea including antiamoebic, antibiotics, anthelmintic, oral rehydration salts (ORS) and zinc (Table 2). Similarly, a wide variety of antimicrobial agents were dispensed and/ or recommended in simulated scenarios. Among the dispensed antibiotics, the most common was Amoxicillin [18] followed by Amoxicillin-clavulanic acid capsule [19], Metronidazole [15] and Azithromycin [15].

Motivation behind non-prescribed sale of antibiotics

Majority of pharmacy staff who were interviewed reaffirmed the finding from the simulated patient visits that non-prescribed sale of antibiotics is a common practice. This malpractice seems to be driven by a variety of factors which are summarized as behavioural belief (perceived financial benefit) and normative beliefs (high expectation of customers and competition among pharmacies).

Perceived financial benefit

The lucrative financial benefit gained from the sale of antimicrobial agents whenever the patient requested

Table 1 Actions and advice in response to SPs in Gondar, Northwest Ethiopia, 2017

Type of action and advice	Total	Childhood diarrhea (n = 50)		URTI (n = 50)	
		Pharmacy (n = 28)	Drug store (n = 22)	Pharmacy (n = 28)	Drug store (n = 22)
Dispensed antimicrobial (s) without prescription	86	21	19	22	24
Asks drug allergies	7	3	–	4	–
Instruction on dose and duration	36	12	7	11	6
Instruction on side effects	24	13		8	3
Queries about past medical and medication history	18	7	1	10	–
Need for prescription	7	4		3	
Advice to visit physician	9	3	2	3	1
Non-pharmacological advice	12	4	2	3	3

Abbreviation: URTIs: Upper Respiratory Tract Infections

them is discussed across all participants. There were also instances where participants indicated that their employers (pharmacy owners) expect them to do what is most profitable to the company including dispensing antibiotics without a valid prescription.

"I am particularly concerned about the financial consequences for my pharmacy. It becomes difficult these days to be a pharmacy owner and gain some financial benefits since everybody even the nurses are taking away our business. So I do whatever it takes to cope up with such financial pressure and this includes handing over antibiotics and other medications without a doctor's prescription (P1)".

"Yes, it is very unprofessional to dispense these drugs (antibiotics) irrationally, but the pressure is very immense...you have an employer here that tells you constantly to dispense without a prescription. I don't want to rescue my job by not doing so. Besides, a nearby

Table 2 Medications dispensed in response to the simulated scenarios, Gondar town, Ethiopia, 2017

Antimicrobial (s) dispensed	Acute diarrhea	URTI
Cotrimoxazole	11	–
Metronidazole	15	–
Mebendazole	10	–
Loperamide	9	–
ORS with Zinc	16	–
Amoxicillin	–	23
Amoxicillin-clavulanic acid capsule	–	19
Azithromycin	–	15
Ciprofloxacin	–	5
Cephalexin	–	1
Cefexime	–	1
Levofloxacin	–	3

Abbreviation: ORT: Oral Rehydration Therapy; URTI: Upper Respiratory Tract Infections

pharmacy is voluntary to dispense even if I said no. Thus I usually sale this products to our customers (P7)".

High expectation of customers and competition among pharmacies

Perceived beliefs regarding customers' expectation and beliefs about the practice of other pharmacies were the two main normative beliefs held by the majority of the participants. One participant pointed out that their pharmacy business model is in such a way that customers satisfaction is the central core value.

"We believe in customer satisfaction, this is something we developed over years of experience. If we insist not selling these products to them, we definitely loss these customers because they will be dissatisfied. Thus, we are usually pretty much encouraging for my employees to give them what they asked with the correct instruction (P8)".

"Everyone comes with a request of either Amoxicillin or Amox/Clav and it looks like they already used it once or twice before and are very much confident about what they are asking for. It's just impossible to say no when over half of your profit comes from selling antibiotics. I would say it is a matter of constant customer demand and financial consequence (P2)".

The perceived belief that customers can easily access antibiotics from neighbouring drug retail outlets appears to be one of the main drivers behind the pharmacists' dispending behaviour.

"It is very simple. If I am not happy to sell them (customers) these products, they will go to the neighboring pharmacy and easily get them easily without a question. So it becomes a matter of competition and retaining customers (P11)".

Discussion

In most of the developing countries, the sale of antimicrobials in community medicine retail outlets is largely unregulated, without involvement of a licensed pharmacy personnel, and is often without a valid medical prescription [3]. This is the first comprehensive sequential mixed-methods study to document the extent and drivers of non-prescribed sale of antimicrobials in community pharmacies in Ethiopia. We employed a simulated patient methodology in phase 1, which is a more reliable approach if pharmacy staffs could be tempted to hide their actual behavior and practice due to a potential desirability bias [20]. Our use of a simulated patient method allowed us to evaluate the actual practice of a pharmacy staff when confronted with the choice of dispensing antimicrobials without a valid prescription, rather than assessing their performance with self-reported surveys, which is subjected to a number of potential biases. We also employed an in-depth interview with the aim of uncovering the drivers/motivations behind OTC sale of antibiotics. Although illegal and prohibited by legal regulatory frameworks, dispensing antibiotics without a valid prescription remains a serious problem in Ethiopia, as in many other African countries such as Zambia, Nigeria and Tanzania [19–21]. During the simulated visits, antibiotics were obtained without a valid prescription with ease from more than two third of pharmacies and drug stores of Gondar town. Furthermore, antibiotics were handed over to simulated patients with negligible queries regarding details of symptoms, past medical and medication history, possible drug allergies and the potential side effects of the dispensed medications. Similar studies conducted in many low and middle income countries (LMICs) also reported comparable findings [19–22]. In Tanzania, antimicrobial agents were dispensed without a prescription to 81% of simulated diarrhea cases and 95% of simulated upper respiratory infection [19]. Similarly, studies conducted in Zambia and Uganda reported that non-prescribed sale of antibiotics is widespread and frequent [20, 22]. Studies conducted in a number of other countries including Greece and Spain also showed that dispensing of antibiotics without a prescription is a common practice [18, 23].

In Ethiopia, as in many other countries [21, 24–26], antimicrobial agents are classified as prescription-only medicines and they can only be accessed, procured, and/ or dispensed with a valid medical prescription. A number of factors could be cited for the higher rate of non-prescribed sale of antibiotics in the study area. One reason could be to the fact that most pharmacy staffs are more engaged with making sales and serving their commercial interests than providing primary healthcare services to the public. This notion is further supported by the study conducted in Saudi Arabia, where pharmacy staffs dispensed antimicrobial agents without even being requested [24]. Similar other studies conducted in Ethiopia and other African countries cited continued client demand as a major reason for perpetuating non-prescribed sales of antibiotics [21, 27, 28]. Another

potential reason for widespread antibiotic dispensing in CMROs could be the market financial incentives where antimicrobial agents may be more profitable than evidence based, better and rational management options for minor ailments such as acute diarrhea and upper respiratory infections [29].

The potential benefits gained from investing in multi-faceted interventions to protect the general public from the consequences of antibiotic misuse/overuse (such as antimicrobial resistance and increased healthcare cost) can outweigh the potential perils. Although a comprehensive pharmacy-based educational intervention is essential to curb inappropriate use of antibiotics [30], it should only be a part of a more comprehensive, multifaceted strategies and measures, which may include increasing awareness of rational use of antibiotics and antimicrobial resistance among the community, strictly implementing national regulations governing OTC sale of antibiotics and promoting pharmacists as antimicrobial stewardship proponents.

While we conducted this study utilizing a simulated patient method, which can be an effective method of deriving valid, reliable outcomes that are difficult to achieve by any other method in pharmacy practice research, our approach may have some limitations. First, the practice behavior in response to some simulated clinical scenarios may not be generalized to other clinical scenarios; this may preclude the evaluation of the pharmacists' non-prescribed sale of antibiotics at pharmacies. As this interventional study recruited smaller amount of pharmacies from one urban area (Gondar town), our study may not be generalized to other practices of drug shops in rural areas, where alternative systems of medicine access may be more popular. The present study was conducted in community medicine retail outlets serving a relatively homogenous population. Future studies should consider recruiting community pharmacies from both rural and urban areas as the dispending behaviour of pharmacists could be affected by the geographical location of the pharmacy premises and the residents it serves. Regardless of the limitations mentioned, this study has significant implications in curbing the emergence of antimicrobial resistance via limiting the sale of antibiotics without a valid prescription in CMROs.

Conclusions

The finding of the present study provides a basis to develop, execute and evaluate various comprehensive educational interventions aimed at providing correct, customized and evidence based information to pharmacists about antibiotic use and management of minor ailments. There is an urgent need of a paradigm shift among community pharmacists in Ethiopia to shift from commercial and business-based interests/practices to the provision of primary healthcare services to the community. Moreover, a stringent law/ policy enforcement regarding the sale of antibiotics without a valid prescription should be in place so as to make sure that pharmacy practices are in line with national guidelines for good dispensing practice.

Abbreviations

AMR: Antimicrobial resistance; FMHACA: Food, Medicine and Healthcare Administration and Control Authority of Ethiopia; OR: Odds ratio; SPSS: Statistical Package for the Social Sciences; WHO: World Health Organization

Acknowledgements

The authors also acknowledge the support of School of pharmacy, University of Gondar in assisting the data collection process.

Funding

No funding from any commercial or government organization was obtained to conduct this study.

Authors' contributions

DAE: Involved in study conceptualization, formal analysis, investigation, methodology, wrote review & edited original draft; SYA: Involved in formal analysis, investigation, methodology, wrote-up, review & edited original draft. Both authors read and approved the final version of the manuscript.

Consent for publication

Not applicable.

Competing interests

The authors declare there is no competing interest.

Author details

[1]School of Pharmacy, University of Gondar, Lideta kebele 16, P.O.Box: 196, Gondar, Ethiopia. [2]College of Medicine and Health Sciences, University of Gondar, Gondar, Ethiopia.

References

1. WHO. The evolving threat of antimicrobial resistance: options for action: World Health Organization; 2012. http://apps.who.int/iris/handle/10665/44812.
2. Leung E, Weil DE, Raviglione M, Nakatani H. The WHO policy package to combat antimicrobial resistance. Bull World Health Organ. 2011;89(5):390–2.
3. Morgan DJ, Okeke IN, Laxminarayan R, Perencevich EN, Weisenberg S. Non-prescription antimicrobial use worldwide: a systematic review. Lancet Infect Dis. 2011;11(9):692–701.
4. WHO. Antibiotic resistance: Multi-country public awareness survey. 2015.
5. Ayalew MB. Self-medication practice in Ethiopia: a systematic review. Patient Prefer Adherence. 2017;11:401.
6. Erku DA, Mekuria AB, Belachew SA. Inappropriate use of antibiotics among communities of Gondar town, Ethiopia: a threat to the development of antimicrobial resistance. Antimicrob Resist Infect Control. 2017;6(1):112.
7. Erku DA, Mekuria AB, Surur AS, Gebresillassie BM. Extent of dispensing prescription-only medications without a prescription in community drug retail outlets in Addis Ababa, Ethiopia: a simulated-patient study. Drug Healthc Patient Saf. 2016;8:65.
8. Dellit TH, Owens RC, McGowan JE, Gerding DN, Weinstein RA, Burke JP, et al. Infectious diseases society of America and the Society for Healthcare Epidemiology of America guidelines for developing an institutional program to enhance antimicrobial stewardship. Clin Infect Dis. 2007;44(2):159–77.
9. Erku DA. Antimicrobial stewardship: a cross-sectional survey assessing the perceptions and practices of community pharmacists in Ethiopia. Interdiscip Perspect Infect Dis. 2016;2016:5686752.
10. Ayele AA, Mekuria AB, Tegegn HG, Gebresillassie BM, Mekonnen AB, Erku DA. Management of minor ailments in a community pharmacy setting: findings from simulated visits and qualitative study in Gondar town, Ethiopia. PloS One. 2018;13(1):e0190583.
11. CSA. Complete report Ethiopian census 2016 Addis Ababa: Central Statistical Agency.; 2016 [Available from: http://www.csa.gov.et/census-report/census-tables/category/301-census-tables.
12. Werner JB, Benrimoj SI. Audio taping simulated patient encounters in community pharmacy to enhance the reliability of assessments. Am J Pharm Educ. 2008;72(6):136.
13. Ajzen I, Lange P, Kruglanski A, Higgins E. Handbook of theories of social psychology: Sage London; 2012 [Available from: http://sk.sagepub.com/reference/hdbk_socialpsychtheories1.
14. Fleming ML, Barner JC, Brown CM, Shepherd MD, Strassels S, Novak S. Using the theory of planned behavior to examine pharmacists' intention to utilize a prescription drug monitoring program database. Res Soc Adm Pharm. 2014;10(2):285–96.
15. Gavaza P, Fleming M, Barner JC. Examination of psychosocial predictors of Virginia pharmacists' intention to utilize a prescription drug monitoring program using the theory of planned behavior. Res Soc Adm Pharm. 2014; 10(2):448–58.
16. Creswell JW, Clark VLP. Designing and conducting mixed methods research. California: Sage publications; 2017.
17. Bowen GA. Naturalistic inquiry and the saturation concept: a research note. Qual Res. 2008;8(1):137–52.
18. Zapata-Cachafeiro M, González-González C, Váquez-Lago JM, López-Vázquez P, López-Durán A, Smyth E, et al. Determinants of antibiotic dispensing without a medical prescription: a cross-sectional study in the north of Spain. J Antimicrob Chemother. 2014;69(11):3156–60.
19. Kagashe GA, Minzi O, Matowe L. An assessment of dispensing practices in private pharmacies in Dar-es-salaam, Tanzania. Int J Pharm Pract. 2011;19(1):30–5.
20. Kalungia AC, Burger J, Godman B, Costa JO, Simuwelu C. Non-prescription sale and dispensing of antibiotics in community pharmacies in Zambia. Expert Rev Anti-Infect Ther. 2016;14(12):1215–23.
21. Akinyandenu O, Akinyandenu A. Irrational use and non-prescription sale of antibiotics in Nigeria, a need for change. J Sci Innov Res. 2014;3(2):251–7.
22. Mukonzo JK, Namuwenge PM, Okure G, Mwesige B, Namusisi OK, Mukanga D. Over-the-counter suboptimal dispensing of antibiotics in Uganda. J Multidiscip Healthc. 2013;6:303.
23. Plachouras D, Kavatha D, Antoniadou A, Giannitsioti E, Poulakou G, Kanellakopoulou K, et al. Dispensing of antibiotics without prescription in Greece, 2008: another link in the antibiotic resistance chain. Eur Secur. 2010;15(7):19488.
24. Abdulhak AAB, Al Tannir MA, Almansor MA, Almohaya MS, Onazi AS, Marei MA, et al. Non prescribed sale of antibiotics in Riyadh, Saudi Arabia: a cross sectional study. BMC Public Health. 2011;11(1):538.
25. Al-Mohamadi A, Badr A, Mahfouz LB, Samargandi D, Al Ahdal A. Dispensing medications without prescription at Saudi community pharmacy: extent and perception. Saudi Pharm J. 2013;21(1):13–8.

26. Moura ML, Boszczowski I, Mortari N, Barrozo LV, Neto FC, Lobo RD, et al. The impact of restricting over-the-counter sales of antimicrobial drugs: preliminary analysis of national data. Medicine. 2015;94(38):e1605.

27. Gebretekle GB, Serbessa MK. Exploration of over the counter sales of antibiotics in community pharmacies of Addis Ababa, Ethiopia: pharmacy professionals' perspective. Antimicrob Resist Infect Control. 2016;5(1):2.

28. Hoffman D, Botha J, Kleinschmidt I. An assessment of factors influencing the prescribing of antibiotics in acute respiratory illness: a questionnaire study. South African Family Practice. 2003;45(6):20–4.

29. Löfgren J, Tao W, Larsson E, Kyakulaga F, Forsberg BC. Treatment patterns of childhood diarrhoea in rural Uganda: a cross-sectional survey. BMC Int Health Hum Rights. 2012;12(1):19.

30. Chalker J, Ratanawijitrasin S, Chuc N, Petzold M, Tomson G. Effectiveness of a multi-component intervention on dispensing practices at private pharmacies in Vietnam and Thailand—a randomized controlled trial. Soc Sci Med. 2005;60(1):131–41.

Permissions

List of Contributors

Regev Cohen
Head of Infectious diseases unit, Sanz Medical Center, Laniado hospital, Neytanya, Israel
Ruth and Bruce Rappaport Faculty of Medicine, Technion, Haifa, Israel

Frida Babushkin, Shoshana Cohen and Marina Afraimov
Infectious diseases unit, Sanz Medical Center, Laniado hospital, Netanya, Israel

Maurice Shapiro and Martina Uda
Medical and Surgical intensive care unit, Sanz Medical Center, Laniado hospital, Netanya, Israel

Efrat Khabra
National Center of Infection Control, Ministry of Health, Tel Aviv, Israel

Amos Adler
National Center of Infection Control, Ministry of Health, Tel Aviv, Israel
Sackler Faculty of Medicine, Tel Aviv University, Tel Aviv, Israel

Ronen Ben Ami
Sackler Faculty of Medicine, Tel Aviv University, Tel Aviv, Israel
Infectious diseases unit Tel Aviv Sourasky Medical Center, Tel Aviv, Israel

Svetlana Paikin
Microbiology Laboratory, Sanz Medical Center, Laniado hospital, Netanya, Israel

Appiah-Korang Labi
Department of Microbiology, Korle-Bu Teaching Hospital, Accra, Ghana

Noah Obeng-Nkrumah
Department of Medical Laboratory Sciences, School of Biomedical and Allied Health Sciences, Accra, Ghana

Edmund Tetteh Nartey
Centre for Tropical Clinical Pharmacology and Therapeutics, School of Medicine and Dentistry, Accra, Ghana

Stephanie Bjerrum
Department of Infectious Diseases, Copenhagen University Hospital, Rigshospitalet, Blegdamsvej 9, 2100 Copenhagen, Denmark

Nii Armah Adu-Aryee
Department of Surgery, University of Ghana School of Medicine and Dentistry, Accra, Ghana

Yaw Adjei Ofori-Adjei
Department of Medicine, Korle-Bu Teaching Hospital, Accra, Ghana

Alfred E. Yawson
Department of Community Health, School of Public Health, College of Health Sciences, University of Ghana, Accra, Ghana

Mercy J. Newman
Department of Medical Microbiology, School of Biomedical and Allied Sciences, Accra, Ghana

Dennis Souverein, Sjoerd M. Euser, Bjorn L. Herpers and Jeroen W. Den Boer
Department of Epidemiology and Infection Prevention, Regional Public Health Laboratory Kennemerland, Boerhaavelaan 26, 2035 RC, Haarlem, The Netherlands

Corry Hattink
Department of Infection Prevention, Rode Kruis Ziekenhuis, Beverwijk, The Netherlands

Patricia Houtman and Amerens Popma
Department of Infection Prevention, Spaarne Gasthuis, Haarlem and Hoofddorp, The Netherlands.

Jan Kluytmans
Laboratory for Microbiology and Infection Control, Amphia Hospital, Breda, The Netherlands.
University Medical Center, Utrecht, The Netherlands

John W. A. Rossen
Department of Medical Microbiology, University of Groningen, University Medical Center Groningen, Groningen, The Netherlands

Li Shen, Xiaoqing Wang, Ning Zhou, Lu Sun and Hong Chen
Department of Infection Control, Xi'an Hospital of Traditional Chinese Medicine, No.69 Feng Cheng 8th Road, Weiyang District, Xi'an 710021, China

Junming An
Department of Acupuncture and Moxibustion, Xi'an Hospital of Traditional Chinese Medicine, No.69 Feng Cheng 8th Road, Weiyang District, Xi'an 710021, China

Jialu An, Jing Han and Xiaorong Liu
Department of Information Consultation, Library of Xi'an Jiaotong University, No.76 Yan Ta West Road, Yanta District, Xi'an 710061, China

Lin Feng
Department of Cadre Health Care, Xi'an Hospital of Traditional Chinese Medicine, No.69 Feng Cheng 8th Road, Weiyang District, Xi'an 710021, China

Tufa Kolola and Takele Gezahegn
Department of public health, Debre Berhan University, Debre Berhan, Ethiopia

Jacqueline Färber, Katja Bauer and Gernot Geginat
Institute of Medical Microbiology, Infection Control and Prevention, Otto-von-Guericke University of Magdeburg, Leipziger Straße 44, 39120 Magdeburg, Germany

Dirk Schlüter
Institute of Medical Microbiology, Infection Control and Prevention, Otto-von-Guericke University of Magdeburg, Leipziger Straße 44, 39120 Magdeburg, Germany
Organ-specific Immune Regulation, Helmholtz Centre for Infection Research, Braunschweig, Germany

Sebastian Illiger and Christoph H. Lohmann
Department of Orthopedic Surgery, Otto-von-Guericke University of Magdeburg, Magdeburg, Germany

Fabian Berger and Barbara Gärtner
Institute of Medical Microbiology and Hygiene, Consultant Laboratory for Clostridium difficile, University of Saarland, Saarland, Germany

Lutz von Müller
Institute for Laboratory Medicine, Microbiology and Hygiene, Christophorus Kliniken, Coesfeld, Germany

Christina Grabau and Stefanie Zibolka
Central pharmacy, Otto-von-Guericke University of Magdeburg, Magdeburg, Germany

Ina Willemsen
Laboratory for Microbiology and Infection Control, Amphia Hospital, 4800, RK, Breda, The Netherlands
Center for Infectious Disease Expertise and Research (CIDER), Tilburg, The Netherlands

Jan Kluytmans
Laboratory for Microbiology and Infection Control, Amphia Hospital, 4800, RK, Breda, The Netherlands
Julius Center for Health Sciences and Primary Care, UMC Utrecht, Utrecht, The Netherlands

Lauren Clack, Manuela Scotoni, Aline Wolfensberger and Hugo Sax
Division of Infectious Diseases and Hospital Epidemiology, University Hospital Zurich, University of Zurich, Raemistrasse 100, CH-8091 Zurich, Switzerland

Anna L. Casey, Tarja J. Karpanen, Peter Nightingale and Tom S. J. Elliott
University Hospitals Birmingham NHS Foundation Trust, Birmingham B15 2TH, UK

Gutema Taressa Tura, Wondwossen Birke Eshete and Gudina Terefe Tucho
Department of Environmental health Sciences and Technology, Jimma University, Jimma, Ethiopia

Dewi Erikawati and Sanarto Santoso
Department of Microbiology, Faculty of Medicine, Brawijaya University/Dr. Saiful Anwar Hospital, Malang, Indonesia

Noorhamdani Noorhamdani
Department of Microbiology, Faculty of Medicine, Brawijaya University/Dr. Saiful Anwar Hospital, Malang, Indonesia
Infection Prevention and Control Committee, Dr. Saiful Anwar Hospital, Malang, Indonesia

Dewi Santosaningsih
Department of Microbiology, Faculty of Medicine, Brawijaya University/Dr. Saiful Anwar Hospital, Malang, Indonesia
Infection Prevention and Control Committee, Dr. Saiful Anwar Hospital, Malang, Indonesia
Department of Medical Microbiology and Infectious Diseases, Erasmus University Medical Center, 's-Gravendijkwal 230, Rotterdam 3015 CE, The Netherlands

Irene Ratridewi, Didi Candradikusuma, Iin N. Chozin and Thomas E. C. J. Huwae
Infection Prevention and Control Committee, Dr. Saiful Anwar Hospital, Malang, Indonesia

Gwen van der Donk, Eva van Boven, Anne F. Voor in 't holt, Henri A. Verbrugh and Juliëtte A. Severin
Department of Medical Microbiology and Infectious Diseases, Erasmus University Medical Center, 's-Gravendijkwal 230, Rotterdam 3015 CE, The Netherlands

Sukhyun Ryu
Division of Infectious Disease Control, Gyeonggi Provincial Government, Suwon, Republic of Korea
Department of Epidemiology and Health Informatics, Graduate School of Public Health, Korea University, Seoul, Republic of Korea

Bryan I. Kim
Department of Epidemiology and Health Informatics, Graduate School of Public Health, Korea University, Seoul, Republic of Korea

Byung Chul Chun
Department of Epidemiology and Health Informatics, Graduate School of Public Health, Korea University, Seoul, Republic of Korea
Department of Preventive Medicine, Korea University College of Medicine, Seoul, Republic of Korea

Sojung Kim
Department of Insurance Benefit, National Health Insurance Service, Seoul, Republic of Korea

Eili Y. Klein
Center for Disease Dynamics, Economics & Policy, Washington D.C., USA
Department of Emergency Medicine, Johns Hopkins University, Baltimore, USA

Young Kyung Yoon
Division of Infectious Diseases, Department of Internal Medicine, Korea University College of Medicine, Seoul, Republic of Korea

Kaitlin F. Mitchell and Anna K. Barker
Department of Population Health Sciences, University of Wisconsin-Madison, Madison, WI, USA
Division of Infectious Diseases, Department of Medicine, University of Wisconsin-Madison, Madison, WI, USA

Nasia Safdar
Division of Infectious Diseases, Department of Medicine, University of Wisconsin-Madison, Madison, WI, USA
William S. Middleton Memorial Veterans Hospital, Madison, WI, USA
Infection Control Department, University of Wisconsin-Madison, 5221 Medical Foundation Centennial Building, 1685 Highland Ave, Madison, WI 53705, USA

Cybele L. Abad
Department of Medicine, Division of Infectious Diseases, The Medical City, Pasig, Philippines

Jocelyn Qi-Min Teo, Samuel Rocky Candra, Shannon Jing-Yi Lee, Hui Leck, Hui-Peng Neo, Kenneth Wei-Liang Leow and Winnie Lee
Department of Pharmacy, Singapore General Hospital, Blk 8 Level 2, Outram Road, Singapore 169608, Singapore

Yiying Cai
Department of Pharmacy, Singapore General Hospital, Blk 8 Level 2, Outram Road, Singapore 169608, Singapore
Department of Pharmacy, National University of Singapore, 18 Science Drive 4, Singapore 117543, Singapore

Andrea Lay-Hoon Kwa
Department of Pharmacy, Singapore General Hospital, Blk 8 Level 2, Outram Road, Singapore 169608, Singapore
Department of Pharmacy, National University of Singapore, 18 Science Drive 4, Singapore 117543, Singapore
Emerging Infectious Diseases, Duke-NUS Medical School, 8 College Rd, Singapore 169857, Singapore

Tze-Peng Lim
Department of Pharmacy, Singapore General Hospital, Blk 8 Level 2, Outram Road, Singapore 169608, Singapore
SingHealth Duke-NUS Medicine Academic Clinical Programme, 20 College Rd, Singapore 169856, Singapore

Shannon Yu-Hng Chia
Department of Pharmacy, Singapore General Hospital, Blk 8 Level 2, Outram Road, Singapore 169608, Singapore
Tan Tock Seng Hospital, 11 Jalan Tan Tock Seng, Singapore 308433, Singapore

Ai-Ling Tan
Department of Microbiology, Singapore General Hospital, Outram Road, Singapore 169608, Singapore

Rachel Pui-Lai Ee
Department of Pharmacy, National University of Singapore, 18 Science Drive 4, Singapore 117543, Singapore

Britta Becker, Florian H. H. Brill, Dajana Paulmann, Birte Bischoff and Jochen Steinmann
Dr. Brill + Partner GmbH Institute for Hygiene and Microbiology, Norderoog 2, DE-28259 Bremen, Germany

Daniel Todt and Eike Steinmann
Institute for Experimental Virology, TWINCORE Centre for Experimental and Clinical Infection Research; a joint venture between the Medical School Hannover (MHH) and the Helmholtz Centre for Infection Research (HZI), Hannover, Germany

Johannes Lenz
Chemische Fabrik Dr. Weigert GmbH & Co.KG, Hamburg, Germany

Vesna Šuljagić
Department of Nosocomial Infections Control, Military Medical Academy, 11 000 Belgrade, Serbia
Faculty of Medicine of Military Medical Academy University of Defence, 11000 Belgrade, Serbia

Srđan Starčević
Faculty of Medicine of Military Medical Academy University of Defence, 11000 Belgrade, Serbia
Clinic for Orthopedic Surgery and Traumatology, Military Medical Academy, 11 000 Belgrade, Serbia

Nenad Stepić
Faculty of Medicine of Military Medical Academy University of Defence, 11000 Belgrade, Serbia
Clinic for Plastic Surgery and Burns, Military Medical Academy, 11 000 Belgrade, Serbia

Zoran Kostić
Faculty of Medicine of Military Medical Academy University of Defence, 11000 Belgrade, Serbia
Clinic for General Surgery, Military Medical Academy, 11000 Belgrade, Serbia

Ivan Miljković
Institute of Epidemiology, Military Medical Academy, 11 000 Belgrade, Serbia

Dragutin Jovanović
Institute of Microbiology Military Medical Academy, 11000 Belgrade, Serbia

Jelena Brusić-Renaud
Sector for Pharmacy, Military Medical Academy, 11 000 Belgrade, Serbia

Biljana Mijović
Faculty of Medicine, University of East Sarajevo, 73300 Foča, Republic of Srpska, Bosnia and Herzegovina

Sandra Šipetić-Grujičić
Institute of Epidemiology, Faculty of Medicine, University of Belgrade, 11000 Belgrade, Serbia

Jean-Winoc Decousser, Paul-Louis Woerther and Claude-James Soussy
University Hospital Henri Mondor, 9400 Creteil, France

Marguerite Fines-Guyon
Caen University Hospital, 14033 Caen, Cedex 9, France

Michael J. Dowzicky
Pfizer Inc, Collegeville, PA, USA

Marie Davat, Lydia Wuarin, Dimitrios Stafylakis and Didier Hannouche
Orthopedic Surgery Service, Geneva University Hospitals, Geneva, Switzerland

Mohamed Abbas and Stephan Harbarth
Infection Control Program, Geneva University Hospitals, Geneva, Switzerland

Ilker Uçkay
Infectiology, Balgrist University Hospital, Forchstrasse 340, 8008 Zürich, Switzerland

Ksenia Ershova
Center for Data-Intensive Biotechnology and Biomedicine, Skolkovo Institute of Science and Technology, Moscow, Russia

Vladimir Zelman
Center for Data-Intensive Biotechnology and Biomedicine, Skolkovo Institute of Science and Technology, Moscow, Russia
Department of Anesthesiology, Keck School of Medicine, University of Southern California, Los Angeles, USA

Ivan Savin, Nataliya Kurdyumova and Ekaterina Sokolova
Department of Intensive Care, Burdenko National Medical Research Center of Neurosurgery, Moscow, Russia

Darren Wong
Division of Infectious Diseases, Keck School of Medicine, University of Southern California, Los Angeles, USA

Gleb Danilov
Laboratory of Biomedical Informatics, Burdenko National Medical Research Center of Neurosurgery, Moscow, Russia

Michael Shifrin
IT Department, Burdenko National Medical Research Center of Neurosurgery, Moscow, Russia

Irina Alexandrova
Department of Microbiology, Burdenko National Medical Research Center of Neurosurgery, Moscow, Russia

Nadezhda Fursova
Federal Budget Institution of Science "State Research Center for Applied Microbiology & Biotechnology" (SRCAMB), Moscow, Russia

Olga Ershova
Department of Epidemiology and Infection Control, Burdenko National Medical Research Center of Neurosurgery, Moscow, Russia

Yu Lü, Min Hong Cai, Jian Cheng, Kun Zou, Qian Xiang, Jia Yu Wu, Dao Qiong Wei, Zhong Hua Zhou, Hui Wang, Chen Wang and Jing Chen
Healthcare-associated Infection Management Office, Sichuan Academy of Medical Sciences and Sichuan People's Hospital, Chengdu 610072, Sichuan, People's Republic of China

Alyssa M West, Carine A Nkemngong, Maxwell G Voorn and Tongyu Wu
Department of Food Science, Purdue University, West Lafayette, IN 47907, USA

Haley F Oliver
Department of Food Science, Purdue University, West Lafayette, IN 47907, USA
Department of Food Science, Purdue University, 745 Agriculture Mall Drive, West Lafayette, IN 47907, USA

Xiaobao Li and Peter J Teska
Diversey Inc., Charlotte, NC 28273, USA

Mayra G. Menegueti, Ana Elisa R. Lopes and Lécio R. Ferreira
Infection Control Service, University Hospital of the Ribeirão Preto Medical School, University of São Paulo, Ribeirão Preto, SP, Brazil

Gilberto G. Gaspar
Infection Control Service, University Hospital of the Ribeirão Preto Medical School, University of São Paulo, Ribeirão Preto, SP, Brazil
University Hospital of Ribeirão Preto Medical School, Avenida Bandeirantes, 3900 – Vila Monte Alegre, Ribeirão Preto, SP 14048-900, Brazil

Roberto O. C. Santos
Department of Surgery and Anatomy, Ribeirão Preto Medical School, University of São Paulo, Ribeirão Preto, SP, Brazil

Thamiris R. de Araújo, Aline Nassiff and Silvia R. M. S. Canini
Department of Fundamental Nursing, Ribeirão Preto College of Nursing, University of São Paulo, Ribeirão Preto, SP, Brazil

Maria Eulalia L. V. Dallora
Hospital Administration, University Hospital of the Ribeirão Preto Medical School, University of São Paulo, Ribeirão Preto, SP, Brazil

Fernando Bellissimo-Rodrigues
Social Medicine Department, Ribeirão Preto Medical School, University of São Paulo, Ribeirão Preto, SP, Brazil

Maria Jurado-Ruiz
Department of Trauma and Orthopaedic Surgery, Hospital Universitari Vall d'Hebron, Universitat Autonoma de Barcelona, Barcelona, Spain

Gerard P. Slobogean, Nathan N. O'Hara and Andrea Howe
R Adams Cowley Shock Trauma Center, Department of Orthopaedics, University of Maryland School of Medicine, Baltimore, MD, USA

Sofia Bzovsky, Alisha Garibaldi and Brad Petrisor
Division of Orthopaedic Surgery, Department of Surgery, McMaster University, Hamilton, ON, Canada

Sheila Sprague
Division of Orthopaedic Surgery, Department of Surgery, McMaster University, Hamilton, ON, Canada
Department of Health Research Methods, Evidence, and Impact, McMaster University, Hamilton, ON, Canada
McMaster University, 293 Wellington Street North, Suite 110, Ontario, Hamilton L8L 8E7, Canada

Daniel Asfaw Erku
School of Pharmacy, University of Gondar, Lideta kebele 16, Gondar, Ethiopia

Sisay Yifru Aberra
College of Medicine and Health Sciences, University of Gondar, Gondar, Ethiopia

Index

www.ingramcontent.com/pod-product-compliance
Lightning Source LLC
Chambersburg PA
CBHW082032190326
41458CB00010B/3343